T3-BQR-800

WITHDRAWN

LIBRARY
College of St. Scholastica
Duluth, Minnesota 55811

THE CESAREAN EXPERIENCE

THEORETICAL AND CLINICAL PERSPECTIVES FOR NURSES

THE CESAREAN EXPERIENCE

THEORETICAL AND CLINICAL PERSPECTIVES FOR NURSES

Edited by

Carole Fitzgerald Kehoe, R.N., M.S.N.

Assistant Professor
The Catholic University of America
School of Nursing

Doctoral Candidate
The American University
Washington, D.C.

Appleton-Century-Crofts/New York

R G
7 6 1
. C 4 6

Copyright © 1981 by APPLETON-CENTURY-CROFTS
A Publishing Division of Prentice-Hall, Inc.

All rights reserved. This book, or any parts thereof, may not be used or reproduced in any manner without written permission. For information, address
Appleton-Century-Crofts, 292 Madison Avenue, New York, N.Y. 10017.

81 82 83 84 85 / 10 9 8 7 6 5 4 3 2 1

Prentice-Hall International, Inc., London
Prentice-Hall of Australia, Pty. Ltd., Sydney
Prentice-Hall of India Private Limited, New Delhi
Prentice-Hall of Japan, Inc., Tokyo
Prentice-Hall of Southeast Asia (Pte.) Ltd., Singapore
Whitehall Books Ltd., Wellington, New Zealand

Library of Congress Cataloging in Publication Data
Main entry under title:

The Cesarean experience.

Includes index.
Contents: Biophysical factors associated with cesarean
birth / B. Louise Murray—Understanding cesarean
birth / Carole Fitzgerald Kehoe—Facilitation of
maternal-infant attachment following cesarean birth /
Margaret R. Spaulding—[etc.]
1. Cesarean section—Nursing. I. Kehoe, Carole
Fitzgerald, 1935-   . [DNLM: 1. Cesarean section—
Nursing texts. WY 157 C421]
RC761.C46   618.8'6   81-10761
ISBN 0-8385-1107-4   AACR2

Text and cover design: Jean M. Sabato

Production Editor: Ina J. Shapiro

PRINTED IN THE UNITED STATES OF AMERICA

To
Elisabeth and Bobby,
my cesarean-born children

Contents

Contributors

Linda S. Birdsong, R.N., M.S.N.
Laurel, Maryland

Dorothy deMoya, R.N., M.S.N.
Clinical Specialist in Reproductive Counseling
Washington, D.C.

Jacqueline Fawcett, Ph.D., F.A.A.N.
Assistant Professor of Nursing
University of Pennsylvania
School of Nursing
Philadelphia, Pennsylvania

Carole F. Kehoe, R.N., M.S.N.
Assistant Professor of Nursing
The Catholic University of America
School of Nursing
Washington, D.C.

Joanne S. Marut, R.N., M.S.N.
Co-ordinator, Labor and Delivery Room
Georgetown University Medical Center
Washington, D.C.

Ramona T. Mercer, R.N., Ph.D., F.A.A.N.
Associate Professor
Department of Family Health Care Nursing
University of California
School of Nursing
San Francisco, California

B. Louise Murray, R.N., Ed.D.
Professor of Nursing
The University of New Mexico
College of Nursing
Albuquerque, New Mexico

Nancy Newport, R.N.
Cesarean Childbirth Education Trainer and Consultant.
Co-founder, Cesarean Families Association of Greater Washington, D.C., Inc.
Washington, D.C.

Cora McGuffie Rodriguez, R.N., M.S.N.
Consultant
Legal/Medical Affairs
Chevy Chase, Maryland

Margaret R. Spaulding, R.N., Ed.D.
Chairman, Maternal-Child Nursing
Virginia Commonwealth University
Richmond, Virginia

Anne Wilson, R.N., M.S.N.
Clinical Nurse Specialist in Women's Health Care
Alexandria, Virginia

Foreword

The technology of the 1970s contributed to lower infant mortality and morbidity rates. Part of the technology that served to lower infant morbidity and mortality affected the mode of delivery at a time when consumers were demanding more conservative maternity care and more family involvement in the entire childbirth cycle. The woman about to deliver has been caught up in the emphasis on the importance of early mother–infant interaction to enhance bonding and the thought of her mate remaining at her side, concomitant with the medical practice that contributes to better infant outcome. Cesarean deliveries are routinely done for certain breech presentations, maternal illness when fetal lung maturity is evidenced, and when the forces of labor impinge on fetal well-being. The woman who wants the advantages of the conservative vaginal delivery is faced with the real probability of an approximately one in six to one in four chance of abdominal delivery, depending on the locale of her care.

Although infant outcome has improved, the mother faces increased morbidity with the higher incidence of cesarean births. The woman who would have ordinarily watched the baby emerge from her vagina, experiencing a sense of euphoria after pushing her baby out, nursing her infant immediately following birth or very shortly thereafter, and then be comfortably up and about within a few hours, may be that one woman in six (or four) who is disappointed and emotionally depleted as she recovers from abdominal surgery.

Nursing has assumed a large role in preparing parents for childbirth through special classes and in promoting the health of families throughout the childbirth cycle. As the largest group of health professionals, and as the health professionals who have perhaps the most sustained and intense interaction with women in the maternity cycle, nurses must assume larger responsibility for, and accountability to, the public for the health care for families who experience cesarean birth.

Historically, nursing practice has been based on theories from other disciplines, judgments based on the observable evidence, and intuition. With increasing research and mounting empirical evidence, that which is unique to nursing practice is being identified and is increasingly more scientifically based. *The Cesarean Experience: Theoretical and Clinical Perspectives for Nurses* presents such a scientific basis for nursing care for the families who for various reasons experience a cesarean birth.

While the debate continues on whether or not the increased rates of cesarean birth are justified, the nursing profession must help families deal with circumstances as they exist. Various questions arise.

How does one prepare the family for the possibility of cesarean birth without increasing the anxiety and vulnerability that all pregnant women experience during the third trimester? How does the nurse help family members to adjust to their loss of expectations? What kinds of counseling needs do these families have? Often the loss of health equilibrium for the mother or the infant has necessitated cesarean delivery, and these losses must also be dealt with. Continuing research is needed for answers to these and other questions. This volume is timely in that it provides scientific and clinical bases for nursing decisions in the cesarean experience. The impetus for Carole Kehoe's interest in and sensitivity to the special needs of the mother experiencing cesarean birth resulted from her personal childbirth experience a decade ago. Since that time her professional activities have focused on the special needs of the cesarean family and in testing a nursing model for delivering care to this family. Whether the reader opts for a Symbolic Interactionist, Crisis, or Roy Adaptation Model as the basis for her practice, this volume will help her to articulate the rationale for her practice and the logic behind her decisions.

Ramona T. Mercer, R.N., Ph.D.
Associate Professor
Department of Family Health
Care Nursing
University of California
San Francisco

Introduction

Until relatively recently, the nursing literature available on cesarean birth emphasized the actual delivery experience and the immediate postpartum period. Admittedly, these are the times that the needs of cesarean clients are acute, immediate, and obvious, and nurses need literature to provide them with a rationale for practice in order to provide safe and relevant care. However, literature with this focus tends to obscure the effects of the cesarean experience which occur at other phases in the maternity cycle, when needs are less acute and more subtle.

During the 1970s the cesarean birth rate increased steadily, and this was accompanied by a concomitant rise in the consumer movement in this country. As a result, cesarean families became increasingly vocal in expressing their perceptions and reactions to this alternative method of birth. Perhaps more important, nurses and other health professionals listened to the concerns expressed and realized that cesarean birth involves the entire family, not only the mother.

As we begin the decade of the 1980s, there is a general awareness among nurses that cesarean birth affects families throughout the childbearing experience, and this has consequences for clinical nursing practice. If nurses are to offer appropriate and relevant care to these clients, current literature must speak to issues from a broader and more inclusive perspective than was formerly the case.

The purpose of this book is to pull together some of the major theoretical issues and a number of relevant clinical nursing strategies applicable to the nursing care of cesarean families. It is intended to be a resource for nurse practitioners, educators, researchers, and students who want to broaden the scope of their understanding of cesarean birth. Although the book is not an exhaustive compilation of all relevant perspectives, it should be a useful supplement to other professional texts.

It is my belief that cesarean birth is a total family experience, and not merely an isolated event that occurs at a particular point in a family's life cycle. This perspective influenced my ideas about the essential content of the book, as well as my approach to developing the content areas. My overall goal was to provide material reflecting a broad range of viewpoints about cesarean birth—before, during, and after the actual delivery in both the acute care and community settings. To accomplish this goal, I drew upon the expertise of a group of nurses actively involved in maternity nursing in selecting the contributing authors for this book. They represent a broad range of clinical interests, educational backgrounds, and nursing expertise, and they function in clinical and academic settings throughout the United States at various professional levels. It is my belief that the strength of this book lies in the diversity of its contributing authors.

We share the assumption that a solid theoretical foundation is central to the design and implementation of nursing intervention in any setting and at all levels of nursing experience and achievement. This philosophical stance is brought to life in the abundant theoretical approaches and creative clinical nursing interventions suggested throughout the book.

Several chapters present empirical data derived from exploratory studies that were developed exclusively for this book. The findings that these authors share are important and exciting, because they enrich our knowledge about the needs of cesarean families and provide an objectively derived rationale for interventions designed to meet these needs.

Because of the diversity in the issues being addressed by the individual authors, I did not provide specific guidelines for the development of the content in the chapters. Each author wrote her chapter independently, using the full range of her creative talents and her own unique writing style. However, a common philosophy of theoretically based clinical nursing strategies prevails in all the chapters.

Many of the chapters focus primarily on the cesarean mother. However, all of the authors are advocates of the family-centered approach to the care of cesarean families. Therefore, in the chapters where the total family is not mentioned directly, the family-centered philosophy of the author can be assumed.

The book is organized into five major sections, each with its own particular theme.

Section I is foundational to understanding the cesarean experience. In Chapter 1, Murray presents biophysical factors which can result in a cesarean birth. I then focus on social–psychological issues in Chapter 2. The symbolic interactionism concept of "the definition of a situation" is an ongoing theme, and I contend that a mother's perceptions and reactions to cesarean birth reflect the definition of the situation that each mother brings with her to the childbearing experience.

Section II draws the reader's attention to the issue of maternal–infant attachment in cesarean parents. Spaulding discusses facilitation of the attachment process in Chapter 3 and offers many practical suggestions. Mercer, in Chapter 4, focuses on the potential effects of anesthesia and analgesia on attachment and suggests that these agents may make the process more difficult for cesarean clients.

The focus of Section III is to illustrate the use of tools for assessing the needs of cesarean parents. Chapter 5, co-authored by myself and Fawcett, discusses the Roy Adaptation Model. We each then describe studies developed for this book in which the Roy Model was used as the organizing framework. In Chapter 6, I report on my study of the nursing needs of cesarean mothers, followed by Fawcett's presentation in Chapter 7 on the cesarean father.

Section IV considers how the nurse can facilitate adjustment in families who experience cesarean birth. Newport, an experienced childbirth educator, describes the nurse's role in preparing expectant parents for cesarean birth in Chapter 8. Birdsong then reports her exploratory study in Chapter 9 on issues of loss and grieving in cesarean mothers, and she offers practical approaches to grief intervention. In Chapter 10, deMoya focuses on the sexual adjustment of postcesarean couples and argues forcefully that nurses should break the "conspiracy of silence" that surrounds the sexual concerns of childbearing couples in general. The extended postpartum concerns of cesarean families are considered by Wilson in Chapter 11, and she focuses upon establishing a network of support through the use of counseling, telephone services, and postpartum support groups. Specific guidelines for the establishment of these support systems are discussed.

The theme of Section V is change. In Chapter 12, Rodriguez reports a study of hospital policies regarding cesarean family care in the area around the District of Columbia and she then presents suggestions on how the nurse can effect change to improve the care of cesarean families. In Chapter 13, Marut focuses on how a staff nurse in a labor and delivery area can bring about change to improve the care of cesarean families. This chapter describes how Marut extended her own study of cesarean mothers to provide in-service education to maternity staff nurses. In the final chapter of the book Murray considers the rights of women in cesarean birth from a bioethical viewpoint. This innovative discussion culminates with a cesarean mother's "Bill of Rights."

Although one person may have overall responsibility for the development of a book, there are many other people whose influence on this process has been profound. I especially want to thank the contributing authors. The dedication with which they pursued the task of writing their chapters—while conducting other aspects of their busy personal and professional lives—was encouraging and supportive. Their willingness to share ideas with me and among themselves stimulated my own efforts and contributed immeasurably to my ongoing enthusiasim for the collective enterprise in which we were all involved.

This book also presented me with the opportunity to become acquainted with nurses whose writings I was familiar with, but whom I had never met personally. In addition, I renewed my acquaintance with two individuals I had met during postmaster's study at the University of Washington several years ago. Both opportunities were personally and professionally enriching and were serendipitous rewards of editing this book.

It has been observed, in this book and elsewhere, that childbearing is an experience that moves to completion within the framework of a family, and not in isolation. Many times the thought has occurred to me that this is equally applicable to writing a book, for that too moves to completion within the framework of a family. I was especially fortunate to have the unceasing support and understanding of my husband, Patrick, during the period of time I worked on this manuscript. His logical and well-organized mind provided a backdrop against which I could consider and clarify my ideas. In addition, his willingness and skill in providing our young children with the care and nurturance they needed allowed me to pursue this creative endeavor without feeling that they were deprived. For this I am especially grateful.

I would be remiss if I did not acknowledge and thank my children, Elisabeth and Bobby, for their patience with a mother who worked on a book while pursuing doctoral study. Patience is always remarkable when seen in persons only 9 and 6½ years old, respectively.

I also thank my graduate students in maternity nursing, past and present, at The Catholic University of America School of Nursing. Their penetrating questions and observations about cesarean birth forced me to rethink my own perceptions and thoughts repeatedly. In addition, their interest in and understanding of my involvement in this project provided great support. It is my hope that their learning was enhanced by my efforts with this book, and that they learned more because of it. I know that I gained a great deal because of them.

I want also to express my gratitude to the many cesarean mothers who have shared with me their thoughts and reactions to the cesarean experience. It was their perceptions which gave impetus to my ongoing interest in the cesarean experience and directly resulted in the development of this book. It is my hope and prayer that those women who expressed difficulty in accepting the reality of their cesarean experiences eventually reconciled their feelings and were able to find happiness and a sense of fulfillment in carrying out the maternal role. It is to these cesarean mothers and their families that this book is also dedicated.

SECTION I

Bio-psycho-social Considerations

CHAPTER 1

Biophysical Factors Associated with Cesarean Birth

B. Louise Murray

According to Bandman and Bandman (1977), hospitals today are highly specialized centers for diagnosis, treatment, training, and research in all of the medical specialities, including obstetrics. This must be considered in light of the facts that approximately 80 percent of human illnesses are self-limiting, approximately 10 percent are amenable to the type of cure available in hospitals, and another 10 percent of human disease is incurable, despite all therapeutic attempts. These facts to the contrary, hospitals have become institutionalized bureaucracies of "curing" and "treatment," regardless of cost; they have become symbols of medical power in which the actual quality of "caring" is given a very low priority.

Because of the great emphasis on the scientific aspects of treatment, the human needs of hospital patients are generally not considered very important and human rights are often disregarded. Once a person enters the hospital he or she often becomes a "nonperson," treated as incapable of intelligent self-determination, denied or given only sketchy information about his or her condition and proposed treatment, and most often, considered unable to give a truly informed consent. Human dignity and humaneness are disregarded and the person's privacy is invaded. According to Bandman and Bandman (1977), consideration of individual needs and desires, at best, ". . . tends to be sporadic and discontinuous" (p. 868).

Unfortunately, the event of childbirth has fallen victim to this "cure" philosophy. Labor and delivery continue to be looked upon as pathological conditions needing complex technical intervention. The fact that childbearing is a natural process, requiring little "curing" intervention has, in most cases, been obscured by today's aggressive practices. The notion of compassionate, supportive care is largely foreign to such a highly complex, technological environment.

One result of this technological, curing orientation to childbirth is the cesarean method, a procedure being used with increasing frequency. The incidence of this type of medical intervention has doubled and perhaps even tripled over the last decade.

Depending on the source, the accepted rate for primary cesarean deliveries prior to 1971 was as low as 2.6 to 4.0 percent, with the total rate of both primary and repeat cesareans ranging from 4.7 to 8.0 percent (Caire 1978, p. 571). Currently, the accepted rate is much higher. It is estimated that the future average rate will range from 10 to 15 percent—some say 20 to 25 percent, or more (Jones 1976).

Thus, more women than ever are being confronted with the probability of a cesarean delivery, perhaps the most traumatic birth experience they will ever encounter.

TRADITIONAL CONSIDERATIONS IN CESAREAN BIRTH

Some classic reasons for childbirth intervention by cesarean are malpresentation of the fetus (e.g., a transverse lie or a brow or breech presentation), fetal abnormalities, and/or multiple pregnancies. Another factor traditionally associated with cesarean intervention is cephalopelvic disproportion (CPD) due to a small or contracted pelvis or an unusually large or malformed fetus. Cesarean birth is considered necessary after an unsuccessful trial labor, or when CPD has been diagnosed prior to labor.

Cesarean delivery is considered a necessary aspect of emergency treatment due to development of severe toxemia or preeclampsia. The diagnosis of placenta previa or abruptio placenta with accompanying severe hemorrhage necessitates emergency operative intervention.

Uterine inertia or dystocia accompanied by marked maternal fatigue and unsatisfactory progress in labor are also significant factors in the rate of cesarean birth. These procedures have frequently been associated with older (beyond the age of 35) primiparous women and grandmultiparous women. Some of the causes of dystocia are abnormalities of the uterus, ovaries, cervix, or vagina, indicating cesarean birth.

Fetal distress due to a variety of maternal and/or intrauterine events during labor is a major reason for emergency cesarean delivery. Prior to the use of electronic fetal monitoring, fetal distress was typically diagnosed by a nurse or midwife using a fetoscope.

In this country, previous delivery by cesarean has almost always been reason for subsequent delivery by this method, especially when the surgery was accomplished through a classic (vertical) uterine incision. Women who have had primary cesareans have been scheduled for repeats with subsequent pregnancies, usually out of fear of rupture of the uterine scar.

FACTORS ASSOCIATED WITH THE
CURRENT RATE OF CESAREAN BIRTHS:
TODAY'S AGGRESSIVE OBSTETRICS

Doering has noted that viewpoints on what constitutes good obstetric practice have changed markedly in recent years. At one time . . .

> *One could judge a physician by his section [cesarean] rate: the lower it was, the better obstetrician he must be. . . . Things have changed a lot since 1956. Now it often appears that hospitals and obstetricians hold the opposite value: the higher their [cesarean] section rate the better their obstetrical care (Stewart and Stewart, 1977, p. 145).*

Use of Electronic Fetal Monitors

Considerable controversy is evident in the obstetric literature over the value of routinely using electronic devices to monitor fetal heart rate (FHR) and maternal uterine contractions during labor. Proponents staunchly proclaim that this procedure improves perinatal outcome and provides little hazard to the mother. Indeed, Quilligan, at the Hastings Center Conference on Values Underlying the New Childbirth Technology (May 1977) proposed that the fetal monitor should be routinely used in all labors (Steinfels 1978).

Recently, however, a possible cause–effect relationship has been suggested between the use of electronic fetal monitors and an increase in early intervention. Two prospective studies have demonstrated a significantly higher rate of cesarean births when "fetal distress" was diagnosed by the fetal monitor.

Haverkamp testified in April, 1978 before the U.S. Senate Subcommittee on Health in regard to this problem. He described his first prospective study (Haverkamp et al. 1976) of 484 high-risk pregnant women, in which he compared the effectiveness of two methods of fetal heart rate monitoring: in one, nurses auscultated with a fetoscope, and in the other method they used an electronic device. In the group monitored by the electronic method, the cesarean rate was 16.5 percent. The rate in the group auscultated by nurses was 6.6 percent. The condition of the neonates was equally good in both groups.

In his second prospective study (Haverkamp et al. 1978) with a tighter research design, 690 selected high-risk patients were randomly assigned to three separate groups, each with a different type of fetal monitoring: auscultation via fetoscope; electronic monitoring alone; and electronic monitoring with an option to analyze fetal scalp blood samples for pH. The results showed no statistically significant differences in perinatal outcome; all outcomes were excellent. However, the cesarean rates were 17.6 percent for the electronically monitored group and 5.6 percent for the auscultated group.

Paul et al. (1977) and Neutra et al. (1978), in retrospective studies with large numbers of cases, found no differences in the respective perinatal or neonatal death rates of monitored and nonmonitored patients, except in the groups of small infants at especially high risk. According to Doering:

> The link between the two—i.e., fetal
> monitoring and cesarean births—
> could be seen as a positive change,
> if one believes that the monitor re-
> veals fetal distress which would
> have gone unnoticed (Stewart and
> Stewart, 1977, p. 146).

Shenker (1973) reported that the fetal monitor produced patterns of late deceleration in 68 percent of cases, when babies were subsequently born without any signs of depression and an Apgar score above seven. He predicted that with high-risk patients, 56 percent of those fetuses with late deceleration patterns would be born in good condition. Caire (1978) states that:

> .... the fetal monitor has been widely
> adopted for routine use in all
> obstetric cases. Its limitations have
> not been well understood and, as a
> result, section [cesarean] rates
> associated with its use have risen
> dramatically without measurable
> increase in fetal salvage.

Others document that use of fetal monitors in labor can result in erroneous messages, a factor which can lead to cesarean intervention. The external ECG monitor is least reliable and internal ECG monitoring with fetal blood sampling is the most reliable, but both are subject to error in measurement or interpretation (Afriat and Schifrin 1976; Lowensohn 1976).

The use of fetal monitoring on all maternity patients and of other procedures in obstetric care was sharply questioned by members of the Hastings

Center Conference (Steinfels 1978). The possible risk or harm and/or the debatable good of such therapies if they have not been extensively tested before use with patients were viewed with great concern. One member of the conference, Ruth Hanft, Deputy Assistant Secretary for Health Policy, Research, and Statistics (HEW), asked:

> *If clinicians advocate routine use of technology and there are no controlled studies demonstrating its effectiveness, nor criteria established for its use, how can policy makers distinguish between procedures that will benefit patients and those that will not? (Steinfels 1978)*

Another member of the conference had another concern. Nancy Amidei, Deputy Assistant Secretary of Welfare Legislation (HEW), raised the question of who would really be paying the cost if electronic monitors were used in all labors?

> *If the decision is to spend the limited sum available for maternal–infant health programs and good prenatal and well-baby care in isolated rural areas and urban ghettos, where it is nonexistent or inaccessible, to provide technology for all those who already have access to hospitals and doctors, are we deciding to provide nothing for those who have little or no access at all? (Steinfels 1978)*

Uterine Dystocia, Inertia, or Failure to Progress

Certain other obstetric procedures are related indirectly to inefficient and ineffective uterine contractions, fetal distress, and other problems in labor, and thus to an increased incidence of cesarean births:

1. The use of drugs (oxytoxics) for induction and augmentation of labor.
2. The artificial rupture of membranes (amniotomy) to attach a fetal electrode and/or to facilitate the descent of the presenting part and hasten the progress of labor.
3. The use of analgesia, sedation, tranquilizers, and anesthesia to reduce the pain and distress of labor and of obstetric operative procedures.

4. The frequent requirement of bed rest in the supine position during labor.
5. The lack of adequate supportive care, human concern, and skilled coaching during labor from persons who are known to and trusted by the laboring woman.

The oxytoxics used to induce or augment labor cause labor contractions to become much stronger and more frequent and to last longer. As a result of these changes in the labor pattern, the mother experiences greatly increased pain and anxiety, causing her to become more fearful and more and more discouraged with her ability to "stay in control" and work with her labor. Eventually, more often than not, she needs more and more obstetric medication (Shenker 1973; Dunn 1976; Cohen and Rosen 1976). In addition, she may be separated from her husband and/or other meaningful persons. As a result, feelings of loneliness, fear, and inability to cope take over. Her energy reserves are soon dissipated, her fatigue increases, and she eventually calls for relief at any cost (Dulock and Herron 1976; Martin and Gingerich 1976). According to Dulock and Herron, "Interfering with the natural physiology of labor and delivery is becoming more and more common in the United States."

These practices can also create many problems for the fetus. Fetal distress (i.e., abnormal fetal heart rate) can result from the use of oxytoxics by interfering with uterine blood flow and/or by causing cord compression. In addition, the fetus may suffer brain trauma because of the great pressure on the head caused by excessively strong contractions, especially after an amniotomy. Women who receive oxytoxics are put in the high-risk category, even though they may have nothing else wrong with them (Shenker 1973; Cohen and Rosen 1976; Gabbe et al. 1976; Ettinger and McCart 1976; Martin and Gingerich 1976).

All of these factors seem to reinforce one another, ultimately making the labor process ineffective. The control of labor is thus transferred from the woman to her physician, who may make a diagnosis of uterine inertia or distocia and fetal distress and decide to deliver the baby by cesarean.

The Classical Cesarean Incision and Repeat Cesarean Births

Another change in obstetric practice which may have had a favorable influence on the incidence of cesarean birth is the abandonment of the classical uterine incision (vertical) in favor of the lower segment incision (transverse). Women who have had the classical incision are routinely scheduled for an elective cesarean because they are considered to be at high risk for uterine scar rupture, while women who have had the lower segment incision can in many cases deliver subsequent children vaginally. According to Doering (1977):

> *Outside the United States, women*
> *who have had one cesarean delivery*

*are not routinely sectioned with
succeeding births. Trial labors are
common and success rates vary
from 37 percent to 69 percent of
women managing a safe vaginal delivery. . . . When nonrepeating indications such as fetal distress or
malpresentation caused the first
section, about 80 percent of both
groups achieved vaginal deliveries.*

Many American physicians, however, are reluctant not to repeat a cesarean with all births following the primary cesarean. McTammany, a physician in private practice, has allowed his patients to attempt vaginal delivery if the cesarean was done with a low cervical incision and there was an uncomplicated postoperative course free of infection (Stewart and Stewart 1979). About half of such patients achieved successful vaginal delivery. The uterine rupture rate was 0.5 percent, without tearing of the scar, bleeding, shock, or other serious sequellae.

Other Obstetric Procedures and More Frequent Cesareans

A fourth development in obstetric practice, hailed as one of the major advances in the field, is the advent of specialized diagnostic tests and procedures. X-ray pelvimetry and ultrasonographic studies have been developed to aid in predicting unsuccessful vaginal delivery due to such complications as cephalopelvic disproportion, malpresentation, and/or fetal immaturity.

More recently, such other procedures as hormonal tests, fetal stress tests, and amniotic fluid analysis have been utilized to aid in evaluating fetal development and maturity. Caire (1978) has stated that these procedures have real value when used properly to obtain data for making a clinical judgment. However, they are expensive and not always reliable as single indicators, and if accepted at face value they can contribute to an increase in operative interference, possible iatrogenic prematurity, and respiratory distress (Baker 1978; Flaksman et al. 1978; Hack et al. 1976).

Another practice prevalent today is intervention by cesarean for all primagravida breech presentations and for premature deliveries. According to Caire (1978), reports of damage and mortality during vaginal delivery of infants with breech presentation vary according to the source of the statistics, the type of population studied, the incidence and degree of prematurity, and the prevailing attitudes of the physicians involved. He concedes that breech presentation makes vaginal delivery more risky, but maintains that, with careful selection, such infants can be delivered safely. In any case, consideration must also be given to the risks incurred by both the mother and the infant in a cesarean delivery.

Amniotomy, Analgesia, Tranquilizers, and Anesthesia

Amniotomy, or artificial rupture of membranes for the purpose of hastening the progress of labor, eliminates the protective cushion of the fluid-filled amniotic sac over the head of the fetus. Thus with each contraction the presenting part is driven hard against the lower uterine segment and cervix, hastening dilatation. In a vertex presentation there is increased danger of fetal brain damage as well as increased maternal discomfort (Liston and Campbell 1974; Dunn 1976).

Analgesia, tranquilizers, and anesthesia are given to reduce the anxiety and pain of labor. Contractions are slowed or even stopped for a period of time, especially with epidural anesthesia. Thus the mother's ability to work with her contractions is interrupted. The descent of the presenting part is slowed or arrested. As a result, the progress of labor may be sufficiently adversely affected to necessitate a cesarean birth. (Dunn, 1976; Ettinger and McCart 1976; Martin and Gingerich 1976; Cohen and Rosen 1976).

In addition, the possible brain trauma suffered by the fetus during labor and birth can result in behavioral problems for the developing infant and child. Brackbill, in testifying before the U.S. Senate Committee on Health and Scientific Research, stated that damage is best evidenced in gross motor abilities and in emerging cognitive functions, such as the development of language and associated cognitive skills. She also stated that studies of infants and children (from 1 day to 7 years old) indicate that these behavioral effects are permanent (Stewart and Stewart 1979, p. 134).

Other Factors Related to the Incidence of Cesarean Births

Another common obstetric practice today is that of giving the mother intravenous infusions of glucose and/or other fluids rather than letting her take fluids by mouth. In such cases a blood pressure cuff is usually wrapped around the mother's uninvolved arm to allow for frequent readings. These practices make it difficult for the mother to assume any other body position than lying flat on her back. Thus the mother cannot utilize gravity or helpful body positions to aid the progress of the fetus through the birth canal. In addition, she is usually not allowed or would find it awkward to walk around with all of the equipment attached to her. Nor can she engage in any other activities, which would serve to distract her and help her to avoid excess tension and fear, thus aiding the progress of labor (Caldeyro–Barcia et al. 1960; Dunn 1976; Baker 1978; Cohen and Rosen 1976).

Another important sequela of intrusive procedures (such as internal monitoring, amniotomy, frequent vaginal exams, and cesarean births) is an increased frequency of maternal and fetal/neonatal infections. These infections can result in such major problems as morbidity, lengthened hospital stay, and separation of mother and baby, among others (Gee and Ledger 1976; Gassner and Ledger 1976).

In consideration of the foregoing practices, participants at the Hastings Conference asked:

> *How suspicious should medicine it-*
> *self be of new forms of treatment*
> *and diagnosis where their effects are*
> *untested, particularly in a normally*
> *non-pathological process like preg-*
> *nancy and childbirth? For instance*
> *drugs, anaesthesia, induced labor,*
> *and restricted oral intake are often*
> *introduced for well-defined thera-*
> *peutic ends and quickly become*
> *routine practices, even in normal*
> *pregnancies. Only when problems*
> *appear are they given the critical*
> *scrutiny they should have had in the*
> *first place (Stenfels 1978).*

Steinfels (1978), a former associate for the humanities at the Hastings Center, concluded that the extension of the "medical model" and the "sick role" to such life experiences as pregnancy and childbirth has a number of question-able consequences:

> *1. It mobilizes the coercive power*
> *of labels. We are more permis-*
> *sive in regard to good/bad or*
> *legal/illegal than toward sick/*
> *healthy or high-risk/low-risk.*
> *2. It shifts authority to the physi-*
> *cian and the setting to the*
> *hospital.*
> *3. It casts the patient in a passive*
> *role and minimizes the patient's*
> *sense of responsibility.*
> *4. It justifies the use of specialized,*
> *technical, and often very ex-*
> *pensive therapies.*
> *5. It isolates the experience from*
> *other realms of meaning, i.e. child-*
> *birth becomes primarily a medical*
> *event, rather than a family event,*
> *a religious event, or a special*
> *moment in the life cycle.*

Laboring women in hospitals are given no food or oral fluids until after de-livery. It is little wonder that they become greatly fatigued during the hard work of labor. Their infants also sometimes show signs of hypoglycemia or other fluid and electrolyte imbalances, especially if they have been stressed by interference in essential blood and oxygen supply (Martin and Gingerich 1976).

All physicians are currently concerned about malpractice suits. Jones (1976) reported the results of a survey of medical school department chairmen, professors, and practicing obstetricians. In almost all of the responses, malpractice suits were mentioned as one of the main reasons for the recent increase in the choice of cesarean birth.

The aggressive practice of obstetrics has a wide range of effects which are not limited to negative influences on the mother and fetus. Most medical students receive obstetric training in hospitals where aggressive obstetrics are practiced. They usually have *no* experience with normal labor and delivery, as, for instance, that which takes place in a supportive home setting. It is little wonder that when they become practicing physicians they continue to practice aggressively, as they have been taught.

In addition, most medical practitioners lack a true awareness of the actual range of time required to complete an uncomplicated labor, for either primagravidae or multigravidae, without aggressive intervention. If the physician has no experience upon which he or she can base a judgment, then frequent premature obstetric intervention can be expected. The mother herself may have sufficient experience or knowledge to better evaluate the need for such intervention, but, as Steinfels said at the Hastings Center Conference (1978), "The nature of obstetrical practice seldom allows women to make choices about medical intervention, and when they do so they are likely to be accused of jeopardizing the lives and well-being of their infants."

PSYCHOLOGICAL EFFECTS OF CESAREAN BIRTH

Mothers who have a cesarean birth, especially if the procedure was necessitated by an obstetric emergency, are often faced with situational as well as developmental crises to which they may have difficulty adapting. Cesarean birth poses special physical and psychological threats, because it is at once a significant surgical procedure and the means of birth of a baby. Many of the physical hazards leading to cesarean birth have already been described. However, the surgery itself constitutes a major bodily intrusion and a threat to the body image over which the parturient has little or no control. There is usually little time for psychological preparation because of the nature of the situation. The physical and psychological reactions to the anesthesia and surgery, to the pain and discomfort, to the difficulty of movement, to medical treatments, to restricted oral intake, and to the not uncommon postoperative complications can be expected to include considerable stress.

The psychological aspects of cesarean childbirth have been covered in detail elsewhere in this book and will therefore not be treated here. Suffice it to say that the sequelae of cesarean birth must be taken into account when a nurse enters into a professional relationship with pregnant women. The physical and emotional experiences of cesarean birth should form the basis of the nurse's responsibility to defend the patient's human rights not only at the time of the cesarean birth, but also before and after it. This responsibility is especially evident at the time of an expected repeat cesarean birth.

REFERENCES

Afriat C, Schifrin BS: Sources of error in fetal heart rate monitoring. JOGN Nurs [Suppl] 5 (5):11s-15s, 1976

Baker RA: Technological intervention in obstetrics. Obstet Gynecol 51 (2): 241-43, 1978

Bandman E, Bandman B: There is nothing automatic about rights. Am J Nurs 77:867-72, 1977

Caire JB: Are current rates of cesarean justified? South Med J 71 (5):571-73, 1978

Caldeyro-Barcia R, Noriega-Guera L, Cibils LA, et al: Effect of position changes on the intensity and frequency of uterine contractions during labor. Am J Obstet Gynecol 80 (2): 284-95, 1960

Cohen WR, Rosen R: Recognition and treatment of fetal distress during labor. JOGN Nurs [Suppl] 5 (5):56s-60s, 1976

Doering J. In Stewart L. Stewart D (eds), Compulsory Hospitalization: Freedom of Choice in Childbirth? Marble Hills, Mo., NAPSAC 1:145, 1979

Dulock H, Herron M: Women's responses to fetal monitoring, JOGN Nurs [Suppl] 5 (5):68s-70s, 1976

Dunn PM: Obstetric delivery today. Lancet 10 (1):790-93, 1976

Ettinger BB, McCart DF: Effects of drugs on the fetal heart rate during labor. JOGN Nurs [Suppl] 5 (5):41s-51s, 1976

Flaksman RJ, Vollman JH, Benfield DG: Iatrogenic prematurity due to elective termination of the uncomplicated pregnancy: A major prenatal health care problem. Am J Obstet Gynecol 13 132 (8):885-88, 1978

Gabbe SG, Ettinger BB, Freeman RK, Martin CB: Umbilical cord compression associated with amniotomy: Laboratory observations. Am J Obstet Gynecol 1 126 (3):353-55, 1976

Gassner CB, Ledger WJ: The relationship of hospital-acquired maternal infection to invasive intrapartum monitoring techniques. Am J Obstet Gynecol 1 126 (1):33-37, 1976

Gee CL, Ledger WJ: Maternal and fetal morbidity associated with intrapartum monitoring. JOGN Nurs [Suppl] 5 (5): 65s-67s, 1976

Hack M, Faranoff AA, Klaus MH, et al: Neonatal respiratory distress following elective delivery: A preventable disease? Am J Obstet Gynecol 1 126 (1):43-47, 1976

Haverkamp AD, et al: Electronic fetal monitoring held no better than auscultation. Ob Gyn News 1, 1978

Haverkamp AD, Thompson HE, McFee JG, Cetrulo C: The evaluation of continuous fetal heart rate monitoring in high-risk pregnancy. Am J Obstet Gynecol 125 (3):310-17, 1976

Jones OH: Cesarean section in present-day obstetrics. Am J Obstet Gynecol 1 126 (5):521–30, 1976

Liston WA, Campbell AJ: Dangers of oxytocin-induced labors to foetuses. Br Med J 3 (7):606–07, 1974

Lowensohn RI: Instrumentation for fetal heart rate monitoring. JOGN Nurs [Suppl] 5 (5): 7s–10s, 1976

Martin CB, Gingerich B: Factors affecting the fetal heart rate: Genesis of FHR patterns. JOGN Nurs [Suppl] 5 (5): 30s–40s, 1976

McTammany J. In Stewart L, Stewart D (eds), Compulsory Hospitalization: Freedom of Choice in Childbirth? Marble Hills, Mo., NAPSAC 1, 1979

Neutra R, Fienberg SE, Friedman E: Effect of fetal monitoring on neonatal death rates. N Engl J Med 299 (7):17, 324–26, 1978

Paul RH, Hughey JR, Yeager CF: Clinical fetal monitoring: Its effect on cesarean rate and perinatal mortality: 5-year trends. Postgrad Med 61:160, 1977

Shenker L: Clinical experiences with fetal heart rate monitoring of 1,000 patients in labor. Am J Obstet Gynecol 115 (8):1112–16, 1973

Stalley RF: Self-determination. J Med Ethics 3 (1):40–41, 1977

Steinfels MO: New childbirth technology: A clash of values. Hastings Cent Rep 8 (1):9–12, 1978

Stewart L, Stewart D (eds): Compulsory Hospitalization: Freedom of Choice in Childbirth? Marble Hill, Mo., NAPSAC, 1979, vol. 1, pp. 134, 145

Stewart L, Stewart D (eds): 21st Century Obstetrics Now! Chapel Hill, NC, NAPSAC, 1977, vol. 1

Stewart L, Stewart D (eds): 21st Century Obstetrics Now! Chapel Hill, NC, NAPSAC, 1977, vol. 2

CHAPTER 2

Understanding Cesarean Birth: A Social-Psychological Perspective

Carole Fitzgerald Kehoe

The purpose of a conceptual framework in nursing is both descriptive and organizational. The real world is so complex that only small portions of it can be conceptualized at any one time. Therefore, a nurse must select a portion of the world that seems relevant to the nursing problem being considered and choose theoretical concepts that are appropriate for describing that problem. This description provides the nurse with a perspective from which she can view and understand the totality of the problems and needs of her client. Using this as a guide, the nurse can then collect and organize data about her client so that the meaning and implications for nursing care are clearly understood. This process forms a logical rationale upon which the nurse can structure intelligent and relevant professional practice (Shaw and Costanzo 1970; Jensen et al. 1977, p. 11.).

Many conceptual frameworks are relevant to understanding the cesarean experience, but no one framework is comprehensive enough to provide all of the knowledge that nurses need in order to meet the nursing needs of cesarean families. The biological sciences provide a rationale for addressing needs which have a physiologic basis. The behavioral sciences present another approach by focusing on the social and cultural aspects of the interaction between the nurse and cesarean clients. This perspective provides a basis for understanding responses to cesarean birth in the psychosocial domain of functioning.

The content of this chapter reflects the latter approach by focusing on psychosocial considerations related to maternity clients who experience cesarean birth. The primary theoretical emphasis is on the social-psychological perspective of symbolic interactionism, and the concept "the definition of a situation" is a recurring theme.

Using a sociological approach to the explanation of human behavior, this chapter describes how definitions of situations emerge, the conditions under which they develop, and the social processes by which they are shaped. Within this framework, the evolution of self, role learning, and the influence of culture, reference groups, and life cycle stresses are considered in light of their relevance to a woman's definitions of cesarean birth.

Although maternal definitions of the situation are emphasized here, it should be noted that the definitions of other family members are no less important. However, constraints of time and space in this chapter do not permit the exploration of issues related to other members of the family. The reader is encouraged to assume a family-centered philosophy of maternity care by this author.

SYMBOLIC INTERACTIONISM: AN OVERVIEW

Symbolic interactionism is a phenomenological or humanistic approach to the study of human behavior. This perspective gives a view of the human experience as a continuous learning process in which patterns of behavior are altered, the meanings attributed to various life experiences change, and the individual's concept of self, in his own eyes and in the eyes of others, is continuously modified. This processual orientation shows human behavior as neither static nor absolute. From the moment of birth to the time of death, humans respond creatively and actively to their environment, changing it and themselves in the process (Lauer and Handel 1977, pp. xvi, 349).

Although George Herbert Mead is considered to be the founder of the symbolic interactionism school of thought within this country, it was one of his students, Herbert Blumer, who actually coined the name "symbolic interactionism" (Kando 1977). Mead's original ideas (1934) have been extended and enlarged upon through the writings and research of many contemporary scholars, such as Blumer, Anselm Strauss, Tamotsu Shibutani, and Erving Goffman (Lauer and Handel 1977, pp. 299-300). These individuals have demonstrated the applicability of the symbolic interactionism approach to a variety of substantive social issues, many of which are health-related.

The theory of symbolic interactionism builds upon three premises:

1. The way humans behave toward objects is based on the meanings these things have for them.
2. These meanings emerge from the process of interaction with others.
3. The meanings which guide behavior are constantly modified through an

ongoing interpretive process used by the individual in dealing with persons and things that he encounters (Lauer and Handel 1977, pp. 303-304).

This ongoing interpretive process is highly subjective and suggests that the nature of social reality for each individual is what he perceives it to be. Therefore, in order to understand why people behave as they do, one must first glean some insight into how people perceive, define, and interpret the situations in which they find themselves (Lauer and Handel 1977, p. 308).

The symbolic interactionist has several conceptual tools for analyzing and explaining human behavior and social processes. One of these concepts—the definition of the situation—is especially relevant to cesarean birth and will be considered throughout this chapter.

THE DEFINITION OF A SITUATION

Many years ago, W. I. Thomas, an American sociologist, proposed the concept of "the definition of a situation" to describe emerging lines of scholarly thought about the causes of social behavior (Thomas and Znaniecki 1918). Several years later, after refining earlier thoughts, he articulated this classic theorem (Thomas and Thomas 1928 p. 572):

> *If men define situations as real,*
> *they are real in their consequences.*

In the early 1900s, when sociology was just beginning to emerge as a separate and unique discipline, Thomas's assertions about the influence of subjective factors in human life gave an innovative approach to the analysis of human behavior. His theorem was one of the first attempts by a social theorist to propose that a causal relationship exists between a person's perceptions and interpretations of an event and his subsequent behavior or reaction (Roach 1967, p. 297).

According to Thomas (1928), a person's definition of a situation reflects not only the observable and verifiable aspects of reality, but also, and perhaps primarily, the subjective meaning of that particular situation. Once an individual has defined a certain event in a certain way, his subsequent reactions will reflect that ascribed definition—be it positive or negative (Merton 1956, p. 422).

Humans live in a symbolic world and they respond to various situations through symbolic mediation. When a person defines a situation he represents it to himself symbolically and responds accordingly. Thus a person's definition of a situation reflects primarily the subjective meaning and interpretation of a particular situation. Objective perceptions and interpretations made by others are less important to the person than his own, because his reality is whatever he perceives it to be. Therefore, the behavior of a person cannot be clearly understood if one relies upon objective factors exclusively. Such objective factors are essentially extrinsic to the person. Subjective perceptions are crucial to the process of defining such events as cesarean birth (Lauer and Handel 1977, pp. 84-85).

The definition that is assigned to any given event incorporates both social and cultural variables. On the social level, events are perceived and defined according to categories of attitudes, meanings, and motives personally derived during the process of anticipatory socialization in childhood. On the cultural level, however, events are perceived and defined on the basis of categories of attitudes, meanings, and motives which are shared with other members of social groups within the environment (Wolff 1964, p. 182).

To understand how a cesarean mother defines the situation of cesarean birth is to understand the meaning that this situation has for her, and thereby to understand why she behaves as she does. Much of the behavior that nurses encounter on a day-to-day basis in their interactions with cesarean clients is understandable if they know the client's definitions of situations. This notion is an important conceptual tool for nurses in other clinical areas as well. It can explain behavior that might otherwise be perplexing and suggests a variable of importance in the assessment phase of the nursing process (Yura and Walsh 1978).

As with other concepts in symbolic interactionism, the definition of the situation is processual and therefore more or less fluid. Definitions of situations change throughout one's life. To understand how this change can occur, it is helpful to be familiar with the processes involved in the emergence and development of definitions of situations. The following section considers these related issues.

EMERGENCE AND DEVELOPMENT OF DEFINITIONS OF SITUATIONS

The Primary Group and Socialization

Every child is born into one of the many subcultural groups which together comprise the society as a whole. The survival and perpetuation of these groups depends in part upon the ability of each of its members to perceive the structure of the group correctly and to have the motivation necessary to conform to the group's norms and prescribed behaviors. The process by which the knowledge, values, attitudes, skills, and other socially relevant behaviors of the group are transmitted to newly born group members is known as "anticipatory socialization" (Goode 1964, p. 10; Folta and Deck 1966, p. 13; Hurley, 1978, p. 31).

A child may be born with the biological capacity to become an effective, functioning member of his social group, but it is through socialization that he really becomes a social being. Through this process the physical and psychological qualities of the newborn child are shaped and molded by the adult members of his primary group or family to conform to the cultural norms adhered to by the society at large (Goode 1964, p. 11).

The social group into which an infant is born has already developed definitions of the general kinds of situations faced on a day-to-day basis. Accordingly, the group develops rules of conduct and moral codes of behavior to which each group member must conform. Socialization processes are designed by the significant others in the child's primary group to help him to internalize these group definitions of situations. It should be noted that a child cannot create his own definitions and follow their implications without adult interference. Conformity to society's definitions is one of the goals of socialization, and deviations from this goal are not well tolerated. Those in charge of the socialization process—the child's significant others—act quickly to enforce conformity when transgressions become apparent, using a system of rewards and punishments (Stryker 1964, p. 131).

The Self

An infant is not born with a consciousness of self. The self, which is the conception that one has of oneself, is a product of social interaction. It begins with the intimate relationship between a child and his significant others, and gradually emerges as communication skills grow and social interactions become more numerous.

One of the most important features of the self is its reflective character, which was referred to initially by Cooley (1902) as the "looking-glass self." He introduced the notion that the interpretation of others' judgments is an essential element in the development of one's own self-conception.

Children are very susceptible to subtle indications of approval and disapproval. At a very early age, an infant learns how to elicit attention from those responsible for his care and he strives for signs of their approval of his behavior. He is equally sensitive to indications of disapproval. A child repeatedly parades himself before the social "looking glasses" that comprise his primary group, seeking positive reinforcement for his behavior.

His interpretation of the image that he *thinks* he sees there determines to a great extent his opinion of himself. This image—be it positive or negative in the child's view—influences his emerging self-identity, and his subsequent behavior is controlled by and reflects this identity. Thus the evolving self is the means by which social control eventually becomes self-control (Lundberg et al. 1968, p. 277; Lauer and Handel 1977, pp. 66-71).

The quest for self-identity is a life-long process. The self is always in a state of emergence in response to interactions with others and is an integral part of the human experience. The self is never complete or finalized. It continues to evolve and is modified throughout the individual's entire life, though to a somewhat lesser degree in adulthood (Kando 1977, pp. 158-159). Cesarean birth is an example of an experience that may modify a woman's sense of self.

It is important to remember that personality structures and biological capacities differ from one person to another. These innate differences, as well as the social and cultural milieu in which each person is socialized, have a profound influence on the emerging self. Ultimately, self-identities vary considerably, and people's definitions of situations always reflect the distinct character of their individually evolving self.

Role Learning

The learning of social roles and the definitions of situations associated with those roles begins with a deep personal attachment between an infant and his mothering person and gradually extends to include others in the infant's primary group.

"Mothering person" is a global term, referring to the person (or persons) who have primary responsibility for meeting the infant's physical and psychological needs. This person may be the infant's biological mother, but this is not necessarily the case. Since the role of the male in providing nurturing care for the children is becoming more accepted in our society, this person may not necessarily even be a female.

The behavior of the mothering person is especially important in the gradual process of learning definitions of situations. She (or he) imparts to the child her own internalized definitions of situations through gestures, voice inflections, and the like. From her behavior the infant infers the mothering person's social definitions of situations. Due to his intellectual immaturity and limited social experiences, the infant accepts the definitions of his significant others without question. As a result, his beginning perspective of social definitions is narrow in scope, because it reflects the definitions of a very restricted, small group of people.

As he matures, the infant becomes aware of the social definitions of situations that are subscribed to by all the members of his primary group. These significant others define the social world for him and become role models for later development of his own definitions of situations.

Although the social definitions of the significant others are paramount during the initial stages of life, the definitions held by others soon assume even greater importance. As his social world expands, the child interacts with others outside of his primary group. The roles and social positions of those persons gradually become apparent to the infant through this contact and contribute to his emerging definitions of situations and social role learning.

Learning social roles involves the learning of elements common to the enactment of roles, such as mothering and childbearing. These elements are role prescriptions, role expectations, and role performance.

Role Prescriptions–The prescriptive aspects of roles refer to the behaviors that somehow "ought to be" or "should be" performed. These are society's norms, or requirements designed to regulate the behavior of its members so that the various functions of the society can proceed in an orderly and predictable manner (Biddle and Thomas 1966).

Role Expectations–Role expectations encompass the knowledge, skills, and attitudes required to perform a particular role successfully. This information serves to set standards for acceptable role performance (Hardy 1978, p. 76).

The complementary nature of role expectations is basic iu all role performance. Role behaviors are designed to mesh with each other. This mutual reliance serves a specific purpose in social life, for each role partner needs to know what to expect of others and what others expect as well, so that interactions may proceed in an orderly and predictable manner.

Through the process of specifying role expectations, the implied definitions of situations are made overt and explicit to the child. When his significant others spell out precise expectations of his role behavior, they also spell out the definitions of situations that they expect him to conform to and adopt. Role expectations, then, are the empirical referents of the theoretical definitions of situations subscribed to by a child's significant others (Stryker 1964, p. 140).

Role Performance–Role performance involves the overt behaviors, verbal and nonverbal, that are evident when a person actually enacts a particular role. The terms "performance" and "behavior" are used interchangeably in the literature to describe this process (Lum 1979, p. 49).

A particular role performance may not always correspond to the expectations of the role occupant, or to the expectations of those observing the role performance. This inconsistency between expectations and performance is often unintentional nonconformity. Role expectations provide a range of acceptable behaviors, all of which reflect a wide range of definitions of situations. Therefore, a role occupant may choose from among several behavioral options. These choices reflect internalized and unconscious definitions of situations. Thus the same social role may be performed slightly differently by different persons. In addition, subcultural differences and biophysical factors over which there may be no control (such as cesarean birth) will influence role behavior. When assessing another's role behavior, these points should be remembered before making hasty conclusions about the adequacy or inadequacy of a particular role performance (Lum 1979, pp. 49-50).

Learning Selected Family Roles

Every child in a society learns the role elements associated with being a mother and a childbearer. These definitions, acquired in childhood, pattern the personal definitions of childbearing and mothering experiences that one has as an adult.

The Mother Role—A female child identifies with the mother role early in life because she is the recipient of activities associated with this role from birth. Societal norms clearly spell out the behaviors appropriate to performing the mother role.

Appropriate mothering behavior involves providing nurturing, loving care for the child. This includes, interestingly, not only the physical care aspects of mothering, but also the "feelings" that a person should have when performing these functions. These feelings are expected to reflect an emotional attachment to the child and a perception of the child as a valued and respected human being. Thus a mothering person is expected to have unconditional positive regard for the child, regardless of his behavior (Rogers 1961; Robischon and Scott 1969).

By observing and interacting with the mothering person, children of both sexes gradually learn and internalize expectations about mothering behaviors that are enacted before their eyes. They learn what mothers are supposed to do, what they should say, how they should feel, and how they should conduct themselves in various situations.

Definitions of mothering are assimilated on a gradual and unconscious level, based on exposure to these definitions from a variety of sources. This is an evolving process that continues into adulthood, when persons actually become parents and enact parental roles.

The Childbearing Role—From earliest childhood, through interaction with the biological mother and/or female mothering person, children learn about the experience of birth. Through stories about their own birth and probably some "old wives' tales," a mental image begins to form about what it is like to have a baby. Depending on the content provided, they undoubtedly hear about the pain, the problems, the inconveniences, and, one hopes, some of the joys that this unique experience can bring to the life of a family.

By the time adulthood is reached, each person has developed a set of expectations to guide role performance during the birth process. It is important to emphasize that these role expectations are part of the definitions of childbearing that couples bring with them when they are actively engaged in the childbearing process.

Throughout the period in which definitions of mothering and childbearing develop, the self continues to evolve, and remains unique to each individual.

Thus the actual performance of the mothering and childbearing roles reflects a combination of "self-definition" and "social definitions" of those roles. The enactment of these family roles, however, differs among adults because of internal motivation, varying attitudes toward the self, and different expectations and response patterns, all of which are derived from each person's self-identity (Lum 1979, p. 50).

Where there is congruence between self, role expectations, and definitions of the mother role and the childbearing role, a more enjoyable, involved, and committed parental role performance is possible. This ultimately affects the happiness and well-being of the entire family unit, because it facilitates orderly and predictable interaction in the role relationships among all family members.

THE SHAPING OF DEFINITIONS OF SITUATIONS

Early definitions of situations are important because they provide a foundation for subsequent adult role behavior. However, the learning of social roles and the process of redefining situations is ongoing and encompasses a person's whole life. The symbolic interactionism perspective emphasizes a processual approach to understanding human behavior and assumes that change is the very essence of social reality. People are continuously modifying their definitions of situations. Their responses reflect these modifications as various circumstances impinge upon their lives and perceptions of reality (Lauer and Handel 1977, pp. 339-340).

Many factors shape and alter the social definitions of childbirth that women bring with them when they are involved in childbearing. Selected factors are described in this section.

The Influence of Culture

A woman is not born *with* a culture, she is born *into* one. Culture is a way of life that is learned, shared with others in the social group, and transmitted from one generation to the next. Culture includes the behaviors, attitudes, values, and beliefs of a particular social group; these elements are common to all cultures. How these elements are interpreted and operationalized define each culture as unique (Folta and Deck 1966, p. 10).

These cultural elements are given life through a series of folkways, mores, and norms, which determine the acceptable limits of behavior and define the behavioral variations that are allowed.

Childbearing is considered an important experience by every culture. In fact, there is no known culture in which childbearing is ignored or treated with total indifference (Newton 1964). This undoubtedly reflects the realization by all people that the survival of the culture and society depends upon the reproductive efforts of its members.

By the time a woman reaches the age when pregnancy and childbirth become physiologically possible, her definitions of this experience have been strongly influenced by the shared definitions of the social and cultural milieu in which she was socialized. The culture determines those aspects of childbearing which will have special meaning to the woman and her family. Against her cultural background, an expectant mother defines and evaluates her entire childbearing performance, before, during, and after the actual birth of the baby. Because the culture identifies for each woman those aspects of her performance which are acceptable and those which are not, it influences how she responds to events that are less-than-ideal in her eyes. In addition, her ability to cope with and adapt to disruptive, unplanned-for situations that occur during the maternity cycle (such as cesarean birth) is dependent upon coping strategies learned within the context of her culture (Anderson 1979; Snyder 1979).

The nurse can observe the influence of cultural definitions in the following aspects of the childbearing experience: the meaning and value of reproduction to the culture; the feelings that pregnancy can evoke in the social group; the feelings of responsibility that are imposed on parents as a result of the pregnancy; the view of birth as either a normal process or a pathological event; the consideration of birth as a private or a social event; the emphasis on birth as a personal achievement of the mother or as an event requiring payment to the birth attendants; and the eating and activity patterns allowed following delivery (Affonso 1979, pp. 107-113).

Cultural definitions of appropriate mothering behavior can be observed in these areas; the meaning and significance of children to the culture; patterns of behavior of caregivers in feeding infants (what, how much, how often, and by what method); grooming of the child; discipline; approaches to meeting the child's needs for psychological nurturance; and parental response to the behaviors and appearance of the infant (Affonso 1979).

There is, of course, considerable cultural variation in the definitions associated with each aspect of the childbearing and mothering roles. In moments of greatest stress associated with the enactment of these roles, a woman can be expected to cling tenaciously to her cultural definitions. Her cultural beliefs and values will have far more influence on her perceptions and reactions than will the intervention of strangers. In the face of anxiety and uncertainty (as regards cesarean birth, for example), cultural definitions provide comforting structure and stability. Therefore, it is advisable to design a plan of nursing intervention which is consistent with the client's basic cultural beliefs, rather than one that contains features contradictory to these persuasions. A mother will appreciate respect for her cultural background and may therefore be more receptive to accepting nursing interventions concerning other aspects of her behavior (Mercer 1977, p. 35).

The Influence of Reference Groups

Reference groups are comprised of others whose attitudes, values, and opinions are considered important enough to influence one's behavior. The perspective of the reference group constitutes a frame of reference that a childbearing woman may use to guide her role performance in situations in which a choice is available to her (Lum, 1978, p. 137).

A reference group may be a psychological construct rather than a membership group. This is not to say that the reference group does not exist. It can, and for many people, does, but the reference point does not have to be a group of people.

Reference groups play a significant part in the socialization of children. As a child matures, his social world expands beyond the boundaries of his primary group to embrace others in peer relationships. The definitions of situations held by peers strongly influence the child's perceptions of his social experiences and the impact that these experiences have upon him.

Zborowski (1952) underscored the importance of reference groups in influencing adult definitions of situations. Patients at a veterans' hospital in New York were studied to ascertain their responses to pain. The sample included Jewish, Italian, and Old American (English, Scandinavian, and other) patients. Although these patients had similar overt reactions *to* pain, the groups had quite different attitudes *about* pain. The findings suggest that the subjects defined pain in very different terms because they did so within the frameworks of different reference groups.

Pregnancy does not occur in total social isolation. A woman is usually a member of some organized social group which shares the experience of her pregnancy with her. Her family, friends, work associates, and others in her social milieu provide supportive relationships which help to sustain her during this period in her life (Snyder 1979).

As a woman advances in her pregnancy and progresses through the psychological work preparatory to achieving the final goal of pregnancy—maternal role attainment—her peer or reference group provides her with models and referents. Through the slow and tedious processes of mimicry, role play, fantasy, and the circular activities of introjection-projection-rejection, the expectant mother accomplishes the tasks necessary for moving into the maternal role after the baby has been born (Rubin 1967).

Peers usually play a much more influential role in these processes than does the woman's own mother. Her own mother may be viewed as too knowledgeable and overwhelmingly competent for this purpose. An expectant mother uses her peers as her role models. In the process of integrating their expectations of how to perform the mother role into her self structure, she also internalizes the group's definitions of appropriate mothering behavior.

In addition to influencing and shaping a woman's definitions of mothering, reference groups shape definitions of the childbearing process. They define those aspects of the experience which may have the most profound impact upon her. If, for example, the group places a high social value on a nonmedicated, participatory, vaginal delivery, then the woman who has a cesarean birth may perceive herself as having violated group norms. This violation casts her into the role of a social deviant, in her own mind.

From a sociological viewpoint, the notion of deviant behavior applies to anyone who fails to conform to the expectations of others—particularly of one's reference group—either intentionally or unintentionally. In violating group expectations, one is also failing to accept the group's definitions of situations, because role expectations reflect the implied definitions of situations of one's social group (Hurley 1978, pp. 67-68).

Blake and Davis (1964, pp. 468-482) identified unintentional deviant behavior as the outcome of physical and environmental conditions outside of a person's control. The cause of the deviance lies in factors over which the individual has no control. In the case of a cesarean mother, the deviance is clearly unintentional, because biophysical factors (see Chapter 1) are not usually within the scope of her control. This notion applies to mothers who expected cesarean birth as well as to mothers for whom cesarean birth was unanticipated. Such deviance is called "felt deviance," because it reflects the mother's self-perceptions rather than the perceptions of others (Bott 1960, p. 447).

Unintentional deviance can be handled by showing acceptance and positive regard for the mother. Interactions which emphasize areas of behavior in which there is obvious conformity can also help the mother to perceive herself as less of a nonconformist. Social acceptance is exceedingly important to a woman who perceives herself as being in a role that is contradictory to the norms of her reference group, a role that may carry with it the social stigma of failure, at least in her own mind.

Reference group influences are particularly relevant for the immature woman who is engaged in childbearing. This woman may or may not be chronologically young, although people do tend to associate immaturity with youthfulness. For the purposes of this discussion, an immature woman is one who shows a lack of psychological or emotional maturity and stability, regardless of her chronological age.

The immature childbearing woman may still be searching for her adult self-identity. This entails a difficult transitional period for anyone, regardless of age, because it is filled with self-doubt. One of the ways a woman may cope with this situation is by closely identifying with her reference group, adopting the group's values, attitudes, and beliefs, as well as various modes of behavior and dress.

A woman unsure of who she is and where she belongs may have considerable difficulty in picturing herself in a new role in which she has to place another's needs before her own, especially if this other is a totally dependent and demanding infant. She will be particularly vulnerable to the judgments of her peer group because of her uncertainty over her own role and her own need for nurturance (Mercer 1979, pp. 369-372).

The immature mother's reference group can provide a supportive and empathetic environment that may ultimately assist an immature mother to cope with the role changes that are an inevitable part of childbearing. The group's influence may provide positive support for the woman who is still questioning her self-worth, regardless of her age (Dyad 1974, pp. 51-55; Welches 1979, p. 33).

The notion of reference groups is relevant to the care of cesarean mothers because it suggests another dimension to assess in identifying the cesarean mother's definitions of the childbearing experience.

The Influence of Stressful Events

Maturational Events—In the developmental continuum stretching between birth and death, stressful events form a common denominator of the human experience. Some stresses occur predictably in life as part of the natural process of growth and development; these carry the potential for becoming maturational crises. Marriage, pregnancy, and parenthood are examples of potential maturational crisis periods. These events usually occur around role shifts, as a person moves from one stage of biological, psychological, and social development to another. Role shifts involve a gradual progression from one level of functioning to a different level (Williams 1974, p. 43).

These periods have a crisis potential because there may be difficulty in making the role changes appropriate to each new maturational level. The psychological and social pressure on the individual to see himself in a new role and to function according to a new set of expectations and a different set of social definitions of situations may evoke stress so intense that former problem-solving and coping skills are inadequate. Thus the individual is unable to deal effectively with the tension resulting from the stress he feels. As a result, a state of disequilibrium occurs, leading to major disruptions in the interaction of reciprocal roles within the family (Baird 1979, p. 299).

Inability to make the role changes necessary to prevent a maturational crisis occurs for the following reasons. First, the person may be unable to picture himself in a new role. Since all social roles are learned, adequate role models and appropriate socialization methods are prerequisite to assuming new roles. If this preparation has been inadequate, perceptions may be distorted and the person may feel threatened and may be reluctant to assume that role. Second, the person in question may not have the personal skills and flexibility needed to change his behaviors and adopt behaviors that are expected in performing a new role. This can interfere with his willingness and ability to cope. Third, this person may not be able to move into a new role because others in his social milieu persist in viewing him from prior social perspectives. They may refuse to see him in a role requiring higher levels of mature functioning. Thus the supports which facilitate the assumption of a new role may be inadequate, ambiguous, or nonexistent (Williams 1974, pp. 44-45).

Situational Events—Whereas potential maturational crisis periods involve an element of predictability, there are other stressful events which occur unexpectedly during the life cycle. These are referred to as potential situational crisis periods and usually occur with minimal or no warning. Their sudden onset renders prior problem-solving and coping skills virtually useless because the problem demands solutions which are novel in view of previous life experiences.

Unlike a potential maturational crisis in which the stress is primarily intrinsic and involves gradual assumption of new roles, the stress in a potential situational crisis is external and is perceived as a sudden threat to self, to role performance, or to social integrity. The birth of a premature infant, the birth of a stillborn, and an unexpected cesarean birth are all examples of situational stressful events that may proceed to crisis (Williams 1974, p. 119; Baird 1979, p. 302).

The processes which lead to a situational crisis are complex, and relate to the notion of self. As described previously, the self-concept which emerges from interactions with significant others is reinforced by the feedback received from others as one learns and enacts social roles. A sense of self-identity is maintained through the continuity of role relationships and a perceived ability to establish new role relationships. When a situational stress arises, the continuity and maintenance of roles considered vital for maintaining self-identity are threatened. Thus a person may question his ability to reestablish role relationships that will make his environment a secure and meaningful place once more. Concurrent feelings of helplessness and hopelessness are aroused. The stress engendered by the perceived loss of roles essential for self-identity and need fulfillment makes such a person vulnerable to experiencing a crisis (Williams 1974, p. 120).

In this chapter, childbirth is assumed to be a potential maturational crisis, whereas cesarean birth is a potential situational crisis. Whether these events actually proceed to the crisis phase or not depends on the mother's perceptions of the event, the availability of support systems, and the mother's learned coping mechanisms. For example, if a cesarean mother perceives the birth in a distorted way, (i.e., as an indication of failure in the enactment of her childbearing role), if she has minimal or no situational supports from significant others to sustain her throughout the stressful period, and if she has ineffective coping mechanisms and problem-solving skills, then she will probably experience a crisis (Caplan 1961; Aguilera and Messick 1978, pp. 70-71).

The Chinese character for "crisis" has a dual meaning: "danger yet opportunity." This is an appropriate symbol, because in every crisis there exists the danger of increased psychological insult and trauma, as well as the opportunity for change, growth, and the attainment of new levels of maturity (Baird 1979, p. 299).

Typically, a crisis is self-limiting and lasts approximately 4 to 6 weeks. This period is a transitional phase in which the individual experiencing the crisis is especially vulnerable to therapeutic intervention. Intervention strategies focus on helping the client to gain intellectual understanding, recognize his feelings, expose past and present coping mechanisms, find and use resources, and carry out anticipatory planning to prevent or reduce the possibility of future crises (Baird 1979, p. 301).

Prior Life Experiences—All persons are products of their prior life experiences. Past stresses which occurred in response to maturational role changes or in unexpected situational events will shape a person's perceptions of present stressful experiences, as well as his adaptive ability (Aguilera and Messick 1978).

A childbearing woman is especially vulnerable to prior stresses. During pregnancy there is a shift in the equilibrium between the ego and the id which allows repressed ideas to surface to the awareness level. This is brought about by the hormonal and metabolic variations that are inherent in the numerous physiological changes of pregnancy. During the second trimester particularly, there is a revival of early childhood memories, fantasies, and unresolved conflicts related to the woman's own mother and siblings in her primary group. At this time a woman will talk with relative ease about prior experiences and interactions that one would ordinarily expect her to feel very anxious about. This willingness to express such thoughts lasts up to the second or third week postpartum. At this point the mother's hormonal structure returns to prepregnant levels and she once again represses this material. If questioned, she may in fact deny that she ever voiced these ideas during her pregnancy (Caplan 1961, pp. 71–81).

The stresses associated with memories of past events have a bearing on a woman's present definitions of situations. However, some of the events in her past are more potent than others in shaping present perceptions and definitions of childbearing and mothering.

Personal experiences in childbearing are important determinants of how the pregnant woman perceives and defines her pregnancy. Experiences which once threatened her self-identity and compromised her childbearing capability are especially relevant. Situational stressful events which proceeded to a crisis that was not completely resolved may impinge upon her present coping and adaptive techniques.

A prior cesarean birth which was perceived as traumatic will shape the definition of cesarean birth that a woman brings to the present pregnancy. Anxiety and tension may be heightened, particularly if the outcome of the prior cesarean birth did not include a healthy, living infant. If she did not receive any supportive intervention aimed at helping her to cope with that event, she will be more likely to be vulnerable to psychological insult if the experience is repeated this time.

There is an abundance of literature which speaks to the issues of stress and crisis as they relate to childbearing. Since the terms "stress" and "crisis" are often used interchangeably, it is obvious that some ambiguity exists regarding their precise meaning. Depending upon the book or article, childbirth is envisioned as a stress, a crisis, or both. Although there may be a lack of conceptual clarity in the use of these terms, one thing is clear. Regardless of the precise term chosen to describe the phenomenon of childbirth, it is certainly a time of transition and of redefining situations related to the enactment of family roles, especially for cesarean families.

A knowledgeable and caring nurse can assist childbearing families to make the role changes necessary to accommodate their new family members. The nurse's assessment of the influence of prior life experiences is one place to begin in the process of designing nursing interventions which support and facilitate a family's efforts to make the inevitable necessary role changes.

SUMMARY AND IMPLICATIONS

The underlying premise of this chapter is that a woman's perception of and reactions to the cesarean experience depend upon how she defines that experience, because her reality is whatever she perceives it to be. If she defines this experience in negative terms, then her reactions to this experience and its impact upon her and her significant others may be negative. Conversely, if she defines cesarean birth more positively than negatively, then it is very likely that the negative impact of this alternative mode of childbearing will be less intense, and a healthy resolution of resulting stresses will more likely occur.

When a woman embarks upon the complex process of bearing a child, she brings with her a whole array of social and cultural definitions about childbearing and motherhood. The implications of Thomas's theorem is that regardless of where the mother is in the maternity cycle, her definitions of situations will influence her behavior and the decisions that she makes. Whether she is considering attending childbirth education classes before the infant's birth or striving to adjust to the physiologic and psychosocial stresses following cesarean birth, her behavior and reactions will reflect how she defines the situation in which she finds herself.

The definition of a situation is one of the major concepts of symbolic interactionism, which is basically a processual theoretical orientation. Definitions of situations should never be viewed as fixed and absolute, but rather as fluid and developmental. One does not continue to define situations the same way throughout life, nor for that matter throughout a specific situation (Lauer and Handel 1977, p. 87).

Because of the transitory nature of a woman's existing definitions of child-bearing, the possibility of change and growth is always present. This suggests that the nurse may be able to help families alter their negative definitions of cesarean birth and to strengthen and encourage positive perceptions of the experience which may already exist.

The final goal in pregnancy is to take on the maternal role along with all of its ongoing and long-term responsibilities. The roles of childbearing and mothering are closely related on the developmental continuum, and the mothering role can be perceived as an extension of the childbearing role. The inability to enact the childbearing role in the expected way can lead the mother to feelings of role failure and frustration. A woman may feel confused and inadequate because of this inability to achieve her childbearing goals. This may adversely affect her desire to move into the mothering role and establish a meaningful reciprocal relationship with her infant, since perceived inadequacy in one role can make an individual reluctant to attempt the enact-ment of a related role. Because of the potential long-range consequences, the nurse's efforts to facilitate a positive cesarean experience assume even greater importance.

Symbolic interactionism offers a wealth of conceptual knowledge that is relevant to the nursing care of cesarean families at all points in the maternity cycle. Perhaps of equal importance is its applicability to the nurse herself, in her interaction with cesarean families, in her personal perceptions of child-bearing, in her own definitions of appropriate maternal and paternal role behavior during this experience, and in her sense of self, both as a woman and as a nurse. These factors cannot fail to influence the nurse's perceptions of cesarean families, the frame of reference in which she assesses their needs and concerns, the quality and relevance of the intervention she designs, as well as the compassion with which she implements her plan of care.

REFERENCES

Affonso DD: Framework for cultural assessment. In Clark A, Affonso D (with TR Harris) (eds), Childbearing: A Nursing Perspective, 2nd ed. Philadelphia, Davis, 1979

Aguilera DC, Messick JM: Crisis Intervention: Theory and Methodology. St. Louis, Mosby, 1978

Anderson D: Cultural strategies. In Johnson SH (ed) High-risk Parenting: Nursing Assessment and Strategies for a Family at Risk. Philadelphia, Lippincott, 1979

Baird SF: Crisis intervention strategies. In Johnson SH (ed), High-risk Parent-ing: Nursing Assessment and Strategies for the Family at Risk. Philadel-phia, Lippincott, 1979

Biddle BJ, Thomas EJ: Role Theory: Concepts and Research. New York, Wiley, 1966

Blake J, Davis K: Norms, values and sanctions. In Faris REL (ed), Handbook of Modern Sociology. Chicago, Rand McNally, 1964

Bott E: Norms and ideology: The normal family. In Bell NW, Vogel EF (eds), A Modern Introduction to the Family. Glencoe, Ill., The Free Press, 1960

Caplan G: An Approach to Community Mental Health. New York, Grune and Stratton, 1961

Cooley CH: Human Nature and the Social Order. New York, Scribner, 1902

Dyad H: How difficult the "I": The adolescent maturation of critical identity. In Hall JE, Weaver BR (eds), Nursing of Families in Crisis. Philadelphia, Lippincott, 1974

Folta JR, Deck ES: A Sociological Framework for Patient Care. New York, Wiley, 1966

Goode WJ: The Family. Englewood Cliffs, NJ, Prentice-Hall, 1964

Hardy ME: Role stress and role strain. In Hardy ME, Conway ME (eds), Role Theory: Perspectives for Health Professionals. New York, Appleton-Century-Crofts, 1978

Hurley BA: Socialization for roles. In Hardy ME, Conway ME (eds), Role Theory: Perspectives for Health Professionals. New York, Appleton-Century-Crofts, 1978

Jensen MD, Benson RC, Bobak IM: Maternity Care, the Nurse and the Family. St. Louis, Mosby, 1977

Kando TM: Social Interaction. St. Louis, Mosby, 1977

Lauer RH, Handel WH: Social Psychology: The Theory and Application of Symbolic Interactionism. Boston, Houghton-Mifflin, 1977

Lum JLJ: Reference groups and professional socialization. In Hardy ME, Conway ME (eds), Role Theory: Perspectives for Health Professionals. New York, Appleton-Century-Crofts, 1978

Lum JLJ: Role theory. In Clark A, Affonso D (with TR Harris) (eds), Childbearing: A Nursing Perspective, 2nd ed. Philadelphia, Davis, 1979

Lundberg GA, Schrag CC, Larsen O, Catton WR: Sociology, 4th ed. New York, Harper and Row, 1968

Mead GH: Mind, Self and Society. Chicago, University of Chicago Press, 1934

Mercer RT: Nursing Care of Patients at Risk. New York, Slack, 1977

Mercer RT: Perspectives on Adolescent Health Care. New York, Lippincott, 1979

Merton RK: Social Theory and Social Structure. New York, The Free Press, 1956

Newton N: Pregnancy, childbirth, and outcome: A review of patterns of culture and future needs. In Richardson S, Guttmacher A (eds), Childbearing: Its Social and Psychological Aspects. Baltimore, Williams and Wilkins, 1964

Roach J: A theory of lower-class behavior. In Gross L (ed), Sociological Theory: Inquiries and Paradigms. New York, Harper and Row, 1967

Robischon P, Scott D: Role theory and its application in family nursing. Nurs Outlook 17 (7):52-57, 1969

Rogers C: On Becoming a Person. Boston, Houghton-Mifflin, 1961

Rubin R: Attainment of the maternal role, part I. Nurs Res 16 (3):237-45, 1967

Shaw ME, Costanzo PR: Theories of Social Psychology. New York, McGraw-Hill, 1970

Snyder DJ; The high-risk mother viewed in relation to a holistic model of the childbearing experience. J Obstet Gynecol Neonat Nurs 8 (3):164-70, 1979

Stryker S: The interactional and situational approaches. In Christensen H (ed), Handbook of Marriage and the Family. Chicago, Rand McNally, 1964

Thomas WI, Thomas DS: The Child in America. New York, Knopf, 1928, p. 572

Thomas WI, Znaniecki F: The Polish Peasant in Europe and America. Boston, Badger, 1918–1920 (5 vols.)

Welches LJ: Adolescent sexuality. In Mercer RT (ed), Perspectives on Adolescent Health Care. New York, Lippincott, 1979

Williams FS: Intervention in maturational crises. In Hall JE, Weaver BR (eds), Nursing of Families in Crisis. Philadelphia, Lippincott, 1974

Wolff KH: Definition of the situation. In Gould J, Kolb WL (eds), Dictionary of the Social Sciences. New York, The Free Press, 1964

Yura H, Walsh M: The Nursing Process, 3rd ed. New York, Appleton–Century–Crofts, 1978

Zborowski M: Cultural components in responses to pain. J Soc Issues 8 (4):16–30, 1952

SECTION II

Maternal-Infant Attachment

CHAPTER 3

Facilitation of Maternal-Infant Attachment Following Cesarean Birth

Margaret R. Spaulding

I am being driven forward
Into an unknown land.
The pass grows steeper,
The air colder and sharper.
A wind from my unknown goal
Stirs the strings
Of expectation.

Still the question:
Shall I ever get there?
There where life resounds,
A clear pure note
In the silence.

—Dag Hammarskjöld, 1965

Every human infant enters the world tethered to his mother. This tether is severed at birth, necessitating a new life line—an attachment of spirit created out of love and caring. The process of creating a maternal–infant attachment requires the active participation of and reciprocal feedback from both mother and infant. Any condition or event that interferes with the timing or attending of the participants may adversely affect the bond that is formed. A cesarean birth can be such an event. Drugs, anesthesia, the condition of mother or infant, increased stress, and separation can all contribute to making the attachment process more difficult. This chapter discusses some of the major factors affecting attachment after cesarean births, factors the nurse will want to consider in planning and providing care so as to enhance the development of a healthy mother–infant attachment. This discussion focuses on management strategies based on the condition of the participants and their development in the attachment process at the time of the intervention.

INTERFERENCE WITH SYNCHRONY

The development of a mother–infant bond is particularly at risk after a cesarean birth because of the disruption of synchronous patterns of mother–infant interaction normally present at birth. These patterns tie physiological, psychological, and behavioral rhythms present in the interacting couple during a particularly sensitive "species specific" acquainting sequence. While some delay in timing of this sequence can be tolerated without permanent disruptive consequences, there is strong evidence that the longer the delay, the greater the likelihood that the mothering behaviors established will be disturbed in some way. Research has linked cesarean birth with later child abuse, failure to thrive, and other disturbances. Helfer (1974) found an incidence of child abuse in families experiencing cesarean birth that was twice that found in families experiencing vaginal births.

The findings of increased mothering disturbances following cesarean birth are particularly upsetting today, since the proportion of cesarean births has risen during the last decade to 22 percent of the total (Evrard and Gold 1978). Furthermore, in some instances the cesarean rate for women who attend prepared childbirth classes is greater than that of the clinic patients who give birth in the same time period (Hughey et al. 1977).

The optimum time for the first mother–infant interaction appears to be within the first 2 hours after birth. A heightened state of awareness has been discovered to exist during this time in both the mother and the infant. At the same time, the mother's sense of time and space is focused on the here and now in much the same manner as a magnifying glass focuses the sun's rays with enough intensity to create fire (Rich 1973). Full concentration of all of the baby's and the mother's senses is brought to bear on identifying and discovering one another. The element of disbelief that what has been awaited for months has finally happened also serves as a powerful orienting force (Gottlieb 1978). In the moment of birth the infant feels for the first time the sensation of air touching his flesh and filling his lungs, an approximate 20° drop in the temperature around him, the sudden removal of limitations on his movement, and bright light impacting on his retina. The only link to his previous existence is his mother. Recent studies foster the belief that multiple synchronized responses between the mother and the infant are present at birth (Rosenblatt 1978).

Prior to birth, both mother and infant have experienced each other through shared bodily warmth, internal touch and movement, hormonal and chemical exchanges, and diurnal rhythms. Brazelton (1978) cites evidence that babies are learning in utero and adapting to information from their mothers, and vice versa. Fetuses are entrained by the mother's metabolic processes and rhythms. They not only respond to auditory and visual stimuli, but can differentiate various stimuli in these modes, showing preferences for certain ones. Far from being strangers at birth, mothers and infants have at that time already interacted for months.

Mothers in the last trimester of pregnancy frequently ascribe personality traits to their fetuses on the basis of behavioral cues they are receiving from them. Fetuses can identify rhythms, as evidenced by one expectant mother's remark: "He likes disco music. He kicks in time to the music." Before studies confirmed the fetus's ability to respond to external stimuli, such remarks would simply have been labeled as fantasy.

The important elements of this first interaction between mother and infant have been teased out by multiple research studies. Consistently, the assumption of an *en face* position by the mother and fingertip touching of the face, arms, and legs have been associated with this initial encounter. The mother pitches her voice to a higher level and uses a sing-song rhythm to which, studies have shown, the newborn is most responsive. Is it coincidence that high-pitched sounds travel best through densities similar to the human abdomen (MacFarlane 1977)? The movement of the mother's face and the sound of her voice lock in the newborn's attention; he can even follow a moving face through a 180° arc during the first hour of life (Klaus 1976). MacFarlane's work (1975) suggests that the sense of smell is also operative at this early point, since babies tested at 10 days of age can already recognize the mother's breast odor and distinguish it from the breast odors of others.

Films of these first interactions show a definite sequence of mutual stimulus-response synchronous behavior patterns, leading to a "dancing together" or falling in love, as Klaus (1976) expresses it. The progression of behavior is orderly and proceeds from fingertip touch to massaging palm contact with the trunk. Holding and encompassing behaviors follow.

Rosenblatt (1978) reports from his work with animals that behavioral synchrony is an important feature of all sustained interaction among animals. This synchrony is more than the sum of the sensory stimuli involved in the interactions. For example, the release of oxytocin merges the mother's psychological and physiological responses to the infant's needs. The infant's cry may provide the initial stimuli for the release of oxytocin, which in turn stimulates milk release into the mammary ducts and also increases the surface temperature of the breast by 1° or 2°.

These synchronized responses form a base on which a communication system can be established. As a stereotype may function for an adult as a "jumping off" place from which to begin a relationship with someone from another cultural background, so this naive synchrony of behavioral, hormonal, physiological, and immunological mechanisms may initiate and cue the interactions between mother and infant which ensure the further development of attachment.

Blauvelt (1964) found many years ago that of the infant's many random movements, those that were responded to were more likely to be repeated than those movements which had passed unnoticed. Since the mother has been schooled by her culture to "see" those movements that have meaning within that culture, she responds only to culturally appropriate movements. Thus the newborn is guided to the intimate interpretation of the cultural environment by his mother. The transmission of cultural values begins with the mother's touch.

When the child makes a fist, for example, the mother's response will differ in accordance with the sex of the infant. If the child is a boy, the mother may close her hand around the fist and refer to the baby as "a fighter," while if the infant is a girl, the mother is more apt to open the fist or ignore it. Films of mother–infant interaction show that the mother only responds to certain of the baby's movements. Thus movements that consistently fit the mother's pattern begin to predominate in the baby's behavior. This mechanism may account for how the infant is transformed from "a" baby to "my" baby for the mother and how a communication system between the two is begun. The mother's positive feedback and the consistency of response serve to reinforce the infant's adaptive responses, while the infant's adaptive responses endear the infant to the mother.

A progressively more individual and complex cyclical system of interactions is created as contacts continue. Psychologically, the identifying and claiming process so well described by Rubin (1963) can now be seen from a behavioral perspective.

It is only recently that the newborn's amazing capacity to interact and adapt has been appreciated. Previously, it was thought that the infant was a blob of protoplasm that could only eat, sleep, cry, and wet. Attachment was seen as being all on the mother's part; if she prevailed for 6 weeks or so, the baby would begin to learn to smile. Klaus's report (1978) on eight studies showed that additional skin-to-skin contact between the mother and infant of as little as 15 minutes' duration in the first 2 hours of life produces differences in attachment behaviors as much as 3 months later. Other studies have shown that additional time together during the first 3 postpartum days can also lead to improved mothering behavior (Carlsson 1978; deChateau 1976; McClellan and Cabianca 1980). The importance of the initial contact during the first 2 hours of life in the initiation of attachment process cannot be argued because of the readiness of physiological, hormonal, and psychological bases.

Factors other than the timing of the initial contact between mother and infant may influence the development of maternal–infant attachment. Delay in the initial contact of the mother and the infant can interfere in the establishment of synchrony in another way as well. The newborn is born primed to interact, if not with the mother then with whomever is available. If he is taken immediately to an incubator, handled only through the medium of cloth, and placed where he can be observed but not touched, then how can he begin adaptation to his new environment? A normal newborn in this predicament will be seen rooting and turning toward the sheet beneath him and making active movements of his limbs, often with a startle response thrown in. There is usually crying, too, as the baby tries to cope with his frustration. His first attempt to relate with his world are gaining him only a series of inanimate features of his environment. His early patterning in response to cues (repetitive stimuli) from his mother is replaced by cues from nurses who are responding to "a" baby according to the rhythms of the nursery routine and without regard for his particular rhythms. We may thus interfere with the establishment of attachment through setting up patterns that don't "fit" with the mother's rhythms. The baby must relearn and readapt to his mother at a later point. The longer hospitalization and the often reduced contact between mother and infant that accompanies cesarean birth may intensify the effects of the relearning process.

Obviously the establishment of synchrony is dependent upon the active and reciprocal behaviors of both mother and infant. Medications and anesthesia may dull or even obliterate the responses of either during the optimum timing for initial contact. Pain or discomfort may distract later contacts. Restrictions in movement or positioning may alter opportunities for eye contact or holding sequences. In addition, fatigue and distress may limit the degree of concentration that the mother brings to the interacting environment.

INTERFERENCE WITH THE MOTHER'S PARTICIPATION

The mother's capacity to interact with her infant following cesarean birth is affected by new psychological and physical recovery needs. She has undergone abdominal surgery, a shock to anyone's system. Further, approximately 50 percent of cesarean births are unplanned prior to labor. In these instances the mother may have no time to assimilate, no control over the decision; she may be tired, and in most situations she suffers loss of the support of her significant other, whom she had expected to be with her for the birth. The suddenness of the decision and the potential threat to the self that these conditions convey are outlined in Table 1.

As discussed in Chapter 1, a life threat to the mother usually involves hemorrhage, rupture of the uterus, or eclampsia. Fortunately in today's obstetrics these threats are seldom seen, but when they are, they occur suddenly. There is little time for explanations and, indeed, the mother is in no condition to hear them. These emergencies are generally accompanied by worsening of the fetal condition as well, so the attachment process is apt to be long delayed until both the mother and the baby are stabilized and out of danger.

TABLE 1.
RELATIONSHIP BETWEEN THE REASON
FOR CESAREAN DELIVERY, THE TIME
AVAILABLE FOR ADJUSTMENT, AND
THE EXTENT OF THREAT

	PRIOR TIME FOR ADJUSTMENT	EXTENT OF THREAT
Reasons for Cesarean Delivery		
Life threat to mother	Emergency	Threat to existence
Life threat to baby	Emergency	Threat to symbiotic self
Failure of powers or progress	Becomes evident in labor (late)	Failure of self-expectations
Cephalopelvic disproportion	Known during labor (early)	Failure of body structure but not of self
Elective or planned	Known during pregnancy	Previous experience

Fetal distress may occur rather suddenly also, and the mother may be acutely aware of and frightened by the rapid changes and the tension of the professionals around her. Explanations may be given and heard but not comprehended. Misinterpretation can easily occur if the mother has an oxygen mask slapped on her face and is moved rapidly to the delivery room. There may be little opportunity for choice and the mother may feel helpless about what is happening to her. Immediate contact is ruled out by the infant's condition. In this instance the attachment process may be further interfered with by the mother's anxiety about the infant's survival. Even if the infant responds well, the mother's perception of him may be that he is a "sick" infant. This "definition of the situation" (as described in Chapter 2) may lead her to question her ability to care for him.

It is important to remember that at this point in time the infant is still not a separate entity in the mother's mind; any threat to the infant is a threat to her. Thus the loss or near loss of the infant reflects upon her adequacy to fulfill her primary initial function as a mother. Feelings of biological incompetence may lessen a mother's self-confidence or at least make her more vulnerable to the situational effects of separation (Seashore et al. 1977).

In some ways it may be easier to accept the need for a cesarean birth when there is a life-threatening situation than when there is a failure to progress. Every woman sets up expectations of what labor will be like. These expectations may be based on information from classes or professionals and/or the experience of other mothers. In addition, the mother's knowledge of her own reactions to pain and discomfort and her confidence in her ability to control her behavioral responses enter into the formation of her expectations. The average pregnant woman seldom entertains the thought that she may need a cesarean, even though this possibility may be discussed in classes (see Chapter 8). It then comes as a shock when, because of failure to progress in labor, a cesarean becomes necessary. Frequently the decision comes after several hours of ineffective labor. The mother may be told that if there is little progress in the next hour or two, a cesarean will be done. Thus there is some time for explanations and questions, time for some awareness of the situation to seep through to consciousness. The parents may even be able to take part in the decision or allowed to make choices about the anesthesia used, the husband's presence at delivery, and so on.

Despite the fact that there is some time for adjustment when a cesarean birth occurs because of lack of progress in labor, it should be noted that the mother's coping abilities are already taxed by the stresses imposed by the continuation of labor and fatigue. She must also deal with her sense of failure to meet her expectations, which may be associated with feelings of guilt. Under these circumstances her readiness to interact with her newborn is apt to be impaired until her self-doubts are resolved.

When cephalopelvic disproportion (CPD) is the reason that a cesarean birth occurs, time for adjusting expectations may be even greater. During late pregnancy or early labor, estimates of size of the fetus and of the pelvis may raise a suspicion that a cesarean birth may be necessary. Sonography can be used to confirm these suspicions, or the mother may be made aware that a trial of labor will be conducted. Thus the time frame for adjustment of expectations can be lengthened. In addition, the knowledge that a time limit for the trial has been set may alter stress and fatigue factors.

Finally, when a cesarean birth is expected because of some existing condition or a previous cesarean, then expectations can be made that correctly coincide with actuality. Previous experiences can be reworked and plans made to relieve anxiety. Questions can be answered in advance and explanations of hospital policies covered. The wishes of the parents can be incorporated in planning for care. These opportunities to relieve anxiety and individualize care are all too frequently neglected. In these instances the unresolved fears and feelings from previous experiences with cesarean births may affect the present birth experience as well and interfere with the mother's capacity to interact with her infant.

According to Caplan (1959), when a stressful event occurs there is a potential for either growth or personality disorganization, depending on the support received at the time and afterward. For some women the cesarean birth is greeted with relief, but for many it is an upheaval that is both physically and emotionally traumatic. One other way that cesarean births may modify the mother's capacity to interact with her infant is in initiating birth prematurely. Mothers who have diabetes, severe preeclampsia, or renal disease or who are expecting a repeat cesarean birth may be scheduled for surgery prior to the normal date of confinement. In this situation the physioendocrine changes involved in the establishment of mothering may not yet have occurred. Work with animals suggests that biochemical changes stimulated by labor and passage of the young through the birth canal trigger maternal behavior (Rosenblatt 1978).

INTERFERENCE WITH THE INFANT'S PARTICIPATION

Let us turn now to the infant and the ways that cesarean birth may interfere with his capacity to interact with his mother. One obvious way is through the drugs and anesthesia given to the mother that pass the placental barrier. The effects of these agents are described by Mercer in Chapter 4. One must also consider the infant's condition at birth. Many cesarean births occur because of such fetal factors as distress, prematurity, abnormal position, or the presence of a disease in the mother (such as diabetes) that is known to affect the fetus. In all of these cases except perhaps abnormal position, the infant's condition is apt to be compromised at birth. Some complications in infants that correlate with cesarean births are anoxia, RDS, and immaturity.

FACTORS WHICH MAY MODIFY
CESAREAN BIRTH EFFECTS

The preceding sections show that there are some potential difficulties inherent in the cesarean birth experience which interfere with the establishment of an emotional tie between the mother and the baby. Despite these difficulties, most mothers and infants are able to establish a firm attachment to each other. Several factors may modify the consequences of delayed contact and these can be used by the nurse to identify those at risk for mothering disturbances. These factors are: (1) prenatal progress in the development of mothering, (2) acceptance of and desire for the infant, (3) the previous and current stress loads of the mother due to other things in her life, and (4) adequacy of the mother's present coping patterns.

The many physiological, psychological, and social changes of pregnancy trigger the development of the mothering process prior to birth. This process is the precursor of the mother's actual assumption of the mothering role. Rubin (1975) has described the stages in the psychological development of mothering during pregnancy as mimicry, role playing, fantasizing, and introjection–projection–rejection. This process normally begins with the first stirrings of life that the mother feels and continues throughout pregnancy. Comments of mothers-to-be can indicate how far along they are with the process. Typical activities of the pregnant woman are: watching over other mothers at every opportunity, asking her own mother about herself as a baby, volunteering for babysitting, and comparing the ways different mothers handle similar situations and thinking about how she would approach similar situations.

The mother usually also fantasizes about what her baby will be like. She may picture what he will look like, his sex, his behavior, and his likes and dislikes. Whole personalities are woven from fantasy. While many women have difficulty accepting the fact that they are pregnant, their acceptance and their desire for their infants usually increase as their pregnancies progress. The way a woman refers to her child can clue the nurse in on the development of the mother's feelings toward the baby. Early in pregnancy the mother typically refers to the baby as "it" or "the fetus." After quickening, the mother begins to identify the infant as the "baby" by sex, or even by a pet name. Later, her fantasies begin. If the expectations expressed in these fantasies are inflexible, then the mother may have problems accepting and responding to reality when it comes. Problems can also arise if the mother always speaks of the infant as being older than a newborn baby (Caplan 1959).

Failure to progress along the normal continuum for the development of mothering should function as a red flag for the nurse, telling her that this mother may have difficulty forming an attachment to her infant. A mother's preoccupation with her own discomforts or evidence of such a high anxiety level that she does not talk about her baby in the third trimester is an indication of potential trouble. Continued referral to the baby as "it" long past quickening is also a warning sign of possible problems.

Feelings of ambivalence or even rejection of the fetus are normal in early pregnancy, but with the first stirrings of life and the hormonal changes of later pregnancy most women come to accept and even look forward to having the baby. Expressions of nonacceptance or negative fantasies about the baby's personality—such as "He's mean." or "He's going to be a troublemaker."—late in pregnancy should alert the nurse to the need for paying special attention to the attachment process.

In those situations in which prenatal mothering, development, and acceptance of the fetus have proceeded on course, delay in interaction opportunities will probably not affect the quality of the attachment that is ultimately formed between mother and infant. However, some intervening situations may lead to less than optimal attachment even when the mother has shown normal development and acceptance. For example, when the mother has had a particularly long and painful labor prior to the cesarean birth or a stormy postpartum course, she may blame the baby for her hardship and have difficulty feeling the motherly love so necessary for long-term attachment. In

other instances, normal patterns of mothering development can be interrupted by disappointment that the infant is not the sex desired or has an appearance or behavior very different from that which the mother fantasized
prenatally. The presence of obvious birth defects can also interfere with the
attachment process.

Pregnancy itself is a health change that challenges the mother's adaptive
capacity physiologically, psychologically, and socially. The woman's own
report of anxiety or stress appears to be the best predictor of complications.
Nuckolls (1977), using a "schedule of recent experiences" scale developed
by Holmes and Rahe (1967), found that life stresses alone could not predict
complications of pregnancy; however, when the mother's adaptive potential
for pregnancy was considered along with life stresses, an interesting relationship was found. Women with high adaptive potential for pregnancy and high
life change scores both before and during pregnancy had one-third the com-
plication rate of women with similar life change scores but low adaptive
potential. The mother's adaptive potential for pregnancy measured "the
subject's feelings or perceptions concerning herself, her pregnancy and her
overall life situation, including her relationships with her husband, her extended family and the community" (Nuckolls 1977). This essentially summarizes the mother's assessment of her coping ability and the support she
feels from her significant others. The importance of this study is that it con-
firms the need to consider stress from the mother's perspective, her capacity
to adapt, and the availability of support in her environment—as *she* perceives
it (Hutchins 1978). The interrelationship of stress, support, and the ability
to cope can be seen as a continuum. It is as important to assess the mother's
strengths as it is to identify problems.

Adolescent mothers comprise one group frequently associated with high
life stress. True to expectation, these mothers are at risk in forming successful attachments to their infants. Pregnancy in this group is often unplanned
and conflicts with the achievement of other personal goals. The adolescent is
forced to assume an independent parental role in which she gives care before
she has relinquished the dependent child's role in which she is the recipient of
care. The abruptness of this role change, the other adjustments occasioned
by pregnancy and her evolving adult identity intensify the young mother's
disequilibrium. At the same time, the adolescent's arsenal of coping mechanisms is often inadequate to resolve the conflicts produced. The more immature the mother's personality development, the more likely she is to be
overwhelmed by the mothering role (Mercer 1979).

There are several factors that contribute to adolescents' high-risk status in
establishing strong attachments with their infants. First, they lack appropriate
coping strategies developed through life experiences. Second, they generally
experience increased and prolonged dependency needs and consequently have
a longer taking-in phase during the postpartum period and a greater expenditure of energy. Third, they have trouble accepting and becoming comfortable

with body image changes and fear a loss of body intactness. The cesarean scar only adds to the trauma of an already vulnerable person. Fourth, the focus of the adolescent is rather intently centered upon herself, and so she brings to motherhood certain deficiencies in perceiving the needs of the infant.

These factors can work to the detriment of maternal–infant attachment. Fortunately, management strategies applied by the nurse may influence the outcome. These strategies will be discussed later. It is sufficient to say at this point that strong support is needed at all phases of the childbearing cycle. Mercer (1979) suggests that accurate assessment of the adolescent's supportive resources, level of psychological and cognitive development, and cultural background is needed to anticipate care needs and to facilitate bonding.

THE NURSING ROLE IN FACILITATING MATERNAL–INFANT ATTACHMENT

A word has been coined for use in research—"max-min-con"—that is a contraction of three words: maximize, minimize, and control (Kerlinger 1973). This word, with a slightly different definition, can be used to describe the objectives of care in facilitating bonding between mother and infant; this is true whether the nurse has contact with the mother prenatally, during labor, at birth, or postpartum. In a nut shell, one should: (1) maximize the mother's choices, her participation in care, her support system, and her coping abilities; (2) minimize stress through anticipatory guidance and support of her decisions and efforts; and (3) control the situation by providing knowledge, focusing the mother's attention (when she is ready) on the baby, timing interactions so that both partners are ready to interact, and decreasing environmental distractions. The following sections will discuss how these principles can be implemented despite some of the interferences introduced by the cesarean birth process.

Since the attachment process begins prenatally, the nurse's role begins there, too. Establishing a warm, open climate in which the prospective mother is treated with respect and concern is essential to implementing a facilitative relationship in the antepartum period. Within such an atmosphere the mother will feel free to share her innermost thoughts and fears. When the mother is able to share her feelings with someone who can accept them without judging her, she can be supported and provided with knowledge that will enable her to cope with each stressful situation as it arises. Caplan (1959) long ago described the way in which the openness of pregnancy allows a reworking of unresolved problems, thus making possible healthier resolutions of these problems. Now it appears that the purpose of such openness may be to disrupt old patterns and permit the mother greater flexibility in adapting to the uniqueness of her infant (Brazelton 1974). Even though the mother has other children and is familiar with childrearing tasks, the attachment formed with each child is based upon the specific interaction between *this* infant and the mother. As the mother successfully copes with each of the multiple crises of pregnancy, she comes to believe in herself and gains confidence in her own ability to cope and to handle the parental role. By supporting and reinforcing the strengths within the mother and her family, the nurse encourages this essential self-development. The nurse should not make decisions for the mother or try to solve her problems for her. Nursing care is of greatest benefit to the mother when she makes her own decisions, for then she grows. The nurse may define the options available, give information or an explanation, and support the mother's concern as normal, but the mother and her family must actively participate in decision making.

While this discussion may seem distant to the actual establishment of attachment, in fact it is not. The more evidence the mother has of her own ability to cope, the more energy she will have at the time of birth for the attachment process. Therefore, in addition to supporting the mother in coping with actual stress during pregnancy, the nurse's role includes providing anticipatory guidance and information so that the mother can form reality-based expectations for the birth experience. Again, the more closely the birth experience comes to the mother's expectations, the less energy is needed to cope with the differences between the fantasized delivery and the actual experience.

A nursing history should be taken as early as possible in the prenatal period. It should include assessment of current and past stressors, of the support system available, and of the mother's own abilities and patterns for coping with stress. Consideration should also be given to the expectant mother's attitudes, feelings, and fears about present and past pregnancies and to her ideas about the kinds of care she expects or wants. It is important that this information be included as a part of the mother's chart so that it will be available to all who have contact with her in the health care system during her childbearing experience.

Another important consideration that is often overlooked is the provision of a primary care nurse who can establish a therapeutic relationship with the mother, provide continuity of care, and monitor the development of mothering throughout pregnancy. Expectant mothers often hesitate to bring up negative feelings or thoughts unless they are sure they can trust the nurse with such information. Having the same nurse throughout can make the mother feel that she can indeed talk about things with "her" nurse. The nurse, on the other hand, also benefits by being able to follow through and detect stresses by evaluating the mother's ongoing response and through previously given information. For example, a mother's continued weight gain after a discussion of nutrition is often a cue to look for stress that is preventing her utilization of the information. If the same nurse is seeing the mother throughout, she can pick up on this much more easily than a nurse seeing the mother for the first time, who might feel compelled to reassess her diet knowledge.

Establishing relationships with people and sharing feelings are very difficult for some expectant mothers, especially those who have limited social contacts. They are the very ones who most need the resources of the nurse to draw them out and help them identify their feelings. These women are often missed in the usual prenatal clinic or office because it may take more than one visit to establish their interacting patterns and to realize there is a problem. When different nurses see the mother at each visit the interacting pattern is not as discernible.

The presence of named support persons provides no guarantee that the expectant mother is being supported; the quality of the relationship is of paramount importance. Does the mother talk over her feelings with her significant other? What is his (or her) response? How does he (or she) help her? One should keep in mind that support is a feeling that only the mother can determine, although there are generally hints in her description of behaviors. For example, one woman who had had repeated prematures had a husband who would go off every weekend with his motorcycle gang, leaving her with the children. The nurse learned that the mother never had shared with him her needs for rest because of rising blood pressure. With the nurse's support she began to tell her husband more about how she felt. On the next visit she reported with some surprise that he had gotten the wives of his buddies to come in and clean for her and had stayed home on the weekend to help her with the children. Later, when she started in early labor, he brought her to the hospital and stayed in the father's waiting room. While this might not be construed by the nurse as particularly supportive, the mother said she felt very supported. He had never stayed around in the hospital during any of her previous births. She appreciated knowing he was there because she knew how afraid he was of hospitals and realized only a strong feeling for her would account for his behavior. It is often possible to build the mother's support system through improving communications and urging the sharing of feelings during pregnancy.

About 50 percent of all cesarean births are performed as a result of the mother having had a previous cesarean birth experience. A small proportion of those having a cesarean birth for the first time will be scheduled without prior labor experience—e.g., diabetic mothers, those with a known contracted pelvis, and those with positive stress tests. For these women, specific plans can be made; the nurse can use her influence to see that the woman and her significant other are given every opportunity to participate in the planning. Wherever possible it is desirable to comply with the couple's wishes. If this is not possible, then a full explanation should be given ahead of time so the couple's expectations can be adjusted to more accurately meet reality. Hospital policies need to be examined in light of their relevance to helping couples achieve their parenting roles with the least amount of stress. Such a perspective often reveals many ways in which greater flexibility or change can be implemented without compromising the safe care of either the mother or the baby.

Women often experience their first cesarean births after a period of labor. This may be a trial of labor in which the possibility of a cesarean exists from the beginning. If the parents have full knowledge of how long the labor trial will last and of what progress will determine the decision to either go on or terminate the trial, then they can begin to modify their expectations and adjust to the decision on the basis of their knowledge of whether or not they are meeting the standard for progress. The nurse can help couples prepare themselves for deviations from their expectations. She can also observe how the prospective parents cope and how they support each other. She can help the parents develop greater consideration for each other's feelings and to re- solve the issue of joint participation in the delivery.

Swanson (1978) has summarized the elements of nursing in the labor room that are most helpful to the process of attachment. The following are impor- tant in all births, whether vaginal or by cesarean:

1. *Recognizing the individual worth of the expectant mother and father.*
2. *Providing comfort measures.*
3. *Providing encouragement and praise.*
4. *Remaining present to lend support to alleviate fears.*
5. *Keeping the expectant couple informed as active participants in the experience. (Swanson 1978)*

If possible, the mother's significant other should be present at the cesarean birth. First of all, in keeping with the principle of maximizing the mother's support system and her coping abilities, the presence of the significant other can decrease the mother's fear and ameliorate her sense of loss of control as she is strapped down, etc. This is particularly important during the prepara- tion stage, when no one else has time to comfort her. Second, by going through this experience together, the parents have the possibility of sharing their feelings and responding to one another with touch and eye contact, thus helping one another to maintain control. Even as a child can tolerate more stress when the parent is present, so the adult can cope better when another's support is available. Having the familiar significant other present has the added advantage of permitting the two to later relive the experience and fill in any gaps or lapses of memory. This is particularly important if the mother is not awake during delivery (Donovan 1977). In addition, the father is thus able to hold the newborn baby and begin the attachment process with him. The father represents a continuity person and is the most culturally appropriate person available with whom the newborn can begin an interaction cycle. He may be able to hold the baby so that the mother can get an *en face* look or even skin-to-skin contact (with her face, at least), or he can take pictures to share with her later.

Many hospitals do not permit the parents to have the choice of being together during the cesarean birth experience. Others permit husbands only; in the husband's absence no one else may be substituted. In some instances the couple may decide against the significant other being present for the cesarean birth. Regardless of the reason, if the mother does not have a significant other with her, it is desirable that the nurse who has established a rapport with the mother substitute as the mother's supporting person. If this is not possible, then the nurse should provide or see that others provide explanations for what is happening to the mother and why.

The mother should be permitted to see the infant as soon as possible after he is born; if she is awake, this can occur while the surgical repair is being done. Care should be taken to hold the baby so that *en face* viewing is possible. No drops should be put in the baby's eyes until after the baby is taken to the nursery. The nurse can facilitate skin contact between the mother and the infant by letting the mother kiss the baby or by brushing the baby's face against the mother's cheek. If one of the mother's arms can be freed to permit her to hold the baby even briefly, then this opportunity should be seized. If the baby's condition warrants and the mother is awake, the baby can be placed in an incubator and placed so that the mother can focus clearly on him. If the mother normally wears glasses, then these should be provided to allow her to really see the infant. The nurse may also uncover the baby briefly so that the mother can see that he is alright and appears normal.

All of the above suggestions fit the criteria for maximizing the support system at the time of increased stress and for allowing the mother to participate in her care to the greatest degree possible. They also follow the principle, established by the previously mentioned research into the attachment process itself, of arranging for mother–infant interaction at the earliest moment permitted by the condition and state (e.g., awake, alert) of mother and infant. Furthermore, these suggestions allow use of the greatest possible number of sensory modalities.

Not all situations allow for both mother and infant participation immediately after a cesarean birth. The mother may be asleep or the infant may require immediate transfer to the nursery. However, even in the latter instance, the baby can be shown to the mother briefly so that she can begin to adjust to the reality of her infant's birth and condition. It is also possible that the father may not be present at the delivery; however, using the same principles described above, it is still better to allow the father to hold his infant than to allow him only a brief look as his baby is taken to the nursery.

The recovery room is the next place where the family can be united. This reunion affords the parents an excellent opportunity for employment of a full range of sensory modalities in establishing the feeling of "this is my baby." Gottlieb (1978) pointed out that the mother uses a discovery process to convince herself that the baby is indeed her own. The presence of the baby activates the mother's sensory apparatus—visual, olfactory, tactile, and auditory/verbal. There are three aspects of the discovery process:

> Identifying *refers to when the mother points out physical characteristics and actions; in other words, what her child looks like and what her baby can do.* . . . Relating *refers to an identified behavior which is related to a familiar event, person, object, or fantasized child.* . . . Interpreting *refers to the infused meaning that the mother gives the baby's actions and needs.* (Gottlieb 1978)

Even if the mother has been permitted to see and even touch the baby during surgery, the use of the recovery room for fuller exploration and development of the discovery process is advisable. More can be accomplished in the way of positioning for *en face* viewing and holding. In addition, the comments of the father as he too begins the discovery process may direct the mother's attention to details of the infant's appearance or behavior that she would otherwise miss.

The use of the recovery room for the initial contact between the mother and the infant is very important, because the baby will most likely still be in the alert stage described in the literature and the mother may still be comfortable as a result of the drugs and anesthesia given for delivery, though still alert enough to interact.

While the family does need some time alone during this phase, the necessity of frequent monitoring of the mother's condition gives the nurse the opportunity of observing parts of the interaction. Observations can be made on the attachment process that will be significant to later nursing intervention. For example, if the mother and father appear to be focused on the baby and are making remarks about the baby's appearance ("Look how red he is!" or "He even has eyebrows!") or are relating his behavior or appearance to something familiar ("She has more hair than I imagined." or "He has your nose.") or are interpreting his behavior ("Look at that fist; he's going to be a fighter!" or "Her mouth is going already; she's going to be a good eater."), then the nurse can conclude that the attachment process is proceeding on target. However, if the parents are ignoring the baby, talking over him but not to or about him, or appear to be disinterested, then the recovery room nurse should communicate this to her colleagues in the postpartum and nursery areas so that they can be on the alert for possible problems with the attachment process.

Other features that can be noticed at this early time are *en face* behaviors, stroking, fingertip or even palm touching (more apt to be seen in later interactions), and speaking to the baby in a high-pitched tone. Particularly relevant are observations of behaviors that are elicited by a cue from one of the interacting partners—e.g., as the mother speaks to the baby he focuses on her face, and she then strokes his cheek. These reciprocal behaviors constitute synchrony between the relating mother and child, with each responding to the other's cues.

Obviously, difficulties in positioning, the effects of drugs and anesthesia, the presence of IVs and a BP cuff, and the general condition of the mother and the infant are hindrances to the achievement of synchronous behaviors in the recovery room. Nevertheless, the importance of a recovery room interaction cannot be minimized. Aside from psychosocial considerations, there are important biophysiological connections that may be made, even though there are some distractions. Many mothers remember that such a meeting took place even though they may not remember what the baby looked like.

While the attachment process may begin in the delivery room or the recovery room, many more encounters are needed to truly establish a lasting emotional tie. Mothers frequently say that they did not feel like mothers for several days. The nurses in the postpartum area are therefore called upon to manage the environment in such a way as to aid attachment behavior following cesarean birth.

Since the needs of postpartum cesarean mothers are discussed at greater length in Chapter 6, the following discussion focuses primarily on facilitation of the attachment process.

The nurse's most important postpartum role is to facilitate attachment by maximizing the attachment potential of each contact between the mother or father and the infant; by minimizing anxiety, discomfort, and the energy drain to other needs; and by controlling the timing and length of contacts between participants in the bonding process. To do this the nurse uses several management strategies, as follows.

1. Support the mother's dependency needs and encourage her to ventilate her feelings about the birth experience.
2. Promote rest by altering the routine so that she can follow natural body rhythms—e.g., sleep longer in the morning, if that is what she is accustomed to.
3. Mother-infant interaction should be arranged as early as the condition and state (awake, alert) of both mother and infant permits. This may involve anticipating the cycles of both the mother and the infant and

timing pain medications so that the mother is provided relief and comfort but is alert enough to concentrate on her baby's behavior. The nurse should allow "getting acquainted" time. If the baby is sleeping, the nurse should suggest that the mother hold the baby upright for a few minutes, play with his hands, and stroke his mouth while talking to him. The mother should be allowed to discover how she can bring her baby to an alert state by her handling. If the baby is crying, the mother should be shown how to quiet him by saying insistently, "Baby, baby, baby, baby. . . ." (Brazelton 1978)

4. Enhance learning through focusing sensory modalities on significant patterns occurring in the interaction and/or in the infant's capabilities for interaction. The nurse can enhance the mother's discovery process by helping her appreciate the infant's state controls and his specific feedback modes and preferences for soothing. One way to enhance the discovery process is to use parts of the Brazelton examination to show the mother how the baby expresses stress, how he consoles himself, and how he habituates himself to repetitive stimuli. The emphasis is on the newborn and his capacities, but the mother is also learning perception of cues for mothering. Gottlieb (1978) pointed out that ". . . sensory mediators are the mother's instruments of discovery. . . . The choice of mediators is related to the mother's personal style of communication and to her feeling of ease with her child." Another way to increase the mother's awareness of her infant may be through comments made during the interaction itself, such as, "See how he looks right at you," or "Look how he has his hand on your breast," or "Feel how soft his skin is."

5. Reduce energy dissipation to other stimuli and decrease the environmental interaction space. For example, the nurse could position the mother for comfort, help move the baby from one side to the other, or burp the baby. The nurse should turn off the TV and put curtains around the interacting couple so as to minimize distractions.

6. Encourage positive synchronized mothering attempts and explain why they are positive. Such comments as "You have him positioned very well: his head is supported well that way," or "You handle him so gently and yet securely. See how he cuddles when you do that? He quiets right down when you care for him," help her to feel positive about what she is doing and serve as guidelines for future mothering behaviors.

7. The identity process should be stimulated through such questions as "Who does the baby look like? Does he have your eyes?"

8. The plane of observation between mother and infant can be kept free of obstruction. For instance, the nurse should keep her hand beneath the baby's head and the blanket between his head and her hand when putting the baby to the mother's breast; in this way the nurse will

not stimulate his skin, which might make him turn to her hand and away from the mother's breast. The mother should be allowed to put the breast in the baby's mouth so that she can maintain direct view of both the baby and the breast. The baby should be placed in the crib near the mother's bed so that she can observe him at any time and even touch him if she likes. However, she should not be expected to lift the baby from the crib, as this is difficult after a cesarean.

9. Contacts between the mother and the baby can be maximized, within the limits of the mother's desire. The mother should be able to have the baby as frequently and for as long as she wishes. However, when she is tired or for any other reason wants the baby to be taken back to the nursery, this desire should be attended to promptly and cheerfully. The nurse should convey the feeling that it is expected that new mothers will want some time to themselves, for rest or other purposes.

10. Involve the father with the baby as much as possible and assist him to establish a bond with the infant.

These management strategies can be employed with considerable variation in suiting individual mothers. The mother's readiness is the key to determining the timing of interactions. For some mothers the trauma (both physical and mental) of labor and delivery is great enough to almost totally incapacitate them for some time (Carlsson 1976).

The nurse in the postpartum area plays a vital role in the establishment of attachment. She must make critical judgments about the progress of attachment on the basis of her knowledge of observable behavior, and manipulate the timing and environmental stimuli to maximize the potential for achieving attachment. The cesarean mother is at risk of not achieving successful maternal–infant attachment. As Rosenblatt (1978) pointed out, "The greater the discrepancy between the mother's condition and the developmental status of the young, the more difficult it is for the two to become synchronized. . . ." It is imperative, then, that the nurse be able to identify the behavioral cues that indicate that attachment is taking place. The cues mentioned in an earlier section of this chapter are applicable here.

In addition to the aforementioned cues, the nurse can observe the phenomenon of entrainment—that is, the timing of movements to coincide with the rhythm of a pattern of speech. Even the baby's breathing or sucking may reflect his concentration on the sing-song rhythm mothers frequently use in speaking to infants. Synchronized movements of the mother and the baby in rhythm appear to the observer as almost a dance in time with the music of the mother's voice. According to Brazelton (1978), the infant's entrainment behaviors comprise a form of feedback that is irresistible to the mother.

Entrainment plays a much more significant role in mother–infant interaction, for it forms the basis for establishing the infant's biorhythms of sleep and alert times according to the mother's routine. The infant's alert states begin to correspond increasingly with the mother's holding times. The nurse can assist in advancing this process by trying to keep the mother's established rhythms and timing the infant's contacts with the mother to coincide with the times that fit best with the mother's routines. When the baby is alert, he is ready to actively participate in interaction with his mother. The timing of contact is a critical variable in achieving the development of entrainment. Increased infant alertness and the initiation of "games"—i.e., repetitive patterns of interaction—between the mother and infant can be observed by the nurse. Games are important, for, as Spitz (1965) pointed out, it is through repetitive patterns that the baby is helped to organize his world by learning to recognize the importance of some stimuli over others in his environment.

In addition to evaluating her observations, the nurse can judge the development of attachment through the mother's comments and questions as she goes through the discovery process. Positive comments, desire for the baby, and interest in what he is doing are indications that the mother is proceeding normally toward attachment. The absence of comments or questions about the baby and expressions of concern for herself and her own condition may be warning signs of impending difficulties in the attachment process.

Because of early delays in establishing attachment, the initiation of mothering behaviors may move at a slower pace following cesarean birth than following vaginal delivery. However, if the nurse can reinforce the parents' strengths most families can be helped to achieve a good attachment. To do this, the nurse must be aware of her own motives and behaviors in working with parents. Most health professionals like to have people depend on them. The nurse may unconsciously devalue the parental role in an effort to see herself as the important caretaker of the newborn. This attitude can negatively affect parental–infant attachment. Only by learning to emphasize and value the parental role can the nurse positively influence the attachment process (Brazelton 1976).

Although the nurse may help new parents have positive interactions with their infant during the postpartum period, some parents still find it difficult to attach to their infants. Accurate charting of the progress of the attachment process can form the basis for a referral for follow-up care, if needed. The child's healthy growth and development depends on the emotional tie that exists between that child and his parents. This tie begins to grow early in the period just following the infant's birth. The postpartum nurse can use her knowledge and observational skills to identify potential problems in the establishment of the strong emotional tie so necessary for a successful and satisfying childrearing experience.

SUMMARY

As the proportion of cesarean births has increased during the last decade, studies on maternal–infant attachment have emphasized the importance of early contacts between mothers and infants in establishing optimum attachment behaviors. Early separation of mother and infant has been found to be related to an increased incidence of disturbed mother-infant relationships. Cesarean births often necessitate such a separation during the early postpartum period. This chapter has focused on how the cesarean birth experience can interfere with the establishment of synchrony, or the capacity of the mother and the infant to interact with one another. Complications, increased stress and energy needs for the mother, and increased recovery needs have been discussed as potential detractors in the establishment of an emotional tie between the cesarean mother and her infant.

Several key factors may modify the influence of cesarean birth on the attachment process. These are the mother's prenatal progress in the development of mothering, her acceptance of and desire for the infant, her stress from other life events, the availability and adequacy of her support system, her developmental level, and her coping patterns.

The nurse's role as a facilitator of attachment following cesarean birth has been delineated. In summary, the nurse can maximize the mother's choices and participation in her own care, strengthen the mother's support system and coping abilities, and minimize stresses by providing knowledge, focusing the mother on the baby, timing interactions, and decreasing environmental distractions. Emphasis should be placed on looking for strengths and offering positive feedback and praise as means of facilitating appropriate mothering behaviors.

REFERENCES

Blauvelt H: Differential latency of oral response on the first day of life. J Genet Psychol 104:199-205, 1964

Brazelton TB: Commenting. In Klaus MH, Kennell JH (eds), Maternal-Infant Bonding. St. Louis, Mosby, 1976, p. 97

Brazelton TB: The remarkable talents of the newborn. Birth Fam J 5 (4): 188, 1978

Brazelton, TB, Kozlowski B, Main M: The origins of reciprocity: The early mother-infant interaction. In Lewis M, Rosenblum L (eds), The Effect of the Infant on its Caregiver. New York, Wiley and Sons, 1974

Caplan G: Concepts of Mental Health and Consultation: Their Application in Public Health Social Work. Washington, D.C., Social and Rehabilitation Service, Children's Bureau. HEW, 1959, pp. 47-55

Carey WB: Psychologic sequelae of early infancy health crisis. In Schwartz JL, Schwartz LH (eds), Vulnerable Infants: A Psychosocial Dilemma. New York, McGraw-Hill, 1977, pp. 136-49

Carlsson SE: The irreality of postpartum: Observations on the subjective experience. J Obstet Gynecol Nurs Sept/Oct.:28-30, 1976

Carlsson SE, et al: Effects of amount of contact between mother and child on the mother's nursing behavior. Dev Psychobiol 11:143-50, 1978

deChateau P: Neonatal care routines: Influences on maternal and infant behavior and on breastfeeding. University Medical Dissertations. Umea, Sweden, 1976

Donovan B: The Cesarean Birth Experience. Boston, Beacon, 1977

Evrard JR, Gold EM: Cesarean section: Risk/benefit. Perinatal Care 2 (8):4–8, 1978

Gottlieb L: Maternal attachment in primiparas. J Obstet Gynecol Neonatal Nurs Jan/Feb:39–44, 1978

Hammarskjöld D: Markings, New York, Knopf, 1965, p. 5

Helfer RE: The relationship between lack of bonding and child abuse and neglect. In Klaus MH, Lejer T, Trause M (eds), Maternal Attachment and Mothering Disorders: A Roundtable. 1974, pp. 21–25

Holmes TA, Rahe RH: The social readjustment rating scale. J Psychosomatic Res 11:213–18, 1967

Hughey MJ, et al: The effect of fetal monitoring on the incidence of cesarean section. Obstet Gynecol 49:513, 1977

Hutchins EA: Sociocultural and other factors related to premature termination of pregnancy. Doctoral Dissertation, University of Washington, 1978

Kerlinger FN: Foundations of Behavioral Research, 2nd ed. New York, Holt, Rinehart, and Winston, 1973

Klaus MH: The biology of parent-to-infant attachment. Birth Family J 5 (4):200, 1978

Klaus MH, Kennell JH: Maternal–Infant Bonding. St. Louis, Mosby, 1976, p. 260

MacFarlane A: Olfaction in the development of social preference in the human neonate. Parent–Infant Interaction. Ciba Foundation Symposium 33. Amsterdam, Association of Scientific Publications, 1975, pp. 103–117

MacFarlane A: The Psychology of Childbirth. Cambridge, Mass., Harvard University Press, 1977, pp. 126

McClellan MS, Cabianca WA: Effects of early mother–infant contact following cesarean birth. Obstet Gynecol 56:52–55, 1980

Mercer RT: Perspectives on Adolescent Health Care. Philadelphia, Lippincott, 1979, p. 411

Nuckolls KB, Cassel J, Kaplan BH: Psychosocial assets, life crisis and the prognosis of pregnancy. In Schwartz JL, Schwartz LH (eds), Vulnerable Infants: A Psychosocial Dilemma, New York, McGraw–Hill, 1977, pp. 62–75

Rich OJ: "Temporal and spacial experience as reflected in the verbalizations of multiparous women during labor. Maternal–Child Nurs J 2 (4):1–320, 1973

Rosenblatt JS: Evolutionary background of human maternal behavior: Animal models. Birth Family J 5 (4):196, 1978

Rubin R: Maternal touch. Nurs Outlook 11:838–41, 1963

Rubin R: Maternal tasks in pregnancy. Maternal–Child Nurs J 4 (3):143–53, 1975

Schwartz JL: A study of the relationship between maternal life change events and premature delivery. In Schwartz JL, Schwartz LH (eds), Vulnerable Infants: A Psychosocial Dilemma. New York, McGraw–Hill, 1977, pp. 47–61

Seashore MJ, Keifer AD, Barnett CR, Liederman PH: The effects of denial of early mother–infant interaction on maternal self-confidence. In Schwartz JL, Schwartz LH (eds), Vulnerable Infants: A Psychosocial Dilemma. New York, McGraw–Hill, 1977, pp. 136–49

Spitz RA: The First Year of Life. New York, International University Press, 1965, p. 285

Swanson J: Nursing intervention to facilitate maternal–infant attachment. J Obstet Gyneco Neonatal Nurs 7:2, 1978

CHAPTER 4

Potential Effects of Anesthesia and Analgesia on the Maternal-Infant Attachment Process of Cesarean Mothers

Ramona T. Mercer

Although it is possible to avoid using chemical agents which produce varying levels of painless states and/or consciousness in vaginal birth, analgesia and anesthesia are largely unavoidable in cesarean birth. Alternatives to this use of chemical agents can be found in hypnosis and acupuncture; however, these methods are used infrequently for cesarean birth in the United States. Due to concern about the effect of drugs used during labor and delivery on infant outcome, the American Academy of Pediatrics Committee on Drugs recommended ". . . that the minimum effective dose of those agents should be administered when indicated. . ." (Committee on Drugs 1978, p. 403). The intervening variables impacting on the effects of analgesia and anesthesia, the potential impact of drugs on the neonate, the potential impact of drugs on the mother, and the consequent impact on the mother–infant attachment process are the focus of this chapter. Attachment as a process and some of the assumptions about the process set the philosophical and operational parameters of the concepts presented.

ATTACHMENT

The terms *attachment* and *bonding* are often used interchangeably. Campbell and Taylor (1979) differentiated between the two terms. They described bonding as unidirectional (parent to infant), occurring rapidly following birth (first few hours or days), and as being facilitated through physical contact. They describe attachment as reciprocal (parent to infant and infant to parent), developing gradually over the first year, and as being influenced by many variables. The term *attachment* is used in this chapter to indicate a bidirectional process (parent to infant, infant to parent) in which an enduring affectional and emotional commitment is formed; it is facilitated by positive feedback to each "partner" through mutually satisfying experiences (Mercer 1977).

Three concepts in this definition merit emphasis. As a process, a progression or development involving change in the attaching dyad occurs over time. This two-way process is not instantaneous. Many subtle affective and cognitive changes occur in both partners as attachment develops over a period of time. This developing commitment of mother to infant and infant to mother proceeds from global and general cognitive and affective responses to more highly differentiated and specific responses made by each to the other. The mother begins this process avidly by identifying and claiming her infant; acquaintance is a part of the attachment process.

In viewing attachment as a process, one should note that no single event will necessarily stop the process or prevent it. Some factors may make the process more difficult, may prolong the formation of the process, or may delay initiation of the process. Analgesia and anesthesia have the potential to impact in all these ways. However, placing all of one's attention on any one factor as a prerequisite to or as essential for the development of attachment ignores the multidimensional nature of the process as well as the effect of the mother's motivation, personality, and adaptability.

The second and third concepts in this definition of attachment which merit emphasis are that attachment is facilitated by positive feedback to each partner and that this positive feedback results in a mutually satisfying experience. Maternal anesthesia and analgesia have the potential to impact on these experiences also. The awake, alert infant who follows his mother's face is learning about his mother as his mother responds with joy in his seeming interest in her. The infant learns from and begins to enjoy the warmth of touch and holding just as the mother is thrilled by the grasp reflex around her finger or the moulding of the soft, cuddly form next to her breast. These are enjoyable experiences for both, and enjoyable experiences lead to each partner's seeking and valuing further contact and interaction. In this reciprocal interaction, each partner begins to respond to the other's cues, effecting the cognitive change in each. The mutually satisfying experiences enhance the emotional commitment of each to the other.

VARIABLES IMPACTING ON THE EFFECTS OF ANALGESIA AND ANESTHESIA

Maternal variables, fetal and placental variables, chemical characteristics of the drug, dosage, and time and route of administration all influence the fetal/ neonatal responses to drugs. Because of this multiplicity of interacting factors, the potential impact of drugs is here addressed. Consideration of all of these variables is important for those providing care for the laboring family, particularly in the care of the woman facing emergency cesarean birth. The enthusiastic consumer's movement for childbirth without undue medical interference reflects the mother's concern that she be awake and aware to absorb the events around her infant's birth, as well as her concern that her infant be able to be awake and to respond to her at this time. An important part of the nurse's role is to help family members resolve their dissonance when faced with an event that is contrary to their desires.

Maternal Variables

The woman's size, sensitivity to the drug, metabolism, and general health all affect the drug's impact on both herself and her fetus. If the woman's physical condition interferes with metabolism of a drug, the fetus tends to receive higher amounts of the drug. For example, if the woman has an abnormally low concentration of blood protein, there is a greater tendency for protein-bound drugs to be more readily available for diffusion across the placenta (Cohen and Olson 1970). In obese women, highly lipid-soluble drugs congregate in the body fat, and the drug that passes to the fetus returns to the mother more rapidly because the concentration of the drug in her blood is lower, favoring transfer from fetus to the mother (Cohen and Olson 1970). These are examples of simple diffusion; drugs tend to pass to the side of the placental membrane with the lowest concentration until the concentration is equal on both sides (O'Brien and McManus 1978).

Any maternal factor—such as supine hypotensive syndrome, hypertonic contractions, or hemorrhage—which results in decreased uterine blood flow leads to fetal asphyxia. The effects of any drugs given to the mother are then accentuated in an asphyxiated infant.

Kraemer et al. (1972) found that maternal drug use varies according to the length of labor and parity. They found that drug use was more extensive with primigravidas and those who had longer labors and that drug administration, parity, and length of labor all affected neonatal behavior simultaneously. This should be kept in mind, because many women receive drugs during a long labor prior to a cesarean birth.

Fetal and Placental Variables

The size and health of the fetus alter the effect drugs have on him. In addition, fetal and newborn circulation are different, and the greater blood flow to the fetal brain means that the fetus may be depressed by maternal medication given shortly before delivery.

The size (including thickness) and functioning of the placenta affect the crossing of a drug across to the fetus. Even though drugs do not cross a poorly functioning placenta, the fetus may be in a state of asphyxia due to to the malfunctioning placenta and therefore more vulnerable to the drugs. Although drug transfer to the fetus occurs largely across placental membranes, it may also occur via the amniotic fluid which the infant swallows (Cohen and Olson 1970).

Chemical Characteristics of Drugs

Drugs cross the placenta largely by simple diffusion, as noted earlier. The rate of diffusion is influenced by all of the factors mentioned above as well as by the drug's molecular weight, lipid solubility, and degree of ionization. All drugs that affect the central nervous system can cross the placenta to the fetus.

Drugs with a molecular weight of 600 readily cross the placenta. The diffusion can be very rapid if the molecular weight is less than 300. If the molecular weight is over 1,000, the drugs will not cross at all.

Lipid-soluble drugs cross the placenta easily; Pentothal is an example of such a drug. Nonlipid-soluble drugs don't diffuse across the placental membrane, since to diffuse they have to be soluble in the placental tissue, which is made up largely of lipids (O'Brien and McManus 1978).

All drugs exist in the ionized state (i.e., the molecules carry electrical charges) to some degree. The ionized portion of a drug cannot diffuse across the placental barrier, so that the less ionized drugs get across more easily. For example, Pentothal, which is 50 percent unionized, gets across easily.

Time and Route of Administration of Drugs

Drugs that are administered intravenously or by inhalation are absorbed instantaneously (Aleksandrowicz 1974). Drugs administered intramuscularly or rectally take up to an hour to reach peak blood concentration, but before the effect occurs, the drug has to diffuse to the tissues of the brain. The permeability of brain membranes varies with different drugs.

The time interval between the administration of a drug to the laboring woman and the birth of the infant is not always indicative of the effect of the drug. Kuhnert et al. (1979 I, II), through the use of gas chromatography and mass spectrometry, quantified the concentrations of meperidine and normeperidine (a metabolite of meperidine) in the infant's umbilical vein and artery at birth and in his urine at 3 days postpartum. They found a definite but nonlinear relationship between the interval of drug administration and the amount of meperidine and normeperidine the infant received. Infants whose mothers received meperidine 1 to 3 hours prior to delivery excreted more meperidine during the first day than those infants who were delivered within 1 hour or more than 3 hours after administration of meperidine. Quantities of both meperidine and normeperidine were high enough in the infants' urine for 3 days to indicate that additional time is needed for clearance of the drug and its metabolite. This also suggests that these chemicals may still be exerting an effect during this period.

POTENTIAL IMPACT OF DRUGS ON THE NEONATE IN THE ATTACHMENT PROCESS

In discussing the potential effect of drugs on the fetus/neonate, one must be careful to avoid the stance that drugs are "all bad" for the parturient woman and her infant. The anxiety and fear experienced by a laboring woman are not innocuous. Anxiety and fear trigger the fight or flight mechanism, releasing endogenous catecholamines. Lederman et al. (1978) found higher plasma epinephrine levels in association with self-reported anxiety and lower uterine contractile activity in women at 3 cm dilation.

When stress is induced in the pregnant monkey, ill effects are observed in the fetus—e.g., bradycardia, hypotension, and asphyxia (Meyers 1975). Morishima et al. (1979) induced stress in pregnant baboons, which resulted in increased uterine activity, reduced uterine blood flow, and lower heart rate as well as lower arterial oxygenation in all fetuses. Fetal recovery was prompt when maternal stressors were removed; however, sedation with pentobarbital or nitrous oxide also achieved fetal recovery. In addition, sedation prevented a subsequent decrease in uterine blood flow when the stressor was reintroduced. Lederman et al. (1977) observed that six of eight women who had received regional anesthesia (regardless of technique) had lower mean plasma epinephrine levels during labor than other women.

The infant's innate attachment behaviors are discussed next to allow the reader to relate the research on drug effects to specific behaviors.

Innate Infant Attachment Behaviors

The newborn possesses many behaviors and responses that serve to capture his parents' full and immediate attention. His power as an elicitor of parental attachment behaviors increases with his cognitive, physical, and social development. The newborn infant has been seen by many researchers to play a large role in creating his own environment through his innate behavioral responses (Aleksandrowicz and Aleksandrowicz 1975; Bennett 1971; Brazelton 1961; Yarrow 1963). The newborn's unique characteristics and responses create unique physical environments, both in the home and in the nursery. A visually alert, easily consolable infant endears his caretaker to him, which in turn entices the caretaker to provide more stimulation and human contact for him. The irritable infant with a short attention span who resists being held is soon labeled as difficult and unpleasant and is not sought out for interaction by either the nursery nurses or his parents when he goes home as often as is the alert, easily consoled infant.

Thomas and Chess (1977) identified 10 categories of infant temperament or behavioral style present at birth: activity level, rhythmicity or regularity, approach or withdrawal, adaptability to new or altered situations, threshold of responsiveness, intensity of reaction, quality of mood, distractability, attention span, and persistence. The infant's behavioral style may be initially affected by drugs administered to the mother during labor and delivery. The Brazelton Neonatal Behavioral Assessment Scale (Brazelton 1973) is helpful in determining the infant's responses to stimuli, motor maturity, cuddliness, consolability, defensive movements, peaks of excitement, irritability, activity, tremulousness, amount of startle, lability of states, self-quieting activity, and smiles, all of which may facilitate or inhibit parental attachment behaviors.

The infant's behavioral style tends to be consistent regardless of situation (Osofsky and Danzer 1974; Thoman 1975). If he is alert and responds to auditory cues, he will also look at his mother intently as he nurses or when he is held.

As with other mammals, the infant's behaviors that facilitate caretaker response have been categorized as triggering, orienting, and sensitizing (Harper 1971). The infant first triggers his parents' responses when he looks into his parents' eyes during the period of alertness that encompasses the first hour or two of life. Although this initial alertness may be due to the endogenous adrenalin secreted as part of the infant's response to the stress of labor and delivery, his parents perceive it as being more personal. His helpless appearance and uncoordinated physical movements may also evoke early parental response (Bell 1974). Visual alertness is soon evoked by maternal care (Korner and Thoman, 1970) and such soothing activities as placement on the mother's shoulder (Korner and Grobstein 1966; Korner and Thoman 1970). Visual alertness and eye-to-eye contact are potent facilitators of maternal attachment during the first 6 months of life (Robson 1968). Parents spend much time in trying to get their infants to look at them.

The infant's orienting responses facilitate early mother-infant synchrony during feeding so that both the mother and infant cue in to each other's response. This cuing in sensitizes the mother and reinforces the mother's feelings of accomplishment and competence in meeting her infant's needs. Call (1964) observed anticipatory approach behaviors in infants as early as the fourth feeding. The experienced nursery nurse has long observed the infant's mouthing and anticipation when she holds him in the position for feeding and places a diaper under his chin.

Brazelton (1979), in describing the behavioral competence of the newborn, noted that the infant turns his head toward human voices, his face becomes alert as he searches for the source of the voice, he listens to and chooses a female vocal pitch over others, he prefers human sounds to pure tones in an equivalent range, he looks at and follows faces and objects, he turns his head a full 90 degrees toward a picture of a human face and looks at it for long periods of time, he turns to and prefers milk smells over those of water or glucose, and he tastes and responds with altered sucking patterns to differences between human and cow's milk. Thus we see that the healthy, term neonate brings many capabilities for interaction to the attachment process. The following section reveals the way in which some of these behaviors are affected by drugs administered to the mother during labor and delivery.

Impact of Drugs and Modes of Anesthesia

Research over the past two decades presents strong evidence about the impact of analgesia and anesthesia on the newborn potential for early attachment behaviors. Bowlby (1969) described the specific attachment-eliciting behaviors as crying, clinging, sucking, following, and smiling. Behavioral impairment has been found following the administration of drugs to the mother during parturition, as measured by alertness and reactivity, EEG, sucking, REM and smiling (smiling occurs during REM sleep), attention, eye-to-eye contact, consolability, and irritability (Aleksandrowicz 1974).

Neurobehavioral tests administered to 274 neonates in the first 2 days of life showed that when the infants' mothers had epidural anesthesia, the infants' overall assessment scores were higher (Hodgkinson et al. 1977). The infants' neurobehavioral scores were intermediate following ketamine induction and were lowest after thiopental. Infants delivered vaginally when bupivacaine was used for epidural anesthesia did not suffer from decreased muscle tone and strength, as was observed earlier in infants born after the use of lidocaine or mepivacaine with continuous epidural anesthesia (Scanlon et al. 1976). McGuinness et al. (1978) found that a dose used in cesarean delivery that was 1.5 times greater than the dose used in vaginal delivery did not affect infants any more than tetracaine spinal anesthesia.

Kivalo et al. (1975) studied a series of 1,915 women who had cesarean births with intravenous thiopentone anesthesia. The Apgar score tended to decline with increased doses of thiopentone; the authors suggested doses of 300 mg or less.

Fox et al. (1979) compared oxygen tension and acid–base balance in umbilical venous and arterial blood samples taken from 20 neonates, 10 of whose mothers had had epidural anesthesia for elective cesarean delivery and 10 of whose mothers had been treated with a modified technique of general anesthesia. No significant differences in blood samples or Apgar scores were found between the two groups of infants immediately after delivery. The modified technique for general anesthesia included positioning the woman in the supine position with a wedge under her right hip and preoxygenation with 100 percent oxygen for at least 3 minutes. General anesthesia was then induced with thiopentone.

Brackbill (1977) compared the heart rate responses of six infants whose mothers had had no anesthesia, six whose mothers had had local infiltration for episiotomy, and six whose mothers had general anesthesia at 1, 4, and 8 months. When she found differences between the groups, she checked the results of liver palpations and found that the potency of the delivery medication was significantly associated with liver abnormality (palpable, spongy livers) at 4 and 12 months. A later report by Brackbill and Broman (1979) suggested that all anesthetic and analgesic drugs used are linked with adverse infant outcome in behavioral and gross motor development. In contrast to regional anesthetic agents, inhalant anesthetics used during delivery were strongly related to adverse outcome in infant neurobehavioral development (particularly gross motor development), and these associations did not seem to dissipate with age—children were followed-up at 4 and 7 years of age. Infants in the sample of 3,528 came from 12 teaching hospitals across the country; 95 percent of the mothers had received drugs during labor. This report is considered controversial, and the methodology used has been questioned. However, some demonstrated effects of maternal analgesia and anesthesia on the neonate will be discussed here in relation to some specific responses—wakefulness and biological rhythms, feeding, and neurobehavioral responses.

Wakefulness and Biological Rhythms

Emde et al. (1975) observed the behavioral states of wakefulness, crying, active rapid eye movement (REM) sleep, quiet (non-REM) sleep, and drowsiness in 20 normal infants for 10 hours following birth. Half of the infants' mothers had been administered some form of sedative during labor; the other half had had none. All infants had an initial wakeful period, fell asleep, awoke, and then fell asleep a second time; 15 awoke and fell asleep a third time. Since there were no feedings during this time, it was assumed that these observations were evidence of a sleep–wakefulness cycle in the first 10 hours after birth. Infants whose mothers had received medication showed decreased amounts of wakefulness and increased amounts of quiet (non-REM) sleep. Neonatal smiling occurs during REM sleep (Aleksandrowicz 1974), which means that such infants also have fewer reflex smiles. Since the infant cannot learn about his environment or have eye contact with his mother while asleep, infants in the medicated group would elicit fewer maternal responses and are less likely to increase self-awareness. Infants of mothers who have had drugs in labor have also been observed to be less attentive to visual stimuli; this response persists beyond the age of 4 days (Stechler 1964). Normal and premature neonates demonstrate what Sugar (1976) calls hunger and feeding reflexes. The hunger reflex occurs in two phases; a search phase occurs first when the infant brings his arms, forearms, and hands to his face midline and explores his surroundings with his fingers and hands. When he finds a part of the caretaker's body with his fingers and hands, the tactile phase begins. The feeding reflex begins as the feeding is started and terminates with satiation. During the feeding reflex, the infant holds his fingers and hands rigidly without any searching or stroking movements, showing active acceptance of the caretaker. The 45 degree to 90 degree abduction of the arms may thus serve as a social releasor. Any drug that depresses other infant reflexes has the potential to depress hunger and feeding reflexes.

In comparing infants of mothers who had had little medication with those whose mothers had had a large amount of medication, Brazelton (1961) found that feedings on the second day were 65 percent effective in the group with little medication. The more heavily medicated group had only 25 percent successful feedings. On the fourth day the low medication group had 87 percent successful feeding situations and the high medication group 55 percent. Infants in the low medication group consequently began gaining weight earlier. Thoman (1975) reported a decrease in the number of feeding intervals in direct relation to the effect of analgesics.

Tryphonopoulou and Doxiadis (1972) observed that infants of mothers who had had a cesarean birth with general anesthesia had lower scores in their sucking behavior for the first 5 days than infants of mothers who were delivered vaginally with only a sedative. Their scores began to rise on the sixth day.

Neurobehavioral Responses

Standley et al. (1974) found that the infants who were most alert and least irritable and who had the most mature motor behaviors had mothers who had received no analgesia or anesthesia. They found that local/regional anesthesia had more influence on the infant than the analgesia. Local/regional anesthesia was correlated with decreased motor maturity and greater irritability. The infants in the anesthesia group showed jerky movements, tremulous motions, frequent state changes, and more frequent crying.

Aleksandrowicz (1974) found correlations in all behaviors of the Brazelton Assessment Scale and Drugs. The observed narcotics and general anesthesia lowered the infants' consolability scores and increased their irritability. Conway and Brackbill (1970) reported muscular, visual, and neural development impairment that continued for as long as 4 weeks after delivery subsequent to maternal anesthesia and analgesia.

POTENTIAL IMPACT OF DRUGS ON THE MOTHERS IN THE ATTACHMENT PROCESS

Research has shown that there are many fixed factors that affect the maternal attachment process. Some examples of these are: the mother's early mothering by her own mother, her genetic endowment and personality traits, social and cultural practices, her experiences during previous pregnancies, the course of events during the current pregnancy and childbirth, and her relationships with her mate and family.

The woman's self-esteem (or how she feels about herself) reflects something of how she is able to feel about others. If her body has failed to perform as other women's bodies do (e.g., failing to deliver her baby vaginally), she experiences disappointment and a sense of shame. In addition to her feelings of disappointment and shame, she usually feels guilty that something she *did* or *did not* do led to her failure to deliver vaginally (Mercer 1977).

Mothering is an active process, one that requires the mother to take control to some degree. If the mother is out of control and is passively dependent upon the environment, it is most difficult for her to begin the task of mothering. She has little energy to direct toward her infant until she is physiologically restored and feels in control of her own body and bodily functions. She also has her own temperamental style, which may not fit her infant's. There is a sensitive, complex interplay of many variables in what the mother brings to the attachment process, and when the mother has experienced an unexpected cesarean birth the chances are greater that one or more of these variables may be distorted or exaggerated.

All gestational illnesses, including cesarean birth, play a role in attachment behaviors (Lynch and Roberts 1977; ten Bensel and Paxton 1977). Cohen (1966) observed that any stressful event during pregnancy or delivery has an impact on how the mother perceives her infant. These factors must be kept in mind in considering the impact of analgesia and anesthesia on the mother's attachment behaviors, because the nature of the cesarean birth often presents as a stressor to the woman, as well as increasing her morbidity.

Pain and the Potential Impact of Analgesia and Anesthesia

The impact of pain upon the attachment process is unknown, although many postulations have been made. Peterson and Mehl (1978) found the birth experience to be the second most significant factor in variance in maternal attachment; disappointment in the delivery experience accounted for 27 percent of the variance. They postulated that fear and pain cause resentment of the infant, if he is associated with the fear and pain. Kitzinger (1978) described pain with a purpose or function as being more readily accepted. A few women in the research of Billewicz–Driemel and Milne (1976) supported the contention that the laboring woman values pain in labor. Some 99 women who had had epidural anesthesia and 95 who had had conventional anesthesia (local, inhalation, pethedine injection) were interviewed at 18 to 24 months after delivery to determine whether women suffered a sense of deprivation as a result of a successful epidural block. Although only four women (4 percent) felt deprived (giving such replies as "Painless labour is unemotional: I would like to feel the whole experience of having a baby." and "Pain is good psychologically."), their remarks supported the findings of Mercer and Marut. Mercer and Marut (in press) observe that women delivering vaginally, and consequently expériencing more pain during the birth process than women having cesarean births, felt that they were better persons for having experienced the "hard, terrible pain." They recalled their endurance of the labor and delivery with much pride and emotional satisfaction, indicating their increased self-esteem. A question can be raised as to how much of the cesarean woman's disappointment in and anger at her birth experience is caused by anesthesia that has prevented her from physically and emotionally experiencing the birth to the fullest?

Marut (1978), in a pilot study on women who had had cesareans, observed a difference in response to infant and birth experience when comparing women who had had regional anesthesia to those who had had general anesthesia. Women who had had general anesthesia were slower in identifying their infants and more focused on themselves. Marut and Mercer (1979) found that women who had experienced cesarean birth and had had regional anesthesia viewed their experiences more positively than those who had had general anesthesia $(P = .05)$.

Marut's pilot study and interviews in the Marut and Mercer (1979) study suggested that the women who had had cesarean births had a much greater hesitancy to name their infants; the name that had been chosen antepartally did not seem "to fit the infant" delivered by cesarean birth. This observation was supported, and in naming their infants the difference between mothers who had delivered vaginally and mothers who had delivered by cesarean was significant at the 0.005 level. Women who had had a cesarean and regional anesthesia named their infants earlier than women who had had general anesthesia; the difference was significant at less than the 0.05 level. The woman's ability to enjoy holding her baby for the first time was related to her partner's help during labor and delivery and her perception of her own degree of control during delivery. Women who had general anesthesia seldom had their mates in the cesarean birth room, while those who had regional anesthesia had their mates with them more often. The woman who was asleep obviously had no awareness and thus felt complete loss of control over her birth experience.

Kimball (1979) reported that the placenta is a source of endorphins which are more potent than morphine in raising pain tolerance. Endorphins are evoked by physiological stress concomitant with adrenocorticotropin. Placental endorphins stimulated during labor and delivery could account for the euphoria of women delivering vaginally. Further, endorphins stimulate the release of prolactin and suppress hostility, irritability, and anxiety. Prolactin not only stimulates milk production but reportedly enhances mothering and nurturing behaviors. Kimball suggests that ". . . endorphins provide the emotional reward to reinforce biological behavior that contributes to propagation of the species and advances cultural evolution." If Kimball's subsequent radioimmunoassays identify endorphins in his samples from unmedicated mothers, this will offer explanation for some of the cesarean mother's postpartum blues and distant feelings toward her infant.

Interactional Behaviors and Analgesia and Anesthesia

Parke et al. (1972) found that women who received more medications during labor vocalized to and rocked their infants more. Conversely, the father's interaction decreased as the maternal medication increased. Observations of 19 Caucasian couples between 6 and 48 hours postpartum suggested that maternal medication altered early parental interactions with the infant. Possibilities postulated for these findings were that fathers prefer active, awake infants and leave lethargic infants to their mothers and that mothers who receive high amounts of medications may be more anxious about the infants' health and may consequently stimulate the infants more in an attempt to increase responsiveness.

Tryphonopoulou and Doxiadis (1972) studied the effect of elective cesarean births on initial mother–infant relationships in ten primiparas delivered by cesarean and ten primiparas who delivered vaginally. They reported that initial mother–infant contact did not begin until the third and fourth days for mothers in the cesarean birth group. Mothers in the vaginal group began interacting with their infants on the first and second days. They also noted that both mothers and infants were depressed by drugs. The timing and length of early maternal–infant interaction is determined in part by institutional practices, so that it is difficult to evaluate the impact of surgery and/or drugs.

POTENTIAL IMPACT OF DRUGS ON THE MOTHER–INFANT ATTACHMENT PROCESS

The impact of cesarean birth on the mother and the attachment process is considered in depth in Chapter 3, so only a few points on this subject addressed here prior to consideration of the impact of anesthesia and analgesia.

The woman who has an emergency cesarean birth has a feeling of unreality about the birth experience, views her labor and childbirth experiences very negatively, has a feeling of defeat about her birth experience and a decreased feeling of self-esteem, and makes hostile remarks about her infant (Marut and Mercer 1979). Affonso and Stichler (1978) noted that many women verbalize feelings of failure and grieve that they have lost their desired mode of delivery. Women's feelings of powerlessness in this situation diminish as they resolve their feelings about the cesarean birth.

The mother who experiences cesarean birth and who has general anesthesia has much difficulty believing the baby is hers. Marut (1978) quoted a mother as saying, "I have this dream where the nurse takes this baby out of the closet in the section room and gives her to me, and my baby is taken away. I'll never really know if she's mine."

In describing her feelings following the emergency cesarean birth of her premature son, Schlosser (1978) wrote, "It was three months before I overcame my negative feelings, experienced bonding with my child, and worked through the resentment with my husband."

These data support the contention that the emotional impact of a cesarean birth influences the woman's initial feelings and perceptions about herself and her infant. Accordingly, one must consider the way in which these responses affect the potential impact of analgesia and anesthesia on the attachment process. It might be helpful at this point to reflect on the definition of attachment stated earlier—a process that is facilitated by positive feedback given to each partner through a mutually satisfying experience—and to briefly consider the early maternal attachment behaviors of identifying and claiming the infant. The infant who has longer periods of quiet, non-REM sleep is not eliciting maternal response by two of the strongest social interaction modes—eye contact and the smile. Parents sometimes plead, "Please look at me." One father saw the eye-to-eye contact following birth as part of perfect functioning (Henwood 1979): "I looked at Mick and he looked back at me, right at me." Eye-to-eye contact seems to be such a strong eliciting contact that some parents withhold naming an infant until he "looks" at them. One mother said (Stacy 1979), "We cannot name the baby until he looks at us; we will not know *who* he is until then. The eyes are the windows to the soul."

The infant who is sleepy does not feed well; consequently, the mother fails in her first attempts at mothering acts. The infant's lack of response may be seen as rejection of the nurturing offered.

If the infant is irritable or difficult to console, a mother may feel incompetent in the task of giving love and comfort measures. Feelings of incompetence lead to lowered self-esteem. Perhaps a mother with a very high self-concept and with a strong support system might not be turned off by a lethargic baby who refuses to suck (and thus accept an offered part of herself—if she is breast-feeding, this can be an emotionally laden act of mothering), or a baby who is irritable and takes an unusually long time to console, or a baby who will not maintain eye contact. But for some women, these characteristics can be real turn-offs; they may be too much for those women who have low self-esteem, weak egos, and/or no social support to reinforce their mothering acts.

Studies show that the infant adapts his motility and his state to the environment if the environment is sensitive to him and his needs. The infant in turn shapes the environment. How does the infant who is handicapped by maternal anesthesia and analgesia begin this early differentiation and shaping? Brazelton (1979), in studying parent–neonate interactions, focused on the reciprocity, affective, and cognitive information that a parent transmits to a newborn infant.

When the parent appears to be too anxious or is insensitive to the infant's homeostatic needs (the demands of the physiological systems of an immature organism), the infant withdraws his attention and keeps the tense parent in his peripheral field, checking back briefly from time to time. Brazelton sees the fine interplay between mother and infant as a precursor of affective development. The growing attachment of both partners and the stimulation and the fueling that each receives as feedback from the other facilitate the infant's learning of each new developmental task.

IMPLICATIONS FOR FACILITATION OF MATERNAL-INFANT ATTACHMENT

What can be done to facilitate attachment when analgesia and anesthesia are unavoidable? Since the impact of maternal anesthesia on the neonate depends on the kind of anesthesia and on the degree of maternal awareness during birth, regional anesthesia should be chosen over general anesthesia when a choice is possible in cesarean birth. Regardless of the anesthesia chosen, having a support person in the delivery room fosters the mother's interaction with her infant: as some mothers have commented (Mercer and Marut, in press), "He could see and feel for me and tell me what happened."

Any medication has potential impact on the newborn. All health professionals should therefore encourage mate participation in the childbirth process and attendance of both parents at childbirth preparation classes; parental participation will permit the necessary awareness of the effects of medication. In addition, parents will learn about sensations they will be experiencing during labor and delivery and something of the technological monitoring that may be expected. Knowing the sequencing, duration, and sensations of events during a threatening experience seems to increase the sense of cognitive control over the situation (Johnson et al. 1978).

To facilitate the cesarean mother's grasp of the reality of her birth experience, it is important to awaken her as soon as possible following birth and show her her infant. She will fall asleep again quickly. Women who have been allowed to sleep without having seen their infants have often expressed a wish that someone had shown them their infants earlier.

Since the mother measures her success in her initial mothering acts so strongly in terms of the infant's response, she should be made aware, in the event of difficulty with feeding, for instance, that *no one* could have gotten her infant to suck at that particular moment if he were drowsy or asleep. When the infant is awake and hungry, he should be taken out to his mother, regardless of whether it is the "usual time." Sucking is a very basic behavior which indicates ability to function. In order for the mother to feel good initially it is important that she ascertain that all of her baby's basic systems are functioning.

With sleepy or irritable infants, it is even more critical that the health professional share the observed infant's behavioral response with the parents. This is crucial in helping parents realize that the observed "difficult" response is not directed to them personally. Furthermore, it promotes earlier sensitization to the infant's cues, thus facilitating the infant's move to more organized behaviors.

It is important to keep in mind the fact that different infants have different impacts on parents, and these individual differences are present from birth. Not all persons express feelings of attachment in the same manner. There are persons who are close physical interactors (touchers, kissers) and there are those who are more distal interactors (vocalizers who sing or talk).

In the study conducted by Marut and Mercer (1979), 40 percent of the women who delivered vaginally elected not to hold their infants in the delivery room, with the following reasons: "I was too tired." "They were sewing me up." "My husband held her for me." These appear to be valid considerations. While it is important to promote togetherness in families and to facilitate parenting and the attachment process, individual styles and differences must be respected. Failure to hold the infant in the delivery room does not always mean rejection of the infant. A mother sometimes is not able to hold her infant. Accurate, meaningful data must be recorded and transmitted to the pediatrician, nurse, or involved professional to enable them to provide supportive follow-up for those parents who need special reinforcement of their potential as well as special help in becoming acquainted with their infants.

Parents are persons with preferences; persons with styles of relating and attaching. The nurse's major role is to interpret infant characteristics and behavior and to help the mother learn to "read" her infant. Even more help should be offered to the mother with an infant who is depressed or "difficult." Through role modeling, the nurse can influence parental behavior so that the mother can see that the infant's response is not a response to *her,* but rather, for the time being, a response toward all. The nurse can then help the mother to see what works best for that particular infant in a particular situation.

Norbert Wiener (1956), credited as the brain behind cybernetics, stated, "One has only one life to live, and there is not time enough in which to master the art of being a parent." The ultimate challenge is to work toward minimizing the amount of maternal medications used during childbirth. When administration of these medications is unavoidable and serves a useful purpose, the nurse's task is to help parents master the art of being a parent in spite of these more difficult situations.

REFERENCES

Affonso DD, Stichler JF: Exploratory study of women's reactions to having a cesarean birth. Birth Family J 5 (2):88–94, 1978

Aleksandrowicz MK: The effect of pain relieving drugs administered during labor and delivery on the behavior of the newborn: A review. Merrill-Palmer Quart 20:121–41, 1974

Aleksandrowicz MK, Aleksandrowicz DR: The moulding of personality: A newborn's innate characteristics in interaction with parents' personalities. Child Psychiatry Hum Dev 5 (4):231–41, 1975

Bell RQ: Contributions of human infants to caregiving and social interaction. In Lewis M, Rosenblum LA (eds), The Effect of the Infant on its Caregiver. New York, Wiley and Sons, 1974

Bennett S: Infant-caretaker interactions. J Am Acad Child Psychiatry 10:321–35, 1971

Billewicz–Driemel AM, Milne MD: Long-term assessment of extradural analgesia for the relief of pain in labour, II: Sense of "deprivation" after extradural analgesia in labour: Relevant or not? Br J Anaesth 48:139–43, 1976

Bowlby J: Attachment and Loss: Vol I, Attachment. New York, Basic Books, 1969

Brackbill Y: Long-term effects of obstetrical anesthesia on infant autonomic function. Dev Psychobiol 10 (6):529–35, 1977

Brackbill Y, Broman SH: Pain-killers in labor: "Caution flag is up." Med World News 20 (3):23–24, 1979

Brazelton TB: Behavioral competence of the newborn infant. Semin Perinatol 3 (1):35–44, 1979

Brazelton TB: Neonatal Behavioral Assessment Scale. Philadelphia, Lippincott, 1973

Brazelton TB: Psychophysiologic reactions in the neonate, I: The value of observation of the neonate. J Pediatr 58 (4):508–12, 1961

Brazelton TB: Psychophysiologic reactions in the neonate, II: Effect of maternal medication on the neonate and his behavior. J Pediatr 58 (4):513–18, 1961

Call JD: Newborn approach behaviour. Int J Psychoanal 45:286–93, 1964

Campbell SBG, Taylor PM: Bonding and attachment: Theoretical issues. Semin Perinatol 3 (1):3–13, 1979

Cohen SN, Olson WA: Drugs that depress the newborn infant. Pediatr Clin North Am 17 (4):835–50, 1970

Committee on Drugs, American Academy of Pediatrics. Effect of medication during labor and delivery on infant outcome. Pediatrics 62 (3):402–403, 1978

Conway E, Brackbill Y: Delivery medication and infant outcome: An empirical study. The Effects of Obstetrical Medication on Fetus and Infant. Monogr Soc Res Child Dev 35 (4), Serial No. 137, 1970

Emde RN, Swedberg J, Suzuki B: Human wakefulness and biological rhythms after birth. Arch Gen Psychiatry 32:780–83, 1975

Fox GS, Smith JB, Namba Y, Johnson RC: Anesthesia for cesarean section: Further studies. Am J Obstet Gynecol 133 (1):15–19, 1979

Haar E, Welkowitz J, Blau A, Cohen J: Personality differentiation of neonates: A nurse rating scale method. J Am Acad Child Psychiatry 3:330–42, 1964

Harper LV: The young as a source of stimuli controlling caretaker behavior. Dev Psychol 4 (1):73–88, 1971

Henwood KC: Case study of a family having a premature by cesarean birth. Unpublished manuscript, 1979

Hodgkinson R, Marx GF, Kim SS, Miclat NM: Neonatal neurobehavioral tests following vaginal delivery under ketamine, thiopental, and extradural anesthesia. Anesth Analg (Cleveland) 56 (4):548–53, 1977

Johnson JE, Rice VH, Fuller SS, Endress MP: Sensory information, instruction in a coping strategy, and recovery from surgery. Res Nurs Health 1 (1): 4–17, 1978

Kimball CD: Do endorphin residues of beta lipotropin in hormone reinforce reproductive functions? Am J Obstet Gynecol 134 (2):127–30, 1979

Kitzinger S: Pain in childbirth. J Med Ethics 4:119-21, 1978

Kivalo I, Timonen S, Castren O: The influence of anaesthesia and the induction-delivery interval on the newborn delivered by caesarean section. Ann Chir Gynaecol Fenn 60:71-75, 1975

Korner AF, Grobstein R: Visual alertness as related to soothing in neonates: Implications for maternal stimulation and early deprivation. Child Dev 37:867-76, 1966

Korner AF, Thoman EB: Visual alertness in neonates as evoked by maternal care. J Exp Child Psychol 10:67-78, 1970

Kraemer HC, Korner AF, Thoman EB: Methodological considerations in evaluating the influence of drugs used during labor and delivery on the behavior of the newborn. Dev Psychol 6 (1): 128-34, 1972

Kuhnert BR, Kuhnert PM, Tu AL, et al: Meperidine and normeperidine levels following meperidine administration during labor, I: Mother. Am J Obstet Gynecol 133 (8):904-908, 1979

Kuhnert BR, Kuhnert PM, Tu AL, Lin DCK: Meperidine and normeperidine levels following meperidine administration during labor, II: Fetus and neonate. Am J Obstet Gynecol 133 (8):909-14, 1979

Lederman RP, Lederman E, Work B Jr., McCann DS: The relationship of maternal anxiety, plasma catecholamines, and plasma cortisol to progress in labor. Am J Obstet Gynecol 132 (5):495-500, 1978

Lederman RP, McCann DS, Work B Jr., Huber MJ: Endogenous plasma epinephrine and norepinephrine in last-trimester pregnancy and labor. Am J Obstet Gynecol 129 (1):5-8, 1977

Lynch MA, Roberts J: Predicting child abuse: Signs of bonding failure in the maternity hospital. Br Med J II:624-26, 1977

Marut JS: The special needs of the cesarean mother. Am J Maternal–Child Nurs 3 (4):202-206, 1978

Marut JS, Mercer RT: A comparison of primiparas' perceptions of vaginal and cesarean birth. Nurs Res 28 (5):260-69, 1979

McGuinness GA, Merkow AJ, Kennedy RL, Erenberg A: Epidural anesthesia with bupivacaine for cesarean section: Neonatal blood levels and neurobehavioral responses. Anesthesiology 49:270-73, 1978

Mercer RT: Nursing Care for Parents at Risk. Thorofare, N.J., Slack, 1977

Mercer RT, Marut JS: Comparative viewpoints: Cesarean versus vaginal birth. In Affonso DD (ed), Impact of Cesarean Birth. Philadelphia, Davis (in press)

Meyers RE: Maternal psychological stress and fetal asphyxia: A study in the monkey. Am J Obstet Gynecol 122 (1): 47-59, 1975

Morishima HO, Yeh M, James LS: Reduced uterine blood flow and fetal hypoxemia with acute maternal stress: Experimental observation in the pregnant baboon. Am J Obstet Gynecol 134 (3):270-75, 1979

O'Brien TE, McManus CE: Drugs and the fetus: A consumer's guide by generic and brand name. Birth Fam J 5 (2):58-86, 1978

Osofsky JD, Danzer B: Relationships between neonatal characteristics and mother–infant interaction. Dev Psychol 10 (1):124-30, 1974

Parke RD, O'Leary SE, West S: Mother–father–newborn interaction effects of maternal medication, labor, and sex of infant. Proceedings, 80th Annual Convention. APA, 1972, pp. 85-86

Peterson GH, Mehl LE: Some determinants of maternal attachment. Am J Psychiatry 135 (10):1168-73, 1978

Robson RB: The role of eye-to-eye contact in maternal–infant attachment. In Chess S, Thomas A (eds), Annual Progress in Child Psychiatry and Child Development 1968. New York, Brunner/Mazel, 1968

Scanlon JW, Ostheimer GW, Lurie AO, et al: Neurobehavioral responses and drug concentrations in newborns after maternal epidural anesthesia with bupivacaine. Anesthesiology 45 (4):400–405, 1976

Schlosser S: The emergency c-section patient: Why she needs help. . . what you can do. RN 41 (9):53–56, 1978

Stacy RS: Case study of a family with a premature delivered by cesarean birth. Unpublished manuscript, 1979

Standley K, Soule AB III, Copans SA, Duchowny MS: Local–regional anesthesia during childbirth: Effect on newborn behaviors. Science 186:634–35, 1974

Stechler G: Newborn attention as affected by medication in labor. Science 144:315-17, 1964

Sugar M: Feeding and hunger reflexes in human neonates. J Am Acad Child Psychiatry 15 (2):269-77, 1976

ten Bensel RW, Paxton CL: Child abuse following early postpartum separation. J Pediatr 90 (3):490–503, 1977

Thoman EB: Development of synchrony in mother–infant interaction in feeding and other situations. Fed Proc 34 (7):1587–92, 1975

Thomas A, Chess S: Temperament and Development. New York, Brunner/Mazel, 1977

Tryphonopoulou Y, Doxiadis S: The effect of elective caesarian section on the initial stage of mother–infant relationship. In Psychosomation Medicine in Obstetrics and Gynaecology. Third International Congress, London, 1971. Basel, Karger, 1972

Wiener N: I Am a Mathematician. New York, Doubleday, 1956, p. 224.

Yarrow LJ: Research in dimensions of early maternal care. Merrill–Palmer Quart 9:101-14, 1963

SECTION III

Assessment Tools for Nurses

CHAPTER 5

An Overview of the Roy Adaptation Model

Carole Fitzgerald Kehoe and Jacqueline Fawcett

Within the past decade, a number of conceptual models of nursing have been developed as guides for nursing education, research, and practice (Riehl and Roy 1980). Each model presents a different perspective on people and their environments, health, goals of nursing, and approaches to meeting clients' nursing needs. While their ideas about nursing differ, the proponents of the various models agree that the special social congruence, significance, and utility of each can be determined only by systematic study of its application in a variety of educational and practice settings. In other words, the results of application must be examined for their generation of nursing actions that: (1) meet the expectations of society, (2) make important differences in clients' health, and (3) represent comprehensive nursing care (Johnson 1974).

Nursing models distinguish nursing from medicine and other disciplines (Roy 1976B, p. 690). The validation of these models through empirical testing is imperative for the continuing development of nursing as an autonomous discipline with its own body of knowledge (Chaska 1978, p. 411).

Presently, no one model has been more convincingly supported than any other. Thus the individual nurse's choice of a model for her own activities must rest on her intuitive judgment of its validity in given situations.

We selected the Roy Adaptation Model as the framework for our studies of the needs and nursing care of cesarean mothers and fathers, as presented in Chapters 6 and 7, for several reasons (Roy 1976A). First, this model has been widely used as a framework for nursing education and practice and has generated some research that has led to tentative confirmation of its basic assumptions. The reports of its application in diverse situations indicate application is not especially problematic (Brower and Baker 1976; Wagner 1976; Roy and Obloy 1978; Galligan 1979; Schmitz 1980; Starr 1980). Second, a textbook presenting each aspect of the model in considerable detail, including assessment variables and intervention strategies, is available and clearly aids application (Roy 1976A). Third, the model encompasses many areas that the literature suggests are relevant in the case of cesarean birth. Fourth, Downey's (1974) success in using the model as a guide for comprehensive nursing care of vaginally delivered mothers suggested it could be extended to the care of cesarean parents. Finally, a test of the model in a new situation would be a contribution to nursing knowledge.

The Roy Adaptation Model was developed by Sister Callista Roy in the mid-1960s. Since that time, it has been clarified and refined through application in diverse nursing educational and clinical practice settings. Further, studies conducted in 1971 and 1976-1977 have validated several elements of the model. Thus Roy's model is regarded as one of the most fully developed conceptual models in nursing today (Roy 1980).

The model combines a systems approach with a symbolic interactionist perspective. People are conceptualized as biopsychosocial beings in constant interaction with an ever-changing environment. The model proposes that people have innate and acquired biological, psychological, and social adaptive mechanisms which they use to cope with environmental changes. Roy (1976A) has claimed that people adapt in relation to their physiological needs, self-concepts, role functions, and interdependence. The physiological mode of adaptation is concerned with basic needs requisite to maintaining the physiological integrity and functioning of the human system. Needs include exercise and rest; nutrition; elimination; fluid and electrolytes; oxygen; circulation; and regulation of temperature, the senses, and the endocrine system. The self-concept mode deals with people's conceptions of their physical and personal selves, which vary throughout life as their bodies change and as they interact with others. Self-concept has a number of component dimensions, including:

1. The physical self, which is one's appraisal of self as a physical being (the self-image). This incorporates the person's capacity to function and the ability to control that functioning. Problems in the body's functioning capacity or in its controlling capacity are perceived as loss (Driever 1976A, pp. 174-75).
2. The moral-ethical self, which involves the person's self-perceptions of good and bad, and right and wrong. Transgressions in this area result in feelings of guilt (Driever 1976A, pp. 176-77).
3. Self-consistency, which concerns the constancy between who the individual is today and who he or she will be tomorrow. Indications of a discrepancy between the self of today and the self of tomorrow are expressed as anxiety (Perley 1976, p. 211).

4. Self-ideal and expectancy. Collectively, these are the components of the personal self dealing with what one would like to be and what one expects oneself to be. Problems in this area are experienced as feelings of powerlessness (Roy 1976C, p. 225).
5. Self-esteem, which reflects the value the person holds of himself, is the core of self-concept. Self-esteem is a part of every emotional response and every feeling. Problems in this area reflect feelings of worthlessness (Driever 1976B, p. 233).

The role function mode of adaptation refers to a person's performance of duties on the basis of his or her position within society. This mode is primarily concerned with the need to know how to act in a variety of situations and encompasses both instrumental and expressive behaviors. The components of this mode include:

1. Role mastery, which deals with the person's ability to perform newly acquired role behaviors in a manner consistent with personal and culturally derived expectations. Inherent in this component is role change—that is, adjusting and changing one's performance to meet new expectations related to enactment and mastery of new roles (Schofield 1976, pp. 267–71).
2. Role distance, which occurs when people do not consider the behaviors associated with a particular role as applying to them because the performance of this role threatens their self-esteem. They therefore belittle the role or ignore it (Schofield 1976, pp. 273–74).
3. Role conflict, which occurs when people reject certain roles and the behaviors associated with performance of these roles. In contrast to role distance, role conflict does not derive from threats to self-esteem. Rather, it occurs when ambiguous or conflicting cues regarding role performance arise (Schofield 1976, p. 274).
4. Role failure, which occurs when anticipated role performance is not consistent with the person's expectations of that performance. This is often due to lack of knowledge about the expected role performance or lack of skill in performing prescribed behaviors (Schofield 1976, p. 282).

The interdependence mode of adaptation embraces dependent and independent behavior. The mode is concerned with the individual's needs to know he or she is loved, supported, nurtured, and able to maintain meaningful relationships with others. The term *dependent behavior* refers to the individual's desire to seek human interaction because relationships with others are perceived as rewarding and satisfying. This need for affiliation is manifested in such behavior as seeking help, attention, and affection. The term *independent behavior,* in contrast, refers to the desire to be self-reliant, self-assertive, and to seek relationships with others infrequently. This kind of behavior indicates the need to accomplish things on one's own, a need for achievement. Two behavioral manifestations of the need for achievement are initiative-taking and obstacle mastery. The balance between a person's need for affiliation and need to achieve things independently is reflected by *interdependent behavior* (McIntier 1976).

Roy (1976A) felt that the needs associated with each mode of adaptation stimulate responses that maintain physiological, psychic, and social integrity. The responses, in turn, are manifested in the person's behavior. Whenever the individual's internal or external environment changes, need satisfaction changes and results in a need deficit or excess. This condition then triggers the adaptive mechanisms of the mode with which the need is connected, bringing forth behavior that is adaptive or maladaptive.

A person's ability to adapt positively is a function of the environmental stimuli to which he or she is exposed. Drawing from Helson's (1964) work on adaptation of the retina of the eye, Roy (1976A) identified three types of stimuli that influence adaptive ability. These are: (1) focal stimuli, or all stimuli immediately confronting the person in question; (2) contextual stimuli, or all other stimuli present that affect behavior (the context of a situation); and (3) residual or nonspecific stimuli, such as the person's attitudes, beliefs, experiences, and expectations.

From the perspective of Roy's Adaptation Model (Roy 1976A), the goal of nursing intervention is to promote positive adaptation in each adaptive mode. In general, this is thought to be accomplished (1) by reinforcement of the client's already adaptive behaviors, or conversion of maladaptive behaviors to adaptive behaviors through removal of the primary, or focal, stimulus, and (2) by changing the secondary and tertiary factors—i.e., the contextual and residual stimuli. Roy advocated use of a systematic nursing process to assess specific need disturbances in each adaptive mode engendered by the stimuli and to prescribe interventions that will promote positive adaptation. This process includes an initial or first-level assessment to identify adaptive and maladaptive behaviors; a second-level assessment to identify the focal, contextual, and residual stimuli that are influencing those behaviors; problem identification, or nursing diagnosis; goal setting in terms of desired behavioral outcomes of nursing intervention; intervention by means of manipulating stimuli to promote positive adaptation; and evaluation of the effectiveness of the interventions.

As noted earlier, we used Roy's model ourselves to organize the findings of our exploratory studies of the postpartum needs of cesarean mothers and cesarean fathers and to organize the discussion of nursing care implications. We found that the structure imposed by the model facilitated data analysis and gave us confidence that our suggestions for the nursing care of cesarean parents had taken into account the totality of the parents' needs, while preserving their individual rights and preferences.

REFERENCES

Brower HT, Baker B: Using the adaptation model in a practitioner curriculum. Nurs Outlook 24:686–90, 1976

Chaska NL: Not crystal clear. In Chaska NL (ed), The Nursing Profession: Views Through the Mist. New York, McGraw-Hill, 1978

Downey C: Adaptation nursing applied to an obstetric patient. In Riehl JP, Roy C (eds), Conceptual Models for Nursing Practice. New York, Appleton–Century–Crofts, 1974

Driever MH: Theory of self concept. In Roy C (ed), Introduction to Nursing: An Adaptation Model. Englewood Cliffs, N.J., Prentice-Hall, 1976A

Driever MH: Problem of low self-esteem. In Roy C (ed), Introduction to Nursing: An Adaptation Model. Englewood Cliffs, N.J., Prentice-Hall, 1976B

Galligan AC: Using Roy's concept of adaptation to care for young children. Am J Maternal–Child Nurs 4 (1):24–28, 1979

Helson H: Adaptation Level Theory. New York, Harper and Row, 1964

Johnson DE: Development of theory: A requisite for nursing as a primary health profession. Nurs Res 23:372–77, 1974

McIntier TM: Theory of interdependence. In Roy C (ed), Introduction to Nursing: An Adaptation Model. Englewood Cliffs, N.J., Prentice-Hall, 1976

Perley NZ: Problems of moral–ethical self: Guilt. In Roy C (ed), Introduction to Nursing: An Adaptation Model. Englewood Cliffs, N.J., Prentice-Hall, 1976

Riehl JP, Roy C: Conceptual Models for Nursing Practice, 2nd ed. New York: Appleton–Century–Crofts, 1980

Roy C: Introduction to Nursing: An Adaptation Model. Englewood Cliffs, N.J., Prentice-Hall, 1976A

Roy C: Comment. Nurs Outlook 24:690–91, 1976B

Roy C: Problem in self-ideal and expectancy: Powerlessness. In Roy C, (ed) Introduction to Nursing: An Adaptation Model. Englewood Cliffs, N.J., Prentice-Hall, 1976C

Roy C: The Roy adaptation model. In Riehl JP, Roy C (eds), Conceptual Models for Nursing Practice, 2nd ed. New York, Appleton–Century–Crofts, 1980

Roy C, Obloy M: The practitioner movement: Toward a science of nursing. Am J Nurs 78:1698–1702, 1978

Schmitz M: The Roy adaptation model: Application in a community setting. In Riehl JP, Roy C (eds), Conceptual Models for Nursing Practice, 2nd ed. New York, Appleton–Century–Crofts, 1980

Schofield A: Problems of role function. In Roy C (ed), Introduction to Nursing: An Adaptation Model. Englewood Cliffs, N.J., Prentice-Hall, 1976

Starr SL: Adaptation applied to the dying client. In Riehl JP, Roy C (eds), Conceptual Models for Nursing Practice, 2nd ed. New York, Appleton–Century–Crofts, 1980

Wagner P: Testing the adaptation model in practice. Nurs Outlook 24:682–85, 1976

CHAPTER 6

Identifying the Nursing Needs of the Postpartum Cesarean Mother

Carole Fitzgerald Kehoe

OVERVIEW OF THE STUDY

Assessment of cesarean clients is central to the development of relevant and appropriate plans of nursing care. The conceptual models available today offer nurses a systematic and rational approach to assessing clients within the clinical setting, as well as providing guidelines for nursing research.

This chapter describes a study in which a conceptual nursing model was used in a clinical setting to gather assessment data and to guide the subsequent data analysis. The study was designed to identify the nursing needs of postpartum mothers who had unexpected cesarean births.

The Roy Adaptation Model was the conceptual nursing model chosen for this exploratory study. The literature suggests that issues of physiological restoration, self-concept, role function, and interdependence are relevant considerations in the nursing care of cesarean mothers (Bampton and Mancini 1973; Cassidy 1974; Cohen 1977; Reynolds 1977; Donovan 1977; Affonso and Stichler 1978; Marut 1978). These factors interrelate as the cesarean mother progresses toward the ultimate goal of pregnancy—attainment of the maternal role (Rubin 1967).

It was assumed that the nursing needs of postpartum cesarean mothers would reflect the mothers' perceptions of and reactions to their unplanned cesarean births. The social–psychological perspective of symbolic interactionism, with its focus on individual perceptions of reality, the self, and the concept of "the definition of the situation," is theoretically relevant to this study (see Chapter 2).

This project had its inception before there were any nursing studies available which used cesarean clients as study subjects. Although the cesarean birth rate has climbed steadily in the last two decades, a "cultural lag" has existed between recognition of this reality in maternity nursing and efforts by nurse-researchers to obtain scientific data about this nursing phenomenon. Thus there has been a gap in the knowledge base that nurses have been using as a basis for their interventions with cesarean clients. This study was developed as an attempt to bridge that knowledge gap.

The study also provided my graduate students in maternity nursing an opportunity to actively participate in research and to learn how a conceptual nursing model is used in the clinical practice setting. Furthermore, the study also "modeled" for them the way in which an empirical investigation can be conducted without special funding by taking a conceptual nursing model available in the literature, and using it as the organizing framework to investigate a substantive problem in maternity nursing.

METHODOLOGY

The data were obtained through the use of unstructured interviews with 11 cesarean mothers who had had unexpected cesarean deliveries. These interviews, conducted by graduate students in maternity nursing, occurred during the clients' first 5 postpartum days in a large metropolitan hospital. Selection of study subjects was based on two criteria: first, the mother had to have expected an uncomplicated vaginal delivery when she was admitted to the labor and delivery suite, and second, the mother's postpartum recovery had to have been proceeding within the expected range of normality, so that she was able to communicate and participate in a discussion of her experience.

Each mother was informed of the reason for the interview, and the confidentiality of her responses was assured. All the mothers approached participated willingly.

Since the sample size was small, generalized extrapolation of the results to other cesarean populations is neither meaningful nor appropriate from a methodological perspective. However, one of the reasons for choosing an exploratory design was to provide information to guide the formulation of more precise research questions which could become the basis for subsequent investigations (Selltiz et al. 1976, pp. 90-92).

The data were reviewed for the purpose of identifying common and recurring themes. The focus was on the qualitative nature of the clients' responses, and not on the frequency with which certain behaviors occurred. This approach to data analysis is consistent with the literature related to exploratory research and the guidelines for research conducted from the symbolic interactionism perspective (Lauer and Handel 1977). On the basis of the themes identified, the data were organized according to the categories suggested by Roy (1976) in the four adaptive modes (see Chapter 5).

In the following narrative sections, the data are presented to highlight the major adaptive and maladaptive behaviors assessed within each mode. More attention is given to verbal and nonverbal indications of maladaptive behaviors because they comprise the basis for the nursing interventions suggested. This emphasis in no way suggests that the nurse's responsibility in reinforcing adaptive behavior is any less important, however.

In this chapter the cesarean mother is considered exclusively because the needs of other family members are discussed elsewhere in this book. When the nursing needs of this key family member are addressed appropriately, the needs of significant others with whom she interacts are also dealt with indirectly.

PRESENTATION OF THE DATA

The Physiological Mode

The mothers in this sample were preoccupied with stressors related to the surgical intervention necessary to accomplish a cesarean delivery. Incisional pain and the pain resulting from intestinal gas were stressors with which all the mothers had to cope during the first 2 or 3 postdelivery days. The need for pain relief predominated, and the mothers displayed appropriate adaptive behaviors by requesting analgesics to ease their discomfort.

Several mothers expressed dismay over the intensity of the discomfort they were experiencing. One mother said, "I never expected to hurt so much!" Another commented, "It even hurts to turn over in bed or reach for something from my table." Another mother summed it up by saying, "I feel as if I have been run over by a truck!"

On the basis of what she has heard or read, every pregnant mother expects that childbirth will entail a certain degree of discomfort and pain. The current popularity of childbirth education classes among expectant parents partially reflects a desire to acquire information about the process of labor and delivery which will help them to cope with the expected physiological stresses. When an unplanned cesarean delivery is necessary, however, the postpartum mother is faced with handling an event for which she has minimal preparation and thus limited resources with which to cope. It is not unusual, therefore, that her perception of pain may be heightened by the unexpected nature and emotional stress of the delivery experience (Jacox 1977, p. 74).

The cesarean mother looks to the nurse for comfort measures and reassurance that the pain she is experiencing is within normal limits and that her discomfort will decrease as she progresses through the postpartum period. Nursing measures include administration of analgesics, application of heat to the abdomen to encourage expulsion of gas, and encouragement of ambulation, when appropriate, to stimulate peristalsis (Clark and Affonso 1979).

Another stressor related to the incisional pain was fear of wound dehiscence. This stressor led to maladaptive behaviors, including avoidance of deep breathing and coughing and a tendency to remain inactive to prevent straining the suture line. These behaviors were identified as maladaptive because they consumed so much psychological energy that the mother had only minimal energy left for other restorative behaviors.

The following comments reflect concerns about dehiscence:

"Can I really get up to take a shower? My incision might pop open."

"How long before I heal? I don't want these stitches to break."

"I must be careful not to put the baby on top of my stitches."

The frequent expressions of concern about wound dehiscence suggests that the cesarean mothers in this sample lacked basic information about the healing process of the body.

The assumption that inactivity was one means to promote wound healing has serious implications. It is a well documented fact that postoperative inactivity can lead to such complications as static pneumonia, thrombophlebitis, and delayed return of intestinal peristalsis (Kinnick 1977, p. 758). It is therefore important for the nurse to provide the cesarean mother with information about the healing process and the consequences of inactivity. Encouragement of appropriate levels of activity will augment the health teaching the nurse provides (Kinnick 1977, p. 759).

It was evident that the mothers in this sample needed basic information about their nutritional needs, as well. Some of the mothers interviewed were apathetic about eating and drinking after intravenous fluids were discontinued. Here again, the need identified was an informational one. Mothers who have had cesarean deliveries should be advised that calories, proteins, and fluids are necessary for the regeneration of body tissue and for healing to take place (Bradford 1977, p. 346).

Another stressor related to the surgical nature of the cesarean delivery concerned elimination. Bowel manipulation during surgery and the presence of an in-dwelling catheter interrupted the mother's usual patterns of elimination. The catheter restricts physical mobility and is probably psychologically intrusive as well. In assessing the mother's activity level, the presence of the catheter could be considered either a focal or a residual stimuli.

Expulsion of gas was a problem for several mothers. Lack of privacy (because of the presence of a roommate) and hemorrhoids interfered with adaptive behaviors related to gas expulsion. Here again, the fear of wound dehiscence played a part in the maladaptive behavior of hesitancy to bear down to rid the lower portion of the large intestine of the gas.

In this situation the teaching role of the nurse again assumes primacy. The nurse can reinforce information about the healing process and offer reassurance that the sutures will not break from abdominal pressure. Moreover, she can teach the mother how to "splint" the incision with her hands, a rolled towel, or a small pillow. This teaching may bear dividends in terms of helping the mother to help herself, thereby enhancing her ability to regain control over her bodily functions.

In teaching the mother about the healing processes, it must be remembered that she is striving to cope with the multiple stressors associated with a surgical delivery. The boundaries of her body have been breached by the intrusion of a catheter and intravenous tubing. The appearance of her body has been permanently altered by the presence of an incision that will leave a scar. Added to these stressors is her disappointment over having lost the type of delivery that she had anticipated. These factors necessitate the mobilization of tremendous amounts of psychological energy in order to cope at even a marginal level. As a result, she has minimal psychological energy left for dealing with other environmental inputs. Thus she limits these inputs to those things that she can handle with the least expenditure of energy, and she perceives on a very selective basis (Mercer 1977, p. 34).

This suggests that the initial postdelivery period is not the ideal time to initiate health teaching. Yet nurses need to provide the mother with factual information about recovering from a surgical delivery so that she can be a cooperative and active participant in her own recovery process.

There are some traditional approaches that nurses have used successfully to carry out health teaching. These include dosing the mother with small amounts of information over an extended time period and using varied methods of repetition to reinforce the learning process. These approaches all have merit and are applicable to cesarean clients. Their success is measured by evaluating the mother's behaviors. If the behavior remains static, then this is a clue to the nurse that the teaching goal has not been reached, and she may either repeat the teaching process or initiate alternative strategies until behavioral change becomes evident.

The behaviors identified in the physiological mode of the Roy Model may have consequences for adaptive or maladaptive behaviors in the other three modes, which focus on the psychosocial aspects of the cesarean experience. If the mother's needs are assessed accurately in this mode and appropriate interventions are designed and implemented, promotion of adaptive responses in the other modes may be augmented.

The Self-Concept Mode

The self-concept is a mental construct that is inferred from verbal and non-verbal responses. It cannot be directly observed by the nurse. The data suggest that cesarean birth threatens a woman's self-concept and feelings of self-worth. This is consistent with the observations made by others on the relationship between bodily functioning and a cesarean mother's self-image (Mercer 1977; Marut 1978; Affonso and Stichler 1980).

In this study, self-concept problems centered around issues related to the physical self (ability to function and to control that functioning), the moral-ethical self (self-perceptions of good or bad), self-consistency (constancy between who one is today and who one is tomorrow), self-ideal and self-expectancy (what one is and what one would like to be), and self-esteem (the value one holds of oneself) (see Chapter 5).

The Physical Self (Problems of Loss)—Mothers in this sample shared very openly the aspects of the childbearing experience which they perceived as being lost to them. The loss of a "normal" delivery was a predominating theme. Not only was the vaginal delivery experience lost to these mothers, but they also lost the self-image of being normal females. Comments such as these reflected this loss:

> "I'm the odd one in my group now. All the others had natural deliveries."

> "My sister had a normal delivery. *Why not me?*"

> "Maybe if I put some lipstick on I'll at least *look* normal."

For couples who have anticipated a participatory, natural childbirth experience, the exclusion of the father from the cesarean delivery presented another loss: the loss of being together to welcome their baby into the world. Some of the comments, spoken while weeping were:

> "My husband wasn't with me. I was all alone."

> "My husband couldn't coach me as we had hoped and planned."

As if to offset a delivery in which they perceived themselves as physiological failures, several mothers were determined to experience functional success through breast-feeding. The need for success in their functional capacity as breast-feeders is suggested by the following comments:

> "At least something is right if I'm able to breast-feed."

> "If I had to choose between the delivery and breast-feeding going right, I'd choose breast-feeding!"

> "I tried to breast-feed her this morning, but I just couldn't do it right." [sob]

Another incident reflected determination to regain control over body function. In this case the mother had unrealistic perceptions of her physical capacities and exhausted herself to the point of tears by trying to take care of her baby in excess of her strength on the second postpartum day. Her anguish over what she perceived as another functional capacity loss led to these self-recriminatory comments:

> *"I can't ever do anything right. I*
> *tried to take care of my baby and I*
> *can't even lift her up. I'm so ex-*
> *hausted. I wanted so badly to be a*
> *good mother. I had planned to feel*
> *really good so that I could take*
> *good care of my baby, and I just*
> *can't do it." [sob, sob.]*

Supportive nursing interventions for the postpartum mother who is experiencing loss because of the cesarean delivery begins with the nurse's self-appraisal of her own feelings about cesarean childbirth. If the nurse perceives the cesarean birth as reflecting abnormal functioning and thus as a loss, she may not be able to provide the systematic support needed to establish a relationship of trust and unconditional positive regard with her client. An understanding and supportive nurse can do much to assure a mother that she is perceived positively. This will encourage the mother to share her feelings of loss and express her grief openly (Mercer 1977).

However, not all women want or are able to verbalize their feelings of loss. In these situations, supportive nursing intervention includes staying with the silent mother, providing privacy for her, and demonstrating respect for her right to be silent by just being there. Regardless of the way in which this mother expresses her feelings, the nurse can be accepting of her behavior and individuality in dealing with her loss and grief. The concept of loss in cesarean mothers has been dealt with in detail in Chapter 9.

The Moral-Ethical Self (Problems Reflecting Guilt)—The mothers in this sample demonstrated feelings of guilt by a variety of overt and covert behaviors. Behaviors which often indicate guilt include insomnia unrelated to physical discomfort, statements about inability to carry out appropriate mothering behaviors, loss of appetite, and any signs of depression, such as crying and/or withdrawal (Perley 1976, pp. 204-205).

The following comments suggest concern that the cesarean delivery may have jeopardized the infant's well-being:

"I'm worried about the baby. Since an emergency cesarean was done, the baby must not *really* be O.K."

"I had to have an amniocentesis several months ago. I hope that didn't hurt him [the baby] too."

"I have to take *really good* care of my baby now, especially after having a cesarean."

The nurse's words of reassurance about the infant's well-being can soothe the mother who feels guilty about the delivery and uncertain about her baby's health. The mother may have limited knowledge of the procedural aspects of cesarean birth and may believe that damage to the infant is one of the outcomes. The nurse should therefore explore the level of the mother's knowledge about this procedure and correct any misinformation (Mercer 1977).

Here again, the encouragement of the nurse can help the mother to share her concerns. An ongoing relationship with a nurse whom she has grown to trust will assist this client in expressing her feelings about the birth.

Self-Consistency, Self-Ideal and Expectancy, and Self-Esteem (Problems Reflecting Anxiety, Powerlessness, and Worthlessness)—In reviewing the data, it was unclear whether the behaviors indicating problems in these areas, could be separately identified. Therefore, the behaviors in these subcategories are combined for presentation.

Anxiety took many forms in the mothers in this sample. Identified concerns centered around physiological function and the body's restorative process. There was also much variability in the mothers' emotions; mothers seemed to have difficulty with simple decision-making and with maintaining an appropriate attention span.

Feelings of powerlessness were suggested by the need to fill in the "missing pieces" of the delivery experience. One mother said, "Is this really my baby? I didn't see her when she was born." Another asked, "What was my baby like when he was born? Were you there?"

Other indicators of powerlessness could be seen in reluctance to participate in decision-making in the care of the baby. One mother asked the nurse to take her baby back to the nursery because she simply didn't have the energy to cope with a crying infant and wasn't able to make him stop crying.

Nursing intervention can be directed toward restoring the mother's feelings of control and power. Factual information about the delivery and the baby help the mother to perceive the birth at a reality level and put the "missing pieces" together (Affonso 1977).

The cesarean mother's lowered self-esteem was suggested by self-depreciating comments about inability to accomplish expected goals in childbirth. Concern was also voiced over the husband's acceptance of the abdominal scar and whether this would affect subsequent sexual performance (see Chapter 10). Many of the previous comments about perceived lack of normality are also suggestive of an image of devalued self-worth.

When a mother's self-concept is shaken, she is particularly vulnerable to the slightest hint that she is less than perfect. She is acutely sensitive to the manner and frequency of others' interactions with her. If the nurse is hurried when she attends to this mother's physical care needs, the mother may perceive her hurry as an indication that the nurse shares the mother's low opinion of her body. This will add to her self-perceived worthlessness (Mercer 1977).

Interaction with a sensitive and caring nurse can help to restore the cesarean mother's feeling of self-worth. The nurse should praise mothering behaviors and focus on the mother's strengths and accomplishments in infant care. Reinforcement and positive feedback from the nurse can be an important first step toward restoring feelings of self-worth and pride.

The Role Function Mode

Before the study began it was assumed that the needs identified in this mode would reflect problems primarily in the area of maternal role function because of the physiological limitations which would interfere with maternal role performance. However, review of the data suggests that postpartum cesarean mothers encountered greater difficulty with the role of being a cesarean-delivered client.

The finding that maladaptive role function behaviors occur in both the maternal role and the cesarean role suggested the approach to the presentation of the data. Therefore, within each of the subcategories in this mode, distinctions are made (where appropriate) between maternal role behaviors and cesarean role behaviors.

Role Mastery

Maternal Role Mastery—Concerns about mastering the maternal role revolved around distress over bodily dysfunction. These concerns were reflected in comments about breast-feeding:

"My sister breast-fed her baby just fine. I just can't seem to do it."

"You'd think that I could at least hold my own baby. I can't even do that. I was so scared that I had to call the nurse." [sob]

These comments suggest that the mothers understood the various facets of mothering behavior. The problems and subsequent frustration of such mothers occur when they see themselves as unable to perform these mothering tasks effectively. The underlying concern may be that if they are unsuccessful with these early mothering tasks, then how can they hope for success with more complex mothering behaviors? This is a valid concern, because role learning involves moving from simple tasks which require a minimal number of new behaviors to the mastery of complex tasks involving more sophisticated and complex behaviors.

Another important aspect of maternal role mastery is the process of role learning through the observation of role models (Rubin 1967; Swendsen et al.

1978). One of the processes that a woman goes through psychologically during the antepartal period as she moves toward attainment of the maternal role is identified as "introjection-projection-rejection."

A pregnant woman will "try on" the mothering behavior of a person whom she selects as a role model in order to see whether the behavior is acceptable to her and "fits" her style. If the behavior "fits," she will accept it; if it doesn't, she will reject it and continue to search for a role model whose mothering behavior is acceptable.

Postpartum cesarean mothers in this study voiced concern over not having had role models of maternal behavior who had also had cesarean deliveries. Perhaps they believed that mastery of the maternal role is different when a mother is recovering from a cesarean delivery. These comments suggest this concern:

"I don't have any friends who have had cesareans. How will I know what to do?"

"My sister didn't have a cesarean, and I'm not sure what to do."

"I don't know how I'll manage now that I've had a cesarean. Maybe my husband can help me figure out what to do."

The cesarean mother who has not had the advantage of knowing other cesarean mothers who could serve as role models for maternal role mastery will turn to the nurse for reassurance that she is successfully achieving her new role. Nursing intervention designed to assist in mastery of the maternal role begins immediately after delivery, as the nurse provides physical care and nurturing emotional support for the new postpartum cesarean client (the client's needs for physical restoration and the suggested nursing interventions have been discussed in the section on physiological mode). If the mother's physiological needs are met satisfactorily she will feel better and will have the ego strength to extend herself to caring for her infant (Mercer 1977, Ruben 1961). She will be motivated to learn about her infant's needs and the approaches that she can use to meet these needs.

Learning theory suggests that deriving satisfaction from the learning experience is basic to being motivated to attempt other learning activities (Redman 1976, p. 90). Therefore, the nurse should begin with a task from which the mother can derive a great deal of personal pleasure. Success in feeding her baby is an example of one of these tasks.

After mastering feeding, teaching can progress to other activities, always moving from the simple to the more complex mothering behaviors. Positive feedback from the nurse is essential during the early stages of acquiring a new skill, since learners have difficulty judging the adequacy of their own performances. Feedback enhances their proficiency because it gives the learners cues to guide the performance of a new skill (Redman 1976, p. 98).

At all times, each client's individual progress should dictate the pace of the nurse's teaching. The goals are to present new information to help the mother increase her repertoire of maternal role behaviors, yet to avoid presenting so much information at one time that the mother is not able to assimilate it. Providing time for return demonstrations should be built-in to the teaching sessions.

Cesarean Role Mastery—In our study, mastery of the cesarean role consumed a large portion of the postpartum mother's energy, both physically and emotionally. Some comments indicating determination to master this role were as follows:

> "I've got to do these exercises that the nurse showed me so I can get better fast."

> "It's important that I eat so I can get better fast."

> "I've got to get strong so that I can take care of my baby."

Concern about physiological restoration suggests a desire to recover so that the cesarean role and its inherent inconveniences can be discarded as soon as possible. The nurse can offer assistance by reassuring the mother that her discomforts will decrease and that her energy level will gradually increase. In effect, the nurse is thus telling the mother that the limitations of the cesarean role are temporary.

Role Distance—Individuals tend to maintain distance from roles that threaten self-esteem. In this subcategory, cesarean role distance was frequently observed in the postpartum cesarean mothers we studied. As noted above, the clients were eager to achieve the maternal role, but they wanted to keep as much distance as possible from the cesarean role. Therefore, the following discussion focuses upon the cesarean role exclusively.

Attempts to maintain distance from the cesarean role were observed in mothers who tried to prove that they had the functional ability to perform, even though the delivery made them feel weak and incapacitated in the first few postpartum days. For example, there was the mother who drove herself to exhaustion trying to prove that she could overcome the temporary disability imposed by the surgical delivery. This mother was mentioned in the section on the self-concept mode, and her maladaptive behavior seems to pertain to this mode, too. Other mothers tried to demonstrate functional capacity through breast-feeding. This, too, has already been discussed, and is mentioned here for emphasis.

This overlapping of behaviors in the self-concept and role function modes points out the fact that self-concept and role performance are intrinsically linked in a reciprocal fashion. In other words, the self-concept influences role performance, and the adequacy of one's role performance influences one's feelings of self-worth (Fitts et al. 1971).

Role Conflict—A person is thought to be in a situation of role conflict when she perceives the cues for guiding her role performance as ambiguous or conflicting. As a result she tries to avoid performing the role because she is unsure of what to do.

Conflict about the cesarean role was observed in mothers who seemed genuinely confused about how to perform this unexpected role. Some cesarean mothers simply did not know what they could do physically. Others were in conflict because they were unsure of what the nursing staff would allow them to do. It was very evident that they perceived cues for guiding performance of the cesarean role as being either ambiguous or altogether absent. These comments should be considered:

"Is it alright for me to get out of bed this *soon!*"

"I'm so weak. Is it still alright to try to breast-feed?"

The nurse has the opportunity and the responsibility to provide supportive intervention for postpartum cesarean mothers, helping them to cope with a role that they perceive as unacceptable and wish to avoid. The nurse's proximity to the mother enables her to establish a trust relationship which will encourage the mother to verbalize her perceptions and feelings about the cesarean role. The opportunity to talk to a caring, empathetic nurse whom she trusts can ease the mother's psychological discomfort with a role that threatens her sense of self.

Role Failure—Role failure is an inconsistency between role expectations and actual performance. In this study, mothers who had had unplanned cesarean deliveries felt a sense of failure about their role performance that was pervasive and devastating. Comments about being "abnormal" or "odd" suggested the despair they felt. The mothers' perception of failure could not be attributed to their lack of knowledge or desire to perform the childbearing role. They were caught in a situation over which they had no control, and this fact undoubtedly contributed considerably to feelings of helplessness.

In an effort to cope with perceptions of role failure, some mothers showed an urgency to assume care for their babies, as reflected in this comment: "I should be the one to be taking care of my baby. Instead the nursery nurses are." Another mother repeatedly demonstrated her proficiency in caring for her baby to her husband. His enthusiasm and approval of her efforts were very important to her.

Some mothers seem so consumed with a sense of failure that they cannot perceive anything positive about themselves. The nurse's emphasis of the mother's strengths and capabilities can promote a more realistic and more positive self-appraisal. The need for giving the mother a great deal of positive reinforcement is central to nursing care. The negative impact of the cesarean experience can be modified by nursing care which gives the mother a feeling that she is cared *about* as well as being cared *for*.

The Interdependence Mode

Interdependence is a concept embracing the notions of dependent and independent behavior. Theoretically, the term *interdependence* refers to the balance that an individual maintains between his dependent and independent relationships with others (McIntier 1976).

In assessing behaviors within this mode, the maternity nurse may use guidelines suggested by the "taking-in" and "taking-hold" phases of the postpartum period (Rubin 1961). These phases can suggest empirical referents of dependent and independent behaviors.

The taking-in phase of the puerperium has a specific beginning—the delivery—and a nonspecific end-point—approximately the third postpartum day. During this time period, the mother focuses upon her own needs for physical and psychological nurturance and care. Her behavior is passive and dependent. She waits for the actions of others, rather than taking the initiative herself. The mother's primary need is to receive rather than to give to others.

On approximately the third day postpartum, the mother begins the transition into the taking-hold phase. Her behavior gradually changes from the passiveness of the immediate postdelivery period. She begins to assert her independence as an initiator and producer of actions. At this point she directs her energy toward someone other than herself—her baby. She reorients her priorities and becomes committed to the immediate present and future, rather than being primarily preoccupied with herself and the past. In this phase, the mother assumes an active role in the care of her new child, within the limits of her physiological recovery from the actual birth.

Knowledge of the taking-in and taking-hold phases served two useful purposes in this study. It guided development of definitions of dependent and independent behavior specific to the postpartum cesarean client, and it helped to verify the assessment of dependent and independent behavior for categorization of the data.

The following theoretical definitions of adaptive and maladaptive behaviors were developed for this study:

Adaptive dependent behavior: Dependent behavior observed from delivery through approximately the third postpartum day.

Adaptive independent behavior: Independent behavior observed from approximately the third postpartum day onward.

Maladaptive dependent behavior: Dependent behavior observed from approximately the third postpartum day onward.

Maladaptive independent behavior: Independent behavior observed from delivery through approximately the third postpartum day.

The time dimension for dependent and independent behavior in postpartum cesarean clients is flexible. The less than ideal delivery circumstances of women who have unplanned cesarean deliveries may extend the taking-in phase and the resulting dependent behavior responses (Mevs 1977). Therefore, the qualifying term "approximately" should be kept in mind when assessing these behaviors as adaptive or maladaptive.

The data are presented in the following subcategories (McIntier 1976, pp. 297-300):

Dependent behavior: Help seeking, attention seeking, and affection seeking.

Independent behavior: Initiative-taking and obstacle mastery.

Dependent Behavior

Help Seeking—Theoretically, the purpose of help-seeking behavior is to seek the assistance of another person in reaching a goal or objective. This type of behavior includes both physical and psychological elements on the empirical level (pp. 297-98).

The majority of the cesarean mothers in our study displayed adaptive behaviors with respect to help seeking. These adaptive behaviors involved asking for assistance when beginning activities requiring new skills, especially baby care, and initiating self-care by the third postpartum day. The latter behavior suggested the beginning of the "taking hold" phase.

A response that was considered to be maladaptive was seen in a mother who spoke bitterly and frequently about her dependency needs, which were heightened because of the delivery circumstances. She repeatedly exclaimed, "I can't stand being a patient!" This was her very first hospitalization. Apparently she had gone to considerable trouble to make sure that she would be able to function independently after her baby's birth. She had planned for an unmedicated delivery and had faithfully attended childbirth education classes. The cesarean delivery, performed with general anesthesia, had necessitated a marked revision in these goals and inevitably in her perceptions of the entire experience. These revisions contributed to this mother's anguish over the amount of help that she required in order to cope with the physical limitations imposed by the cesarean delivery.

Another example of maladaptive help seeking was observed in a mother who repeatedly asked for and expected assistance from the nurse each time her baby was brought out to her. She stated with obvious frustration, "I keep calling for the nurse, but she is so slow in coming!" This client was in her fourth postpartum day and had received a great deal of help and support from the nursing staff prior to this day.

This mother revealed that she had a very close and dependent relationship with her own mother, who lived in another state. This client's repeated requests for help suggest a coping style that included the need for validation and praise from a "mother figure." The nurse was the person whom this particular client looked to as a substitute for her own mother, who lived too far away to visit her in the hospital.

Interventions for a very dependent mother should include much reassurance and verbal praise to reinforce independent behavior (pp. 319-20). Movement toward independent decision making can be encouraged by telling the mother the options that are available to her in self-care and infant care and allowing her to choose. Involvement with other cesarean clients (possible role models) on the maternity unit who are appropriately independent may encourage the mother to function more independently (Swendsen 1978).

Attention Seeking—Attention-seeking behavior reflects a need to be noticed by others. A client may display this behavior by requesting extra services or engaging in behavior that focuses attention upon herself (McIntier 1976, p. 298). Crying is an effective strategy for meeting this need. Mothers in our study frequently wept when their husbands visited. One mother repeatedly telephoned her husband and dissolved into tears while talking to him.

The nursing goal is to make the attention-seeking mother feel that she is a valued person in the nurse's eyes by showing her that she is "cared for" and "cared about." This type of positive reinforcement demonstrates approval rather than hostility toward her and increases her ego strength. If the mother perceives herself more favorably, then her need for attention may diminish, and her inappropriate means of eliciting attention may also cease (Mercer 1977, p. 91).

Affection Seeking—This behavior reflects the need to establish in-depth interaction with another and also the need to be responded to by others. Involved here is the need for actual physical contact and proximity, recognition, praise, and approval (McIntier 1976, p. 298).

Postpartum cesarean mothers in our study showed evidence of being concerned about expressions of affection from spouses and their own mothers. The women made recurrent comments showing a constant desire for their husbands' presence and attention, as well as a need to talk to their own mothers.

The mother who has anticipated a vaginal delivery may be overwhelmed by the stress imposed by catheters, intravenous tubing, a painful incision, a feeling of extreme fatigue, and disappointment in herself as a childbearer. Prior coping styles for handling stress may seem ineffective in meeting the demands of this unexpectedly hostile environment. Expressions of reassurance from those in her life with whom she has affectional bonds are particularly important to the mother, who may be questioning her capabilities in many behavioral domains.

In caring for the cesarean client who is seeking affection, the nurse should focus on establishing an empathetic relationship with the client, so that she is assured of support on all fronts—in the hospital as well as from her family at home. Spending time with this mother and being organized and unhurried when providing physical care also show the nurse's regard for the mother as an individual (Mercer 1977, p. 91).

A consideration of the needs of new parents as couples is another way of meeting the affection needs of postpartum cesarean clients. The mother needs time alone with her spouse to talk and share perceptions of the delivery experience, of their new baby, and of their future life together. Because of the unexpected nature of the delivery, cesarean couples may need more time than other couples to work through disappointments and unfulfilled expectations. Their need for privacy in order to accomplish this important psychological work should be acknowledged and provided for by the staff. Some hospitals, for example, have a "meal for two" available for the couple, consisting of steak with all the trimmings and a bottle of wine.

This type of special service for new parents reflects recognition of their ongoing relationship as husband-and-wife by providing an environment in which they can celebrate the birth of their child and renew ties of affection that they share with each other.

Independent Behavior

Initiative Taking—This type of independent behavior reflects a desire to engage in activities on one's own, without the stimulus for that activity coming from someone else. The motivation for initiative taking is the need to regain control of one's life situation (McIntier 1976, p. 299).

The postpartum mothers in this study did indeed demonstrate a need to regain control of their life situations. As discussed in the section on the self-concept mode, their concern about being successful in breast-feeding suggested this need and the psychological importance that this particular activity had for them.

The mothers' urgency to regain a normal activity level so that they could engage in initiative-taking actions was suggested by these comments:

"I have to do everything right, so that I'll get my strength back."

"I don't want any more of that pain medication. It makes me feel so tired that I can't do anything."

The latter comment could be assessed as maladaptive initiative taking because this particular mother was in her second postpartum day, when she would be expected to need some pain relief. In this kind of situation, the nurse can emphasize the normality of the mother's pain and point out that the relaxation brought on by the medication is an important part of the recovery process (Mercer 1977, p. 91). This information helps the mother to reorganize her priorities so that they are consistent with the reality of recovering from a cesarean delivery.

Another example of maladaptive behavior was seen in the mother who panicked and cried uncontrollably because her baby had soiled the diaper. In tears, she explained her behavior with the following words: "No one was here to help me. The baby was screaming because she needed to be changed. I just couldn't seem to figure out what to do first or how to stop her from crying. I'm so embarrassed." [sob]

This mother had been caring for her baby for 2 days and was in the evening of her fourth postpartum day. She seemed torn between her desire to care for her baby independently and her need for additional guidance, which surfaced during this moment of stress.

Maladaptive initiative-taking behavior was observed in a mother who, on her fifth postpartum day, insisted repeatedly that the nursing staff care completely for her and her baby. She said firmly, "I'm just too tired to take care of anyone." The nursing intervention appropriate for a client who refuses to engage in any self-care activity when she has been progressing within normal limits begins by exploring the reasons for this behavior. The mother may doubt her functional ability. Rather than trying an activity and failing, the safer alternative is to avoid attempting anything at all. Here again, providing the mother with information and encouragement about her functional ability may be an appropriate and beneficial nursing measure (Mercer 1977, pp. 92–93).

Obstacle Mastery—This behavior reflects a desire to complete a task by oneself through persistence and repeated effort.

The mothers in this study demonstrated many adaptive behaviors that reflected persistence and effort. Efforts to actively participate in the responsibility for their recovery from the cesarean delivery were considered to be examples of this. Behaviors mentioned in the section on the physiological mode are also applicable here. Some mothers seemed to be willing to do almost anything to overcome blockages to their recovery and subsequent functioning.

When mothers are reluctant to engage in activity which is in their best interest, it can be frustrating. However, a postpartum cesarean mother may not "hear" the nurse's advice because of emotional preoccupation with her feelings about the cesarean delivery. In addition, analgesics may interfere with the mother's comprehension of the nurse's words, and this necessitates repetition of advice by the nurse.

Behaviors in the interdependence mode underscored the struggle between the mother's need for nurturance and her need to independently mother her new baby. In a sense, all of the problems of physiological adaptation, diminished self-esteem, and distortions in role function behaviors blended together and were seen in the mother's interdependence struggle.

DISCUSSION

The data in this study support the impression that an unplanned cesarean birth has a profound and pervasive effect on a postpartum cesarean mother. This impression is consistent with the findings reported by other investigators (Affonso and Stichler 1978; Marut and Mercer 1979; Affonso and Stichler 1980).

The Roy Adaptation Model proved to be a rational and systematic approach to assessing a mother's responses following an unexpected cesarean birth. However, in the psychosocial domain, the constructs of self-concept, role function, and aspects of interdependent behavior are difficult to sort out and separate because of the conceptual overlap. The use of these modes would be greatly enhanced by further refinement so as to allow determination of the empirical referents of these constructs. Through this study, it was possible to identify client-specific categories from the Roy Adaptation Model which may be used by the nurse for assessing postpartum cesarean clients (Appendix A). Composite nursing care prototypes were also developed for each of the four adaptive modes on the basis of data from selected mothers (Appendix B).

Although the Roy Adaptation Model was chosen as the organizing framework for the study, this does not mean that other conceptual nursing models would not have been appropriate.

The adaptive and maladaptive behaviors described in this chapter are not absolute in any sense. There is too much variation in human behavior for any aspect of adaptation or expression of human needs to be viewed as final and complete. While range and intensity of specific needs of postpartum cesarean mothers undoubtedly vary, the general themes of adaptive and maladaptive behavior described in this study could probably be seen in similar samples elsewhere.

INTERPRETATION OF THE DATA:
THE DEVELOPMENTAL TASKS OF THE
POSTPARTUM CESAREAN MOTHER

In reviewing the data for purposes of analysis, one theme appeared consistently. This theme involved the mothers' intense preoccupation with self as they attempted to regroup their internal resources and cope with the stress

of the cesarean birth. These mothers were intensely concerned about themselves and the perceived functional incapacity of their bodies which resulted
in their cesarean deliveries.

I have observed similar behavior many times in other postpartum cesarean
mothers. Formerly, I explained the behavior in terms of an extended adjustment period, an elongated "taking-in" phase of the postpartum. However,
this explanation seems too obvious and I here propose an alternative.

The internalized focus of cesarean mothers and their pervasive concern over
their functioning ability suggest that a complex psychological process is in
progress. This intense psychological "work" seems to be an integral part of
the physical and psychological recovery from a cesarean birth. I suggest that
this activity is an expression of a series of developmental tasks unique to the
postpartum cesarean mother.

The concept of developmental tasks is a familiar one to maternity nurses.
Many authors have described the developmental tasks of families and pregnancy in detail (Colman and Colman 1971; Rubin 1970; Duvall 1977; Clark
and Affonso 1979). In general terms, developmental tasks are attempts to
satisfy perceived needs that arise at certain points in the life cycle of every
individual. Such needs occur during the transition from an old and familiar
role to a new role. Developmental tasks are akin to "growth responsibilities"
that must be achieved in order to progress successfully from one stage of
growth to the next (Duvall 1977, pp. 167-68).

These growth responsibilities contain both personal and cultural expectations. With each task in the life cycle, specific behaviors are expected to be
demonstrated as the new task is achieved. These behavioral expectations develop over time and become such an integral part of the self-structure that
developmental tasks are not perceived as chores or duties. The motivation to
achieve a particular task emerges from unconscious forces within the individual, as he responds and adapts to new life situations and prepares to assume
new roles and levels of functioning (Duvall 1977).

Theoretically, the developmental tasks of the postpartum cesarean mother
emerge from her internalized and culturally derived need to achieve or take
on the maternal role (Rubin 1967). So very strong is the need for maternal
role attainment, which begins antepartally, that the cesarean mother engages
in intense and unconscious psychological work directed at achieving this
ultimate goal. It is very likely that the mother's "work" is more difficult when
she is simultaneously dealing with the stress of an *unexpected* cesarean
delivery.

The process begins shortly after the cesarean birth, when the mother becomes fully aware of the delivery circumstances. This is a tiring and time-
consuming activity and may account for some of the exhaustion seen in
postpartum cesarean mothers that cannot be attributed to an exhausting labor
prior to the cesarean birth or to the residual effects of anesthesia and analgesia. The tasks occur in an evolving sequence, and the achievement of each

task described in necessary before movement toward achievement of the next one in the sequence can begin.

The developmental tasks proposed here are derived directly from the data in this study, in terms of both the specific task and the sequence suggested. Therefore this discussion is hypothetical, since there has been no effort as yet to validate this proposal. Until the developmental tasks have been tested empirically, they are only speculations about the nature of reality, and are not assumed to be valid constructs by this author.

Developmental Task 1:
The Need for Physiological Restoration

An unplanned cesarean delivery impacts on a mother physiologically in terms of functional incapacity from the absence of peristalsis, the presence of a catheter, the inability to digest solid food, incisional pain, and immobility imposed by the intravenous tubing and urinary catheter.

The first task of the postpartum cesarean mother is to regain normal physiological functioning so that she can actively participate in the care of her baby. Mothering is an active and time-consuming mode of behavior. For that reason, physical incapacity and mothering do not often occur simultaneously and are viewed as mutually exclusive variables. Thus the cesarean mother cannot achieve the maternal role unless the physiological recovery needs are achieved first.

The nurse can facilitate achievement of the first developmental task through the interventions suggested in the section of the physiologic mode. The support of the nurse supplements the mother's own strengths and bolsters her efforts to move into and achieve her first task.

Developmental Task 2:
Regaining a Positive Self-concept

As the mother's functional capabilities return, she begins to feel in control of her body again and is ready to move into the psychosocial tasks. The first of these is the need to regain a positive self-concept.

The mother's self-concept is intertwined with her self-esteem and is, in turn, influenced by her role performance. If her role performance exceeds or at least meets prior expectations during the delivery, the mother will have a sense of heightened self-esteem. When a mother feels "good" about herself and confident about the adequacy of her role performance, she will perceive herself positively and have a positive self-concept as a childbearer.

However, the mother who has an unplanned cesarean delivery may not be pleased with her role performance, and she may not feel "good" about herself. The gap between her anticipated vaginal delivery and the reality of the cesarean delivery diminishes self-esteem and is perceived as a threat to her self-concept. When a mother does not perceive herself in positive terms, she may not have the energy to extend herself to another and to develop positive feelings toward that other. In other words, the mother does not have the ego expansion needed to incorporate her baby into her personal sphere of concern and caring and establish a warm, nurturing relationship with him.

The nurse contributes to the achievement of the second developmental task by helping the mother to regain her self-esteem. The nurse can review with the mother the positive aspects of her behavior during the delivery and emphasize her strengths. This intervention will be even more effective if the nurse has actually observed the birth. If not, another member of the health team who did attend the birth may be brought in to assist the mother in her review of the delivery experience. If the mother is able to reconstruct her role performance during delivery, the discrepancy between her expectations and actual performance may be narrowed. She may begin to feel better about herself in general as she deals with the reality of what actually happened (Affonso 1977; Marut 1978). Regaining feelings of self-worth and self-respect is fundamental to achieving the second developmental task.

Developmental Task 3:
Acceptance of the Cesarean Role

After the mother has begun to perceive herself in more positive terms, she is ready to move toward an acceptance of the fact that she is a cesarean-delivered client and not a vaginally-delivered, as she had anticipated. The data suggest that this is probably the most difficult task of all.

Planning for any new role includes a strategy known as "role rehearsal." In role rehearsal a person imagines or enacts experiences that may take place when he actually performs that role. By acting out the role mentally and having an internal dialogue, the person anticipates what he will say and do and how others will respond. This preliminary enactment or "worry work" enables the person to identify the various ways that he will deal with specific situations before they occur (Janis 1958; Swendsen et al. 1978).

A woman who anticipates a normal vaginal delivery will mentally rehearse the performance of that role many times during her pregnancy. Although role rehearsal does not rigidly structure role performance, this process does outline rather precisely in a mother's mind the dimensions of that role. When she begins labor, her mind-set is geared for the vaginal-delivery role performance that she has rehearsed mentally so many times during the preceding months. Because of the current popularity of childbirth education, the mental process of role rehearsal is augmented by the preparation for labor and delivery that couples practice during these classes.

The mothers in this study had difficulty accepting the reality of the cesarean role. This may have reflected prior preparation for a vaginal delivery.

These mothers also expended great amounts of psychological energy maintaining as much distance from the cesarean role as possible in the ear_y postpartum period, according to the data.

The attempts at cesarean role mastery, which were made by all mothers eventually, reflected the mothers' efforts to achieve the third developmental task. Apparently, once a mother has psychologically resigned herself to the reality of the cesarean birth, she is able to actively pursue achievement of this third task. There is probably a time-specific dimension to the mother's efforts, and this may be an individual factor. The data suggest that the role distance gap must be narrowed first, before role mastery attempts can be initiated. When behaviors reflecting an attempt to cope with and master the cesarean role are observed, one can assume that the mother is moving toward psychological acceptance of that role.

Nursing behaviors which support the cesarean client's efforts in achieving the third developmental task were discussed in the section on the role function mode and are applicable here. Empathetic emotional support and understanding appear to be key factors in helping the mother move toward acceptance of the cesarean role.

Until the mother can face the reality of the cesarean birth, it is unlikely that she will be able to achieve full functioning in the maternal role. So much energy will be consumed trying to resolve the conflict between "what might have been" and "what really is" that she will not have the emotional strength to establish a meaningful relationship with her baby. For this reason, achievement of the third developmental task appears to be crucial for attainment and enactment of the maternal role.

Developmental Task 4:
Integration of the Cesarean Birth
into the Mother's Life-Experiences

Acceptance of the reality of the cesarean role is an essential step for achievement of the fourth developmental task. The mother's ability to achieve this task reflects acceptance of the reality of the overall birth experience.

Achievement of the fourth task indicates that the mother's physiological functioning has been restored, her self-concept has been regained, the reality of the birth has been accepted, and the threat to self has been resolved. At this point, painful perceptions and unfulfilled expectations are finally laid to rest. The mother's self-structure has been reorganized and the birth experience has been successfully assimilated. As a result, she can mother her child without negative perceptions of the cesarean experience interfering in their relationship with each other.

The achievement of this fourth developmental task may not occur during the mother's hospitalized postpartum period. For that matter, the third developmental task may not be completely achieved before the mother's discharge, either. Because of the possible delay in achieving both these tasks while hospitalized, the presence of support systems within the family and the community are crucial when viewed in context of developmental tasks (see Chapter 11).

Before the mother's discharge, the nurse within the clinical setting can facilitate movement toward achievement of the fourth developmental task. To begin to examine threatening life experiences at the awareness level, a person first needs a nonthreatening environment. This environment consists of places and persons where feelings can be expressed without the self being threatened by another's reactions (Rogers 1977, pp. 128-29).

By giving the mother unconditional positive regard and empathetic understanding, the nurse can provide a therapeutic helping environment in which the mother can begin dealing with the cesarean experience by expressing her perceptions and feelings. Many of the nursing interventions discussed previously can help the mother to integrate the cesarean birth into her self-structure and make it part of her life experiences.

Perhaps a cesarean mother would find it easier to integrate her birth experience if other couples and society in general viewed this experience as a normal, alternative birthing method (Affonso 1977). Without meaning to, health professionals at many levels may have contributed to the mother's perception that this is an unnatural, deviant mode of delivery and a threat to self. All those who interact with cesarean families have a responsibility to assist them in modifying their perceptions. This can be done by emphasizing that cesarean birth is simply another way to have a baby and has the potential for being as joyful and fulfilling as vaginal birth. If cesarean birth is viewed as abnormal, then it is very likely that the cesarean mother will be perceived as abnormal, too, both in her own eyes and in the eyes of others. Such a negative perception makes the achievement of the developmental tasks all the more difficult.

The series of developmental tasks proposed here are in an early stage of conceptualization. It should be pointed out that the four tasks presented have broad dimensions. Within major task categories there are usually subtasks that must be worked on before the broader task can be completely achieved (Duvall 1977). These subtasks could not be identified from the data in this study, however.

CONCLUSIONS

During the past decade, maternity care has changed dramatically in this country. Gone are the days when expectant parents approach labor and delivery as passive nonparticipants. Couples today prepare for birth by reading the lay literature and/or attending childbirth education classes. When they approach the delivery experience, many couples expect and want to actively participate in the birth of their children. They assume that they have this right—and indeed they do.

However, if an unexpected cesarean birth becomes necessary because of jeopardy to the maternal–infant dyad, expectant parents are often assigned separate and passive roles during the actual delivery. In some locales, hospital policies are such that the parents and their new infant may not be reunited for several hours. For many new families this is a shattering emotional experience, with the potential for psychological sequelae that last far beyond the actual birth.

The postpartum period offers parents the opportunity to gradually assume parental roles and prepare for the responsibilities inherent in those roles in a protective hospital setting. Ideally, a postpartum unit provides a physically and emotionally supportive environment where the mother may recover from the stresses of labor and delivery, where the parents may become acquainted with their new infant before assuming total responsibility for meeting his needs, and where a couple can share the joy and fulfillment derived from a childbearing experience consistent with their hopes, dreams, and expectations. Unfortunately, for many cesarean families this ideal postpartum experience never becomes a reality. All too often, the cesarean birth is perceived by new parents as an event to be "coped with" and forgotten, rather than an experience to be savored and remembered with joy.

Postpartum cesarean mothers have a unique set of nursing needs as a result of the physiological and psychological impact of this birthing experience. Traditional postpartum nursing approaches may not offer these mothers the extensive nurturing and supportive care that this study indicates they need.

The nurse has an opportunity to mitigate the impact of cesarean birth by providing care that is based on her awareness of each mother's own perceptions and definition of the cesarean experience. The nurse can observe verbal and nonverbal behavior and identify early signs of adaptation problems. She can hear voiced concerns and look for indications of potential difficulties in attaining and enacting the maternal role. The nurse, as teacher, caregiver, and role model, can assist the mother in assuming gradual responsibility for the infant and can encourage appropriate mothering behaviors.

Through the continuing use of the nursing process, the nurse assesses, plans, implements, and evaluates her nursing strategies. By this method, she constantly adjusts her intervention as the cesarean mother's needs in the physiological and psychosocial domains change, which they inevitably do. This postpartum nursing approach to the care of cesarean mothers recognizes differences, respects rights, and facilitates individualized adaptation to the cesarean experience.

ACKNOWLEDGMENTS

I want to thank the following individuals for contributing the data in this study: Maria Ahaghotu, Saundra Albrite, Linda Birdsong, Barbara DeLong, Judy Hogan, Mary Matthews, Cora Rodriguez, Gail Turley, Margaret Ugbor, Mercy Williams, and Anne Wilson. Special credit is due to Saundra Albrite and Linda Birdsong, whose efforts led to the development of the Assessment Guides for the Postpartum Cesarean Mother (Appendix A) and the Nursing Care Prototypes (Appendix B).

REFERENCES

Affonso DD: Missing pieces: A story of postpartum feelings. Birth Fam J 4 (4):159–64, 1977
Affonso DD, Stichler JF: Cesarean birth: Women's reactions. Am J Nurs 3:468–70, 1980
Affonso DD, Stichler JF: Exploratory study of women's reactions to having a cesarean birth. Birth Fam J 5 (2):88–94, 1978
Bampton BA, Mancini JA: The cesarean patient is a new mother too. J Obstet Gynecol Neonatal Nurs 2 (4):58–61, 1973
Bradford RLJ: Nutrition during pregnancy and the postpartum. In Clausen JP, Flook MH, Ford B (eds), Maternity Nursing Today, 2nd ed. New York, McGraw-Hill, 1977
Cassidy JE: A nurse looks at childbirth anxiety. J Obstet Gynecol Neonatal Nurs 3 (1):52–54, 1974
Clark A, Affonso DD: Childbearing: A Nursing Perspective, 2nd ed. Philadelphia, Davis, 1979
Cohen NW: Minimizing emotional sequelae of cesarean childbirth. Birth Fam J 4 (3):114–19, 1977
Colman AD, Colman LL: Pregnancy: The Psychological Experience. New York, Seabury, 1971
Donovan B: The Cesarean Birth Experience. Boston, Beacon, 1977
Duvall EM: Marriage and Family Development, 5th ed. Philadelphia, Lippincott, 1977
Fitts W, Adams J, Radford G, et al: The Self-concept and Self-actualization. Nashville, Dede Wallace Center, 1971
Jacox AK: Pain: A Source Book for Nurses and Other Health Professionals. Boston, Little, Brown, 1977
Janis I: Psychological Stress. New York, Wiley and Sons, 1958
Kinnick VG: Postpartum care of the high risk mother. In Clasen JP, Flook MH, Ford B (eds), Maternity Nursing Today, 2nd ed. New York, McGraw-Hill, 1977
Lauer RH, Handel WH: Social Psychology, the Theory and Application of Symbolic Interactionism. Boston, Houghton Mifflin, 1977
Marut JS: The special needs of the cesarean mother. Am J Maternal–Child Nurs 3 (4):202–206, 1978
Marut JS, Mercer RT: Comparison of primiparas' perceptions of vaginal and cesarean births. Nurs Res 28 (5):260–66, 1979

McIntier TM: Theory of interdependence. In Roy C (ed), Introduction to Nursing: An Adaptation Model. Englewood Cliffs, N.J. Prentice-Hall, 1976

Mercer RT: Nursing Care of Parents at Risk. Thorofare, N.J., Slack, 1977

Mevs L: The current status of cesarean section and today's maternity patient. J Obstet Gynecol Neonatal Nurs 6:44-7, 1977

Perley NZ: Problems of moral–ethical self: Guilt. In Roy C (ed), Introduction to Nursing: An Adaptation Model. Englewood Cliffs, N.J., Prentice-Hall, 1976

Redman BK: The Process of Patient Teaching in Nursing, 3rd ed. St. Louis, Mosby, 1976

Reynolds CB: Updating care of cesarean section patients. J Obstet Gynecol Neonatal Nurs 6 (4):48-51, 1977

Rogers CR: In Hansen JC, Stevic RR, Warner RW, Jr. (eds), Counseling: Theory and Process. Boston, Allyn and Bacon, 1977

Roy C: Introduction to Nursing: An Adaptation Model. Englewood Cliffs, NJ, Prentice-Hall, 1976

Rubin R: Attainment of the maternal role, Part I: Processes. Nurs Res 16 (3): 237–45, 1967

Rubin R: Cognitive style in pregnancy. Am J Nurs 3:502–508, 1970

Rubin R: Puerperal change. Nurs Outlook 9 (12):753–55, 1961

Selltiz C, Wrightsman LS, Cook SW: Research Methods in Social Relations, 3rd ed. New York, Holt, Rinehart, and Winston, 1976

Swendsen L, Meleis A, Jones D: Role supplementation for new parents: A role mastery plan. Am J Maternal Child Nurs 3 (2):84–91, 1978

APPENDIX A.
ASSESSMENT GUIDES FOR THE POSTPARTUM
CESAREAN MOTHER

PHYSIOLOGICAL MODE	
Client-Specific Assessment Categories	Assessment Data—Behaviors and Comments Related To:

A. Exercise and rest
  1. Sleep patterns
  2. Body alignment
  3. Leisure activity
  4. Oxygen and circulatory
    needs
  5. Exercise
	1. Sleep and rest patterns
	2. Physical activity
	3. Exercises
	4. Deep breathing and
	   coughing
	5. Body posture
	6. Fatigue or lethargy

B. Nutrition
  1. Fluid and electrolytes
  2. Food intake
	1. Intravenous feedings
	2. Lack of or decrease in
	   appetite
	3. Distribution of body fat;
	   weight
	4. Thirst

C. Body structure
  1. Age, weight, stature
  2. General appearance
	1. Comments regarding
	   changing body appearance
	   (weight, scarring, increased
	   breast size)
	2. Personal hygiene

D. Elimination
  1. Stools; flatus
  2. Urine
  3. Diaphoresis
  4. Nausea and vomiting
	1. Abdominal discomfort
	   (flatus, constipation)
	2. Stools
	3. Perspiration
	4. Nausea and vomiting
	5. Hemorrhoidal discomfort

E. Healing and Restorative
  Processes
  1. Wound healing
  2. Uterine involution
	1. Incisional drainage,
	   healing, odor, tenderness
	2. Lochia (color, amount, odor)

PHYSIOLOGICAL MODE (*Continued*)

Client-Specific Assessment Categories	Assessment Data—Behaviors and Comments Related To:
	3. Uterine fundus (height, consistency)
	4. Perineum (hematoma, bruising, sutures, edema)
F. Body Regulation	
1. Sensory	1. Body temperature; vital signs
2. Endocrine	2. Pain (wound, uterine, breast, abdominal)
	3. Sensory deprivation/overload
	4. Body warmth and relaxation
	5. Ventilation
	5. Bathing
	7. Lactation
	8. Breast engorgement, tenderness, warmth
	9. Environmental heat, light, noise, odors
	10. Perspiration; "hot flashes"
	11. Mood swings

SELF-CONCEPT MODE

Client-Specific Assessment Categories	Assessment Data—Behaviors and Comments Related To:
A. Physical self	
1. Loss and grief	1. Desire for normal delivery
2. General physical appearance	2. Concern over body functions
3. Restoration of bodily function	3. Loss of self-control
4. Sleep	4. Changes in body appearance
5. Appetite	5. Pain
	6. Healing ability
	7. Ability to lactate
	8. Activity level
	9. Elimination
B. Moral-ethical self	
1. Attitude toward self	1. Guilt and self-blame
2. Physiological components	2. Sleep

SELF-CONCEPT MODE (*Continued*)

Client-Specific Assessment Categories	Assessment Data—Behaviors and Comments Related To:
3. Utilization of defense mechanisms 4. Emotional status 5. Feelings of guilt	3. Depleted energy 4. Mood swings 5. Reality level 6. Sexual identity 7. Interpersonal patterns 8. Moods (depressed)

C. Self-consistency
  1. Physiological function
  2. Restorative processes
  3. Emotional level
  4. Utilization of defense mechanisms
	1. Bladder and bowel functions
	2. Fatigue
	3. Pain
	4. Lactation
	5. Sleep
	6. Eating pattern
	7. Activity level
	8. Return to normalcy
	9. Level of attention
	10. Reality testing
	11. Decision making
	12. Mood
	13. Sexual identity

D. Self-ideal and expectancy
  1. Role adaptation level
  2. Physical self
  3. Psychosocial self
	1. Problem solving
	2. Decision making
	3. Role expectation vs. role performance
	4. Energy level
	5. Body integrity
	6. Mood
	7. Utilization of defense mechanisms
	8. Anger
	9. Loss and grief

E. Self-esteem
  1. Emotional level
  2. Physiological component
	1. Loss and grief
	2. Mood
	3. Feeling too weak to make decisions
	4. Eating patterns
	5. Use of defense mechanisms
	6. Appearance

ROLE FUNCTION MODE

Client-Specific Assessment Categories	Assessment Data—Behaviors and Comments Related To:
A. Role mastery	
1. Young adult female role	1. Cultural expectations in young adult female role; relationships with family and friends
2. Mother role	2. Self-expectations regarding ideal delivery, breast feeding, postpartum experience; ideal vs. real mother.
3. Wife role	3. Husband's expectations; sexual behaviors, fears
B. Role distance	
1. Acknowledgement of roles	1. Being in a "patient" or "sick" role
2. Role performance vs. role expectation	2. Expected vs. actual role performance (as patient, mother, wife, etc.)
	3. Tasks of mothering
C. Role conflict	
1. Interrole conflict	1. Inability to balance duties as wife and mother and business or professional goals, etc.
2. Intrarole conflict	2. Inability to fulfill incompatible expectations from "significant others," health personnel, and self
D. Role failure	
1. Acknowledgement of role	1. Lack of interest in baby, husband, self
2. Performance of role	2. Inability or lack of desire to "mother" the baby
	3. Lack of meaningful communication with husband/family
	4. Profound depression; lack of appropriate affect

INTERDEPENDENCE MODE

Client-Specific Assessment Categories	Assessment Data—Behaviors and Comments Related To:

A. Help-seeking
  1. Self-help
  2. Utilization of support systems
	1. Mothering abilities
	2. Pain, pain relief
	3. Physical disability
	4. Fatigue
	5. Fear of handling baby
	6. Personal inadequacies

B. Attention seeking
  1. Dependency needs
  2. Real/perceived utilization of sources of attention
	1. Relationship with husband, family, staff
	2. Cesarean delivery; the baby
	3. Sociable/nonsociable behavior

C. Affection seeking
  1. Coping styles
  2. Support systems available and utilized
	1. Client's need for approval and love
	2. Fears of postpartum sexual activity
	3. Loss of shared birth experience with husband
	4. Relationship with family members

D. Initiative taking
  1. Physical self-care
  2. Mothering behaviors
  3. Restoration/strengthening of family life
	1. Inability to "do anything" for self or baby
	2. Dependency needs

E. Obstacle mastery
  1. Physical restoration
  2. Psychosocial stability/ability
	1. Inability to relate to baby
	2. Sense of failure due to cesarean delivery
	3. Breast-feeding difficulty

F. Defense mechanisms
  1. Coping styles
  2. Use of crying and laughter
  3. Frequency/appropriateness of use
	1. Crying
	2. Panic
	3. Blaming/guilt
	4. Delivery experience

APPENDIX B.
NURSING CARE PROTOTYPES BASED ON THE ROY ADAPTATION MODEL

PHYSIOLOGICAL MODE

Category	Behaviors	Adaptation Status*	Stimuli	
			Focal	Contextual
Exercise and rest				
Sleep patterns	*"I'm looking forward to exercising and losing this tummy."*	*A*		
Body alignment	*Walked to the bathroom on the second postpartum day*	*A*		
Leisure activity	*"I'm doing the exercises the nurse taught me to do in bed."*	*A*		
O_2 and circulatory needs	*Felt faint when arising on first postpartum day*	*M*	*Cesarean delivery* *Incisional pain* *Decreased circulatory activity*	*Room warm and daily lighted* *No nurse support*
Exercise	*Inability to sleep comfortably or for long durations*	*M*	*Pain* *Anxiety about condition (or baby)* *Refuses medication for pain or sleeping needs*	*Noisy roommate* *Warm environment, noisy*

PHYSIOLOGICAL MODE			
Stimuli Residual	Nursing Diagnosis	Nursing Goals for Clients	Nursing Intervention†
		Maintain adaptive behavior	Support adaptive behavior
		Maintain adaptive behavior	Support adaptive behavior
		Maintain adaptive behavior	Support adaptive behavior
Unaccustomed to sick role	Postural hypotension	Absence of dizziness and fainting	Instruct client to call for assistance when ready to get OOB
			Teach client how to splint incision when moving
Dependent upon home environment and husband	Sleep deprivation due to pain and anxiety	Acquire normal rest and sleep patterns	Assist client with relaxation techniques
			Make environment conducive to rest
			Provide client with information on side effects of medication on herself and baby

(Continued on page 118)

APPENDIX B.
NURSING CARE PROTOTYPES BASED ON THE ROY ADAPTATION MODEL

PHYSIOLOGICAL MODE				
			Stimuli	
Category	Behaviors	Adaptation Status*	Focal	Contextual
	Fear of deep breathing	M	Fear of incision tearing	Intrusive apparatus: Foley catheter, IV infusion
			Abdominal pain	Interruption of normal routine
Nutrition				
Fluid and electrolytes	Appetite increasing	A		
Food intake	Thirst	M	Postpartum diuresis and diaphoresis	Warm environment
Tissue regeneration and healing			Increasing breast milk	Lack of preferred liquids
			Copious amounts of fluid released postdelivery as retained tissue fluids are released	
			Element of the "taking-in" phase	
Body structure				
General appearance	Appears clean, well-groomed	A	Short stature; small frame	

PHYSIOLOGICAL MODE			
Stimuli Residual	Nursing Diagnosis	Nursing Goals for Clients	Nursing Intervention†
Separation anxiety: away from home and husband	Lacks information about the healing process and the need to deep breathe and cough	Realize the importance of deep breathing Understand the healing process of the body	Teach client about importance of coughing and deep breathing to prevent post-operative complications
			Teach client how to "splint" the incision when coughing to minimize pain
			Encourage and praise client for her efforts to cough and deep breathe
		Maintain adaptive behavior	Support adaptive behavior
Habitual low fluid intake	Inadequate fluid and electrolyte balance	Restore fluid and electrolyte balance	Instruct client on importance of fluid intake for restoration of fluid balance and for lactation
			Offer fluids the client prefers.
			Have fluids readily available at bedside
		Maintain adaptive behavior	Support adaptive behavior

(Continued on page 120)

APPENDIX B.
NURSING CARE PROTOTYPES BASED ON THE ROY ADAPTATION MODEL

			PHYSIOLOGICAL MODE	
			Stimuli	
Category	Behaviors	Adaptation Status*	Focal	Contextual
Age, weight, stature	Height 5 ft. Weight 140 lb.	M	Gained 50 lb during pregnancy	Husband bringing in snacks and candy
Elimination				
Stool and flatus	Voids without difficulty after catheter removal	A		
Urination Diaphoresis Nausea and vomiting	"I've had so much gas and abdominal pain that I'm afraid to have a bowel movement."	M	Decreased exercise Surgical bowel manipulation NPO before surgery Full liquid diet	Lack of nursing explanation, support, and teaching Nonprivate environment Fear of wound dehiscence
Healing and restorative processes				
Wound Uterine involution	Incision dry and intact Lochia rubra: moderate Fundus: firm 1 fb under umbilicus	A		
Body regulation				
Sensory	Colostrum present	A		

PHYSIOLOGICAL MODE			
Stimuli Residual	Nursing Diagnosis	Nursing Goals for Clients	Nursing Intervention†
Poor eating habits	*Overweight*	*Weight proportional to height*	*Correct dietary deficiencies, if present*
			Improve the family's nutritional knowledge and status
		Maintain adaptive behavior	*Support adaptive behavior*
Habitual difficulty with flatus and constipation	*Flatus— postsurgical*	*Absence of flatus*	*Encourage exercise and ambulation*
			Roughage in diet, if tolerated
			Provide fluids
			Apply heat to abdomen
		Maintain adaptive behavior	*Support adaptive behavior*
Habitual difficulty with flatus and constipation	*Flatus— postsurgical*	*Absence of flatus*	*Encourage exercise and ambulation*
			Roughage in diet, if tolerated
			Provide fluids
			Apply heat to abdomen
		Maintain adaptive behavior	*Support adaptive behavior*

(Continued on page 122)

APPENDIX B.
NURSING CARE PROTOTYPES BASED ON THE ROY ADAPTATION MODEL

PHYSIOLOGICAL MODE

Category	Behaviors	Adaptation Status*	Stimuli	
			Focal	Contextual
Endocrine	"I go from being depressed to happy." (mood swings)	M	Hormonal changes	Anxiety regarding baby
			Sensory overload (environmental stimuli, including noise, heat, light, strangers)	Information regarding infant and self-care deficient
				Separation from baby, husband, and home
			Physical discomfort	Interruption of communication with family
	Experiencing incisional pain and discomfort	M	Cesarean delivery	Refused pain medication because breast feeding
				Attempted independent handling of baby too soon post–delivery

SELF-CONCEPT MODE

Category	Behaviors	Adaptation Status*	Stimuli	
			Focal	Contextual
Physical self				
Loss: grief	"I looked forward to a normal delivery, but at least my baby is O.K."	A		
General appearance				
Restoration of bodily function	"I'm really trying to exercise and walk."	A		
Sleep				
Appetite (loss)	Increasing appetite	A		

PHYSIOLOGICAL MODE			
Stimuli _____ Residual	Nursing Diagnosis	Nursing Goals for Clients	Nursing Intervention†
Attended childbirth classes and looked forward to a vaginal delivery with husband	Emotionally labile "taking-in" phase	Emotional stability regained	Encourage client to verbalize about birth experience
			Encourage husband participation and interaction
			Offer adequate explanation and teaching to the couple
			Make client as physically comfortable as possible
Decreased pain tolerance No prior surgery	Postoperative pain	Minimize pain or absence of pain	Encourage client to take pain medication p.r.n.
			Explain to client minimal effects pain medication has on infant

SELF-CONCEPT MODE			
Stimuli _____ Residual	Nursing Diagnosis	Nursing Goals for Clients	Nursing Intervention†
		Maintain adaptive behavior.	Support adaptive behavior.
		Maintain adaptive behavior.	Support adaptive behavior.
		Maintain adaptive behavior.	Support adaptive behavior.

(Continued on page 124)

APPENDIX B.
NURSING CARE PROTOTYPES BASED ON THE ROY ADAPTATION MODEL

SELF-CONCEPT MODE				
			Stimuli	
Category	Behaviors	Adaptation Status*	Focal	Contextual
Self-image	"I can't sleep well, but I won't take any medication."	M	Pain due to surgery Fears pain and sleep medication may be harmful to breast-fed baby.	Anxiety over baby
	"I know I will always be depressed about not having a vaginal delivery."	M	Cesarean delivery Husband not allowed to be present at the delivery	Separation from baby Anxiety over baby.
Moral-ethical self				
Attitude toward self	"I'm sorry I had to have surgery, but I know it was best for my baby."	A		

SELF-CONCEPT MODE			
Stimuli Residual	Nursing Diagnosis	Nursing Goals for Clients	Nursing Intervention†
Determined to be a "good mother" Couple has post-graduate education in health sciences	Sleep deprivation and lowered self-concept	Restoration of normal sleep patterns	Use relaxation techniques and comfort measures to encourage sleep. Provide information on effects of medication on self and infant
Wanted ideal vaginal delivery	Lowered self-concept and unmet need to be "normal"	Congruence between real and ideal self	Encourage client to express feelings of concern and accept dependent behaviors. Encourage husband's support and allow the couple privacy. Accept client's grief and mourning for ideal delivery. Support client by your presence, listening, and touch. Strengthen client's problem-solving skills.
		Maintain adaptive behavior	Support adaptive behavior

(Continued on page 126)

APPENDIX B.
NURSING CARE PROTOTYPES BASED ON THE ROY ADAPTATION MODEL

			SELF-CONCEPT MODE	
			Stimuli	
Category	Behaviors	Adaptation Status*	Focal	Contextual
Psychosociological components *Utilization of defense mechanisms* *Emotional status (guilt)*	*"I feel so guilty about being too tired to take care of my baby."*	*M*	*Cesarean delivery* *Decreased exercise and circulatory activity* *Lack of sleep*	*Uncomfortable environment (noise, surgery, strangers)*
Self-consistency *Physiological function*	*"Things are better now. The baby is eating well and I am more together."*	*A*		

SELF-CONCEPT MODE			
Stimuli ——— Residual	Nursing Diagnosis	Nursing Clients for Clients	Nursing Intervention†
Strong desire to mother baby High self-expectations Expected to have vaginal delivery and to be able to care for baby soon after	Guilt	Resolution of guilt feelings	Recognize and convey to client the fact that guilt is normal response
			Maintain beneficial nurse–patient relation ship that promotes trust
			Help client to see that her behavior is acceptable
			Provide support and encouragement
			Let her know that cesarean birth is an acceptable way to deliver
		Maintain adaptive behavior	Support adaptive behavior

(Continued on page 128)

APPENDIX B.
NURSING CARE PROTOTYPES BASED ON THE ROY ADAPTATION MODEL

			SELF–CONCEPT MODE	
			Stimuli	
Category	Behaviors	Adaptation Status*	Focal	Contextual
Restorative processes Emotional level Utilization of defense mechanism (anxiety)	"The baby had a loose stool last night and I freaked out."	M	Anxiety regarding baby Lack of mothering skills	Strange environment Lack of support system
Self-ideal and self-expectations				
Role adaptation level Physical self Psychosocial self (powerlessness)	"No one is ever here when I need them. The baby is just pushed in and we are left. I get angry with myself for not knowing what to do."	M	Anxiety about caring for the baby Lack of mothering skills	Lack of support system Lack of teaching and guidance from nursing staff Lack of self-confidence

SELF-CONCEPT MODE			
Stimuli Residual	Nursing Diagnosis	Nursing Goals for Clients	Nursing Intervention†
No previous mothering experience High self-expectations	Unrealistic self-expectations	Realistic expectation of self and of mothering skills	Give information about restoration to pre-pregnant state Provide a comfortable, non-threatening environment Mother is "taking-in." Be accepting of dependent needs Provide information regarding infant care Remain with the mother while infant is in the room; assist mother with care Promote attachment to infant
No previous experience in caring for baby High self-expectation	Poor role adaptation	Realistic adaptation to mothering role	Provide factual data to help her fill in the "missing pieces." Encourage verbalization about the discrepancy between the mother's expectations and her actual performance Offer mother and father necessary teaching Compliment and encourage the mother on tasks well done

(Continued on page 130)

APPENDIX B.
NURSING CARE PROTOTYPES BASED ON THE ROY ADAPTATION MODEL

SELF–CONCEPT MODE				
		Adaptation	Stimuli	
Category	Behaviors	Status*	Focal	Contextual
Self-esteem				
Emotional level	*Attentive, well-groomed*	*A*		
Physiological component	*"I feel ex- tremely badly that my hus- band missed seeing our baby born."*	*M*	*Emergency cesarean birth*	*Husband sup- portive during labor, but un- able to attend the delivery*

ROLE–FUNCTION MODE				
		Adaptation	Stimuli	
Category	Behaviors	Status*	Focal	Contextual
Role Mastery				
Young adult female role	*"I feel so guilty about not being able to take care of my baby properly" (con- cern over ma- ternal role)*	*M*	*Unplanned cesarean*	*Separation from baby*
Mother role			*Decreased energy level*	*Lack of nurs- ing support for mothering tasks*
Wife role				*Nursery nurses reluctant to let mother care for baby*

SELF–CONCEPT MODE

Stimuli Residual	Nursing Diagnosis	Nursing Goals for Clients	Nursing Intervention†
		Maintain adaptive behavior	*Support adaptive behavior*
Close relationship with husband *Attended childbirth preparation class and expected a vaginal delivery*	*Client experiencing guilt and lowered self-esteem*	*Resolution of guilt and increased self-esteem*	*Encourage verbalization and reliving of labor and delivery experience* *Encourage couple to share feelings about labor and delivery with each other* *Promote attachment to infant* *Focus on client's strengths and accomplishments*

ROLE–FUNCTION MODE

Stimuli Residual	Nursing Diagnosis	Nursing Goals for Clients	Nursing Intervention†
High self-expectations of mother role based on cultural values	*Client experiencing feelings of inadequacy and failure in attaining maternal role*	*Attain mastery of the mothering role*	*Assist mother in caring for infant* *Coordinate mother/infant care with nursery and postpartum nurses* *Meet mother's own dependency needs* *Promote physical rest, nutrition, exercise, relaxation* *Praise mother's skills and accomplishments in infant care*

(Continued on page 132)

APPENDIX B.
NURSING CARE PROTOTYPES BASED ON THE ROY ADAPTATION MODEL

			ROLE-FUNCTION MODE	
			Stimuli	
Category	Behaviors	Adaptation Status*	Focal	Contextual
	Expresses fear about renewal of sexual activity	M	Fears related to rupture of incision Presence of abdominal scars	Feels sexually unattractive
Role distance				
Acknowledg- ment of roles Role perform- ance vs. role expectation	"I can't stand being a patient." (concern over cesarean role)	M	Increased feel- ings of depen- dency due to physiological limitations from cesarean delivery	Needs fulfilled by persons other than self

ROLE–FUNCTION MODE			
Stimuli / Residual	Nursing Diagnosis	Nursing Goals for Clients	Nursing Intervention†
Prepregnant concerns about sexual adequacy	Feels inadequate in her sexual role	Develop feelings of sexual adequacy	Encourage verbalization of client's concern
			Provide information about healing process and strength of scar tissue
			Focus on client's strengths and abilities in other areas of role performance to promote self-confidence
			Encourage sharing of fears and/or feelings of sexual inadequacy with spouse
Very independent person Has never been hospitalized Cultural expectations regarding independent behavior	Unable to cope with unexpected dependency postpartum	Client independence	Help client deal with uneasiness she feels in patient role by clarifying client's expected vs. real experiences in this role
			Encourage verbalization of feelings
			Emphasize client's strengths
			Assist in caring for baby
			Encourage self-care and mothering of baby within client's capabilities, both physically and emotionally

(Continued on page 134)

APPENDIX B.
NURSING CARE PROTOTYPES BASED ON THE ROY ADAPTATION MODEL

			ROLE-FUNCTION MODE	
			Stimuli	
Category	Behaviors	Adaptation Status*	Focal	Contextual
Role conflict				
Interrole conflict	"I am looking forward to going home and being a good wife and mother."	A		
Intrarole conflict				
Role failure				
Acknowledge-ment of role	"I should be caring for my baby but instead the nursery nurses are." (concern over maternal role)	M	Cesarean delivery Separated from baby	Nursery nurses possessive of infant
Performance of role				

ROLE-FUNCTION MODE			
Stimuli Residual	Nursing Diagnosis	Nursing Goals for Clients	Nursing Intervention†
		Maintain adaptive behavior	*Support adaptive behavior*
Very high self-expectations as mother	*Perceives self as a failure in her mother role*	*Success in mothering role*	*Coordinate mother/infant care with nursery and postpartum nurses*
			Assist mother in learning and practicing infant care skills
			Reinforce client's strengths
			Encourage mother to hold and cuddle baby if too tired to perform caretaking activities
			Assist client in discovering that she as "mother" is the most important person in her baby's life now
			Allow time for mother, father, and baby to be together in privacy
			Encourage realistic perception of physical/psychological expectations following surgical delivery

(Continued on page 136)

APPENDIX B.
NURSING CARE PROTOTYPES BASED ON THE ROY ADAPTATION MODEL

			Stimuli	
INTERDEPENDENCE MODE				
Category	Behaviors	Adaptation Status*	Focal	Contextual
Help seeking				
Self-help	*Seeks assistance when beginning new mothering activities*	*A*		
Utilization of support systems				
Affection seeking				
Coping styles	*"I told my husband not to go and leave me all alone."*	*M*	*Increased dependency needs*	*Separated from husband*
Support systems available and utilized				*Unfamiliar environment*
				Disappointed that husband could not share birth experience

INTERDEPENDENCE MODE			
Stimuli Residual	Nursing Diagnosis	Nursing Goals for Clients	Nursing Intervention†
		Maintain adaptive behavior	*Support adaptive behavior*
Very close relationship with her husband	*Increased dependency needs in "taking-in" phase of postpartum period*	*Fulfillment of needs for affection within appropriate limits*	*Establish a trusting relationship with the client* *Provide privacy for couple and baby to promote attachment* *Assess and encourage interaction with husband* *Assist client in exploring her feelings of need for affection* *Promote affection seeking and affection giving between mother and baby* *Plan to spend time with this new mother* *Emphasize the normalcy of affection-seeking behavior during the "taking-in" phase*

(Continued on page 138)

APPENDIX B.
NURSING CARE PROTOTYPES BASED ON THE ROY ADAPTATION MODEL

			INTERDEPENDENCE MODE	
			Stimuli	
Category	Behaviors	Adaptation Status*	Focal	Contextual
Attention seeking				
Dependency needs *Real/perceived utilization of sources of attention*	*Frequent crying spells; call light on continuously*	*M*	*Increased dependency needs in "taking-in" phase*	*Lack of support and assistance from nurses* *Unfamiliar environment* *Roomate talks about her "ideal" vaginal delivery.*
Initiative taking				
Physical self-care *Mothering behaviors* *Restoration/ strengthening of family life*	*"I'm trying to get my strength back. I want to take good care of my baby."*	*A*		

INTERDEPENDENCE MODE			
Stimuli	Nursing Diagnosis	Nursing Goals for Clients	Nursing Intervention†
Residual			
Close ties to family	*Unmet increased dependency needs*	*Fulfillment of dependency needs . . . or client independence*	*Encourage verbalization of feelings*
Family located 400 miles away			*Offer assistance in such a way as to maintain feelings of self-confidence and self-esteem*
Recently moved to this area			
			Plan to spend time with the client, both alone and when baby is present
			Praise mother's accomplishments
			Provide complete information regarding feelings during the postpartum period as well as "normal disappointment" experienced with cesarian delivery
			Encourage appropriate use of support systems
	Maintain adaptive behavior		*Support adaptive behavior*

(Continued on page 140)

APPENDIX B.
NURSING CARE PROTOTYPES BASED ON THE ROY ADAPTATION MODEL

			INTERDEPENDENCE MODE	
			Stimuli	
Category	Behaviors	Adaptation Status*	Focal	Contextual
Obstacle mastery				
Physical restoration	"I tried different positions for breast feeding until we found one that worked."	A		
Psychosocial stability				
Defense mechanisms				
Coping styles	"I've cried on and off for 2 days."	M	Loss of ideal experience	Lack of nursing support and encouragement
Use of crying and laughter			Hormonal changes	
Frequency and appropriateness of use	Withdrawal: sends baby back to nursery and goes to sleep		Feelings of inadequacy as mother	Husband absent during days because of work schedule
			Fatigue from third trimester sleep deficit	

*A = adaptive, M = maladaptive.
†Evaluation of interventions would involve noting the behavioral shift to adaptive responses.

INTERDEPENDENCE MODE			
Stimuli Residual	Nursing Diagnosis	Nursing Goals for Clients	Nursing Intervention†
		Maintain adaptive behavior	*Support adaptive behavior*
Uses crying as a coping mechanism (may be culturally determined behavior)	*Experiencing depression and guilt*	*Resolution of guilt feelings and restoration of emotional stability*	*Accept and meet new mother's dependency needs*
			Encourage expression of feelings and assure mother that such feelings are normal and acceptable
			Encourage visits by husband
			Offer comfort measures (back rubs, fluids, pain medication, nurse's presence, quiet environment, etc.),
			Provide information about baby
			Verbally reward progress in mothering behaviors
			Observe and reinforce maternal/ infant touching to promote attachment

CHAPTER 7

Assessing and Understanding the Cesarean Father

Jacqueline Fawcett

This chapter deals with the special needs of the father involved in a cesarean birth experience. The focus is on identification of his needs and specific nursing actions suggested by the Roy Adaptation Model of Nursing (Roy 1976). Thus consideration is given to assessment and intervention in the areas of physiological status, self-concept, role function, and interdependence relations. Throughout the chapter, attention is given to the differences for the father between a cesarean birth experience and an uneventful vaginal delivery. Additional distinctions are drawn between reactions to planned versus emergency cesarean birth.

REVIEW OF THE LITERATURE

The effects of the cesarean birth on the mother have been reasonably well documented and are discussed in other chapters. However, little is known of the father's response. It is therefore incumbent upon nurses to identify the specific needs of the father and to devise nursing interventions that will meet those needs.

A search of the literature revealed few books or articles containing references to men during pregnancy and childbirth, and even fewer comments about cesarean fathers. One question that is considered is whether or not the cesarean father should be allowed in the delivery room (Persson et al, 1978). Arguments sound strikingly similar to those advanced over the past several years by proponents and opponents of the father's presence during vaginal delivery. Thus the current controversy revolves around such familiar points as family bonding, the stabilizing force and calming influence a man can exert on his partner at this time, and the loss of fees from patients who go to physicians who are affiliated with hospitals permitting the father's presence. Other aspects of the issue focus on breaching of infection control barriers and the potential increase in malpractice suits if fathers are allowed to attend the cesarian birth. However, these latter points are minimized by those who maintain that ". . . properly suited, booted, capped and masked, [the father] appears to be no more or less a contaminant than any other person in the room" (Donovan 1977, p. 123), and that there is no evidence of more lawsuits. In fact, although there have been no objective studies of malpractice suits in cesarean deliveries, the prevailing impression is that there are fewer legal problems when the father is present for the birth.

Another element in the literature focuses on the reactions and needs of cesarean parents, with some attention given to the father. Although mainly concerned with the cesarean mother, Reynolds (1977) did note the father's need for support throughout the intrapartal and postpartal periods. As part of a family-centered approach to the care of these childbearing couples, she advocated:

1. Continued verbal communication to inform the father of his partner's progress through surgery.
2. The father's presence in the operating room, if hospital policy permits.
3. Initiation of father–infant bonding immediately after delivery, if the baby's condition is stable.
4. Reuniting the new parents and their baby in the recovery room as soon as possible.
5. Helping the couple relive the experience later in the postpartum period so as to promote integration of the cesarean birth into their lives and to clear up any misconceptions of events.
6. Facilitating recognition that such reactions as a sense of loss, anger, sadness, bitterness, and guilt are normal responses to the forced change in the parents' plan for the "perfect childbirth experience."

Contemporary maternity nursing textbooks pay little attention to the cesarean father, despite claims of family-centered approaches. Reeder et al. (1976, p. 456) devoted just one sentence to the father: "The father should be permitted to visit [his partner] as soon as it is feasible [after the birth]." Moore (1978) superficially focused on the couple as a unit, noting the feelings of disappointment, loss, and abnormality expressed by some cesarean parents and the enforced separation of parents from the newborn if the baby is placed in a special care nursery. However, she made no direct references to the specific nursing care needs of either cesarean parent other than the following admonishment (Moore 1978, p. 430): "Time must be found to allow both parents to ask questions and to express their feelings about abdominal delivery."

Affonso (1979) made two explicit comments about the cesarean father, both gleaned from interviews with the cesarean wives. In one, she noted the positive influence the father exerted on the mother's recuperation by visiting her during the postpartal hospital stay. In the other, she stated that the women described their husbands as being fearful for them and their babies during the delivery. These wives also reported that their husbands' feelings included happiness about the baby's birth, relief that the labor and delivery were over, disappointment, and anger. Affonso (1979, p. 724) concluded by saying, "The obvious nursing implication is to include the husband in the care of the women by offering emotional support, explanations, keeping him informed, and advocating hospital policies which will allow more male participation."

In the most comprehensive references to cesarean birth experiences, Donovan (1977) and Donovan and Allen (1977) identified the numerous reactions parents may have when they learn that an emergency cesarean birth is imminent. These responses include relief that the baby's birth is near; anxiety about or even dread of what will happen to both mother and baby; confusion; a feeling of helplessness; and disillusionment. They further noted that elective and repeat cesareans give rise to many of the same responses, as well as to feelings of inadequacy, shame, and frustration over not being able to have a "normal" vaginal birth.

While many of the feelings cited here are experienced by the cesarean mother to a greater degree than by the father, Donovan and Allen (1977) highlighted the father's anxiety, confusion, and sense of helplessness. Furthermore, Donovan (1977) pointed out that if he is not permitted to be with his partner during their child's birth, the cesarean father may feel alone and ignored. She also noted that as a consequence of his isolation, he worries, fantasizes, and agonizes about what is happening in the operating room.

Although these reactions are similar to those experienced by any man separated from his partner during their baby's birth, they can certainly be intensified by a cesarean delivery. Thus there is even more reason for hospitals not to be, as Donovan (1977, p. 9) said, ". . . remiss in their responsibility to act as a liaison between the doctor, mother-to-be, and expectant father." Clearly, as all authors have emphasized, the father's need for accurate and up-to-date information is crucial. Indeed, since fear of the unknown is a major component of cesarean births, there is a need for a continual flow of information to both parents. To facilitate this, Donovan and Allen (1977, p. 38) proposed a program of ". . . antenatal education, intrapartum nursing intervention, and postpartum support. . . weaving together the surgical and emotional aspects of the cesarean experience in a way that is factual and, of equal importance, reassuring."

The literature review also revealed that authors have a strong tendency to view the father solely as provider of emotional support for his partner. Donovan's comments clearly reflect this perspective, as exemplified by the following statements:

> *The best preoperative "tranquilizer" for a cesarean mother is the presence of the baby's father to support and reassure her. (Donovan 1977, p. 91)*

> *If the father is present for the birth, he can comfort the mother, describe to her what is happening, and reassure her that all is well. (Donovan 1977, p. 98)*

> *The elective cesarean father will know in advance when the delivery is scheduled, which will enable him to make plans so he can spend as much time as possible with his wife and baby in the hospital and during the first week or two at home. (Donovan 1977, p. 22)*

Carrying the theme further, Donovan (1977, p. 51), challenged cesarean fathers to understand the mothers' situation after delivery, asking, "How would they feel being uncomfortable physically and almost totally dependent on others for help?"

Marut (1978) and Harris (1980) reinforced many of Donovan's statements and added others that elaborate on the man's traditional supportive role. They maintained that the man's presence during all phases of the cesarean birth seems to reduce the mother's anxiety and allows him to help the mother claim her child by welcoming the baby, to fill informational gaps in the mother's memory of labor and delivery, and to explain details she did not understand as they relive the experience throughout the postpartum.

Undoubtedly, the cesarean mother requires the father's support. Unfortunately, this orientation to the man's role during childbirth denies his individual needs for nursing care. For, as Kiernan and Scoloveno (1977, p. 488) put it, "Family-centered nursing means more than logistically allowing the father entrance to a particular [hospital] unit." They advocated specific attention to the father by:

1. Nursing assessment of his individual needs.
2. Not generalizing or stereotyping his roles and behaviors as typically male or female.

3. Allowing demonstration of his expressive as well as instrumental functions.
4. Providing a supportive other for him.

A SURVEY OF CESAREAN FATHERS

The literature review revealed that most of the cesarean fathers' responses were identified through interviews with wives and that their needs were inferred by authors relying on these indirect sources of data. Thus the few suggested nursing interventions were based upon third-party perception of needs. Such an approach lacks the advantage of direct client identification of problem areas and suggestions as to how the nurse might help him solve those problems. Indirect data clearly do not provide information about the client's definition of the situation.

An exploratory study was therefore undertaken to determine the expressed needs of cesarean fathers and to elicit suggestions from these men about what could be done to make the cesarean birth a more positive experience for them. The sample for this study was composed of 24 married men. All were husbands of women receiving private obstetrical care. Three men were the investigator's professional colleagues or their spouses. The remainder of the sample was recruited from an obstetrical group practice in southern New England. Potential subjects were contacted by the office nurse practitioner, who explained the purpose of the study and requested their assistance. She then mailed a questionnaire to those who agreed to participate, along with a stamped return envelope addressed to the investigator. Thus identity of these study subjects was known to the investigator only if they chose to include their return addresses on the envelope, which they were instructed to do if a summary of the study findings was desired.

The sample represents a response rate of 46 percent of all subjects who told the nurse practitioner they were willing to participate in the study. Since all of the potential and actual subjects were drawn from the same obstetrical practice, there is no reason to assume meaningful demographic differences between those who did and those who did not finally participate.

Fathers ranged in age from 23 to 42 years of age ($\overline{X}$ = 30.8) and were predominantly middle class. Seventeen were husbands of primiparas; 13 of these men's wives experienced emergency cesarean births, usually after long periods of labor, while four had cesareans that were planned anywhere from the onset of pregnancy to 1 day before the delivery. The 7 husbands of multiparas included 1 whose wife had 2 planned cesareans, 4 who had primary emergency and subsequent planned cesarean deliveries, 1 who had an emergency cesarean for the second child, and 1 whose wife delivered their third child by emergency cesarean and their fourth by planned cesarean.

The births occurred between 1973 and 1980, with all but four occurring after 1977. Reasons given for the cesarean births were cephalopelvic disproportion (N = 15), dystocia (N = 4), fetal distress (N = 2), placenta previa (N = 1), toxemia (N = 1), and genital herpes (N = 1).

Thirteen of the 15 men whose wives experienced labor were present during that time; however, only 6 of these men were allowed in the delivery room. Seventeen men attended Lamaze prepared childbirth classes with their wives. Of these, 14 indicated the classes included some information about cesarean birth. One man attended cesarean birth preparation classes with his wife.

The questionnaire was open ended and was designed to elicit comments regarding the father's physical and emotional responses to finding out the baby would be born by the cesarean method, to the actual birth experience, and the early postpartum period. In addition, the father was asked to identify his greatest needs during the time surrounding the birth and what could have been done by whom to improve the experience for him. This questionnaire is shown in Figure 1.

The responses were classified according to Roy's four adaptive modes: physiological needs, self-concept, role function, and interdependence relations (Roy 1976). Analysis of the data focused on identification of need deficits and excesses in each mode. In addition, the data were examined for indications of behavior necessary to cope with the particular elements of the cesarean birth experience—behavior either initiated by the men or suggested by them as actions that might be helpful to others.

The survey revealed only a few expressed need deficits in the physiological mode. Those fathers who stayed with their wives during the long labors preceding emergency cesarean births noted a need for sleep. For example, one father stated he was physically tired after 30 hours of labor. Food was also mentioned by some fathers. The statement that his greatest need during the entire cesarean experience was for "a cup of coffee," coupled with the comment that he was "a nervous, anxious father," suggests that food may have been viewed more as a means to relaxation than an actual nutritional need for this man. Several fathers also noted a feeling of physical tenseness throughout the experience, while others indicated they felt physically "fine," but emotionally "drained." One father stated he felt "extreme terror" and severe anxiety throughout the entire cesarean experience.

The fathers expressed few, if any, deficits of need in the self-concept mode. The data indicated that many men were disappointed their wives would not have the "normal childbirth" they had "trained for." This suggests that the fathers' self-concept needs were not compromised, but that they believed their wives' views of their childbearing capabilities were threatened. One man, apparently in an effort to make the cesarean experience more consistent with expectations, said, "Don't make such a big deal out of the natural occurrence of childbirth." This man also stated that during the time his child was being born (he was not in the delivery room), he felt ". . . confident that come

Your age:
Your occupation:
Your education (highest grade completed):
Did you attend childbirth preparation classes?
If yes, did they include information on cesarean birth?

PLEASE ANSWER THE FOLLOWING QUESTIONS IN
AS MUCH DETAIL AS YOU CAN PROVIDE. USE THE
BACK OF THIS PAGE IF NECESSARY.

How did you feel, physically and emotionally, when you found out your wife was to have your baby by the cesarean method?

How did you feel, physically and emotionally, during the actual birth experience?

Were you with your wife during labor and/or in the delivery room?

What happened after the baby was born? How did you feel, physically and emotionally, during that time?

What were your greatest needs during the entire experience?

What could have been done, and by whom, to make this experience better for you?

Additional comments:

FIGURE 1.   *Cesarean Birth Experience Questionnaire.*

what may, healthy baby or otherwise, God's will would be done. . . ." and was ". . . very happy, awestruck at the miracle of new life."

The survey data indicated several need deficits in the role function adaptive mode. The event of cesarean birth appears to create need deficits, especially in the area of role failure, for the fathers. That is, fathers often cannot perform the supportive, coaching role they "trained for" during childbirth classes. This was especially noted by the men who had been with their wives during labor but were denied the opportunity to share the baby's birth. For example, one expectant father said he was ". . . extremely nervous as well as wishing I could watch the operation [and] disappointed probably since we were prepared for vaginal birth." Another man commented that he felt "left out and with no control over outcome, especially [since he was] unable to comfort [his] wife, as taught in Lamaze class."

The data also indicated that some men were able to successfully perform the usual roles as husbands and fathers, especially if they knew of the cesarean birth in advance. For example, one father noted that while the first cesarean experience was ". . . frightening and frustrating, . . . knowing ahead of time [with their second child] was better for me. It gave me time to prepare myself." This father, who was present for his second child's birth, expressed reactions similar to those of men present during vaginal births, saying that he felt ". . . apprehensive at first, wondering how I would react, and how everything would go. That gave way to excitement when I could see the baby being taken out of my wife. No picture or explanation could ever convey the emotion of that moment." Similarly, another cesarean father who was also present for the delivery wrote, "Baby was cleaned and given to me to hold and to show my wife. Physically I felt fine. Emotionally I was nervous holding the baby—self-conscious." Another father indicated that after the baby was born, he felt a "natural high" and was "happy, exuberant." He also stated, as do many new fathers, that he ". . . wanted to have a get-together to let everyone we love, know, even acquaintances share the joy."

Comments made by many of the cesarean fathers in the survey indicated they wanted detailed information about the reasons for and events connected with this method of childbirth. Typical of these comments are the following:

"A longer and more thorough explanation by the doctor as to the need for the cesarean. Everything moved along too rapidly with too little communication."

"I think that if our doctor took a little more time to explain things to us, I would have felt more secure."

These statements suggest that such knowledge would provide clues for appropriate behavior in the role of cesarean father.

Many comments made by the fathers indicated need deficits in the interdependence mode. Feelings mentioned earlier, such as "no control" and a desire for detailed explanations, indicate deficits in the area of obstacle mastery. Other statements clearly express these fathers' needs for closer relations with their wives during the cesarean experience. One man noted that his greatest need was to be with his wife during delivery and with both wife and baby after the birth. Another similar need was expressed in this statement: "To be with my wife and share with her what she was going through physically and emotionally, making the entire experience, including the decision to go cesarean, something we shared *together*." Still another comment sums up the need to love and be loved: "I wanted to have more physical contact with my wife to let her know how much I love her and make her more aware of my presence." This father, who witnessed his child's birth, further indicated affiliative needs when he said, "After the baby was born, I felt excited, to say the least. I wanted to kiss everyone in the room for making this experience possible."

Other comments suggested the cesarean fathers were forced into dependent behavior by the situation. Manifestations of this included mention of feeling nervous, drained, or numb, as well as noting that there was a great need for patience.

In summary, the data obtained from this survey revealed that these cesarean fathers' reactions echoed those reported in the literature.

NURSING ASSESSMENT AND INTERVENTION

The paucity of research on the cesarean father prohibits development of what Haller et al. (1979) call "innovation protocols"—that is, nursing care interventions based on findings of sound clinical nursing research. However, the few data that are available permit advancement of some general suggestions for nursing. While use of Roy's model to structure assessment and intervention strategies provides some assurance of a comprehensive approach to the nursing care of cesarean fathers (Roy 1976), more specific prescriptions for nursing actions must await development of knowledge that has been tested and validated in clinical settings.

While the cesarean father is not a patient in the usual sense, he should be regarded as a client in need of nursing care. Assessment of his needs can be accomplished by carefully noting his responses to the entire cesarean birth experience. All sources of data, including the literature review and the survey findings reported earlier, indicate similarities in most cesarean fathers' behavior and in the influencing factors. Since the focal stimulus for most men is the cesarean birth itself, and since it is obviously not possible to eliminate that event, the other stimuli must be modified so that the man is better able to cope with this experience in a positive manner. Indeed, the father's ability to cope with the cesarean experience appears to be most strongly influenced by the events surrounding the birth (the contextual stimuli). The data suggest that the most important elements here are:

1. Whether the cesarean birth is anticipated or an emergency.
2. Whether the parents are together during the experience.
3. The amount of information given to the couple before, during, and after the cesarean.

The data further suggest that the primary residual stimulus is the father's specific expectations regarding his participation in the birth.

Within the category of the physiological adaptive mode, the nurse can expect a nervous, tense man who is worried about the mother and child. He may also need rest or sleep and food. When the cesarean birth is planned in advance, it is important to encourage the man to get adequate sleep the night before and to eat a good breakfast, so that he will be prepared for the events of the day to come. In the case of an emergency cesarean, provision for rest, sleep, and nutrition is especially warranted, since much of the father's energy reserve may have been used up during the mother's labor or by the rush to the hospital. Although the data do not indicate disturbances in other physiological needs, the nurse should be alert to the possibility of such disturbances in her observations of and communication with the cesarean father. The nurse's attention to the cesarean father's needs in the physiological mode is especially important because many men do not expect the nurse to consider or meet their needs in this area (MacLaughlin 1980).

Assessment of the cesarean father's self-concept is likely to reveal a person who is disappointed about the disparity between his expectations of childbirth and the reality of the cesarean birth. In addition, many men are anxious and concerned about the physical and emotional impact of a cesarean on the mother, viewing this method of childbirth as a major insult to the woman's concept of herself as a bearer of children. Thus the cesarean father may have to deal with his own and the mother's feelings of failure, disappointment, and anger about the surgical birth. The genesis of such feelings appears to be, at least in part, the current emphasis on prepared, family-centered childbirth. Any deviation from the idealized experience is regarded as a failure on the part of all participants—mother, father, nurses, physicians, and even the baby. Nurses can play a major role in altering this type of response by helping the man to discuss his feelings, by answering his questions, and by clarifying any misconceptions. Even more, they can encourage those who teach prepared childbirth classes to explain the realities of childbirth and to emphasize the idea that deviations are not failures.

Also in the self-concept mode, and in direct conflict with his usual perception of himself as a "take-charge" person, the cesarean father may feel helpless or powerless as he tries to deal with hospital personnel. Furthermore, the father's feelings of helplessness may extend into the postpartal period as a response to the mother's behavior. For example, while many reactions of the cesarean mother are typical of any woman who is trying to cope with a new baby, her physical and emotional condition may magnify these postpartal responses. She may thus feel markedly exhausted for the first several days at home and cry frequently, especially when the baby begins his or her seemingly incessant demands for attention. This type of reaction often gives rise to bewilderment on the part of the father, who cannot understand why the mother cries every time the baby cries. In this situation, the nurse can help both new parents to realize this is a common, time-limited response during the "settling in" period. Moreover, she can suggest that the couple arrange for outside help as soon as the new mother is ready to venture out of the house.

In addition, the cesarean father may have to cope with the mother's delayed reactions to the birth. In fact, since the ". . . cesarean mother may harbor resentment . . . against the baby's father for making her pregnant in the first place, or for not coaching and supporting her well enough. . . ." (Donovan 1977, p. 54), it is important to tell the father to anticipate this reaction and to encourage him to express his feelings about this undeserved hostility, if it occurs. Since this reaction may be delayed for some time, the nurse should plan to maintain continued contact with the family for several months after hospital discharge.

In the area of role function, the data indicate both positive and negative stimuli and resultant behavior. Usually, the cesarean father is able to fulfill his role expectations as a new parent by announcing his child's birth and reporting the mother's condition to relatives and friends. However, the demands of cesarean birth may dampen the joy usually felt by a new father, especially if he is given only the barest details about mother and child. Indeed, the data indicate that some men have had to wait several hours for more than cursory news. The nurse should make certain all information is trasnmitted as soon as possible.

The data also indicate that all too frequently the cesarean father is excluded from the delivery room and prevented from performing his anticipated role as coach. This seems to create a feeling of disappointment and frustration, especially since the reasons for the cesarean birth are often not made clear. Conversely, when the father is with the mother during labor and delivery he may be in a state of need excess in his roles as husband and father. Although the man may lack sufficient information about his wife's progress, he is still expected to support her and initiate attachment with the newborn and, like all new fathers, notify relatives and friends of the baby's birth and the mother's postoperative condition. As pointed out earlier, this situation denies the man's need for nursing care.

All sources of data strongly indicate the parents' need for information about cesarean births. While the decision to deliver a baby by the cesarean method is properly made by the physician, nurses must take responsibility for explaining the reasons for this decision and for providing detailed information about ensuing events. They must also make sure the information is comprehended. The explanations should include what is presently happening and what will happen during the intrapartum and postpartum. This information is best given as a step-by-step description of events as soon as the possibility of a cesarean is known. Ideally, the information should be given to all couples during the antenatal period, since the occurrence of emergency cesarean births has escalated in recent years.

In addition to the description of the factual events surrounding a cesarean birth, there should be discussion of the sensations both the father and the mother are likely to experience and of coping mechanisms they can use to adapt positively to the cesarean. This type of information seems especially important in light of recent research findings. Johnson et al. (1978) have repeatedly found that if discussion of the objective aspects of an experience is coupled with descriptions of typical subjective sensory experiences and appropriate coping behaviors, patients' negative responses to such threatening events as endoscopic examination, breast and pelvic examination, orthopedic cast removal, cholecystectomy, and herniorrhaphy are markedly reduced. In fact, their most recent research revealed that the combined objective and subjective information given to cholecystectomy patients significantly reduced the length of the postoperative hospital stay and the amount of time elapsing before patients ventured from home after discharge. Moreover, sensory information that focused on when, for how long, and how frequently an event would happen reduced the patients' feelings of helplessness during the postoperative period.

While the effects of combined information on cesarean parents has not yet been studied, the consistency of the findings of Johnson et al. and the repeated requests for information noted in the survey sample suggest that giving such information is an appropriate nursing intervention for this client population. Furthermore, it is probable that this type of information will be of great help to cesarean fathers in overcoming need disturbances in all adaptive modes.

Assessment of needs in the interdependence adaptive mode is likely to reveal the father's desire for close and continued contact with his wife as well as his wish to begin a relationship with his newborn child. While the contemporary view of the ideal childbirth experience is often shattered by a cesarean birth, the data indicate that this does not have to be so. Those men who were able to stay with their wives and witness the births of their children expressed a great deal of satisfaction with their experiences. Thus adaptation to loss of the ideal and to other interdependence need deficits can be facilitated by promoting the father's presence throughout the cesarean experience. As patient advocates, nurses have a mandate to encourage any changes in hospital policies required to allow maximum participation in cesarean births.

If conditions are such that the father's presence is at times prohibited or counterindicated by the mother's or baby's health status, the couple should still be together as much as possible throughout the experience. The question of whether or not the father should be present in the case of fetal death is a difficult one. Although no objective research is available upon which to base an answer, informal evidence suggests that his presence helps him to see that everything possible was done to save the baby's life and allows him to comfort and receive comfort from his wife.

Despite the lack of rigorous research, most parents, many health professionals, and almost all authors of books about childbirth advocate parent-infant contact immediately after the baby's birth, to promote bonding. Obviously, this is greatly facilitated by the father's presence during the cesarean birth. However, some anecdotal material indicates that the current emphasis on bonding may result in parental worry and even guilt if immediate contact is not made with the newborn. This situation seems to arise from confusion of the bonding process, which occurs immediately after birth, with the attachment process, which occurs over time. Thus it is crucial that the nurse explain the reality of the situation to the parents, with emphasis on the place of immediate contact in the parents' overall process of establishing a relationship with their child. Again, this discussion could be initiated during the antenatal period, especially during prepared childbirth classes.

CONCLUSION

The central thesis of this chapter is that the cesarean father is a legitimate client in need of nursing care. The Roy Adaptation Model provides one framework for organizing knowledge needed by nurses who wish to deliver high-quality health care to these men. Analysis from this conceptual perspective of data from various sources on the cesarean father suggests several possible need disturbances as well as general strategies for promoting positive adaptation. Systematic nursing research is now needed to determine specific innovations in the nursing care of this client population.

ACKNOWLEDGMENT

The assistance of Billie Carlson, RN in the recruitment of subjects and collection of data for the survey reported in this chapter is gratefully acknowledged.

REFERENCES

Affonso DD: Complications of labor and delivery. In Clark AL, Affonso DD (eds), Childbearing: A Nursing Perspective, 2nd ed. Philadelphia, Davis, 1979.
Donovan B: The Cesarean Birth Experience. Boston, Beacon, 1977

Donovan B, Allen RM: The cesarean birth method. Obstet Gynecol Neonatal Nurs 6 (6):37–48, 1977

Haller KB, Reynolds MA, Horsley JA: Developing research-based innovation protocols: Process, criteria, and issues. Res Nurs Health 2:45–51, 1979

Harris JK: Self-care is possible after cesarean delivery. Nurs Clin North Am 15:191–204, 1980

Johnson JE, Fuller SS, Endress MP, Rice VH: Altering patients' responses to surgery: An extension and replication. Res Nurs Health 1:111–21, 1978

Kiernan B, Scoloveno MA: Fathering. Nurs Clin North Am 12:481–90, 1977

MacLaughlin L: First-time fathers' childbirth experience. J Nurse Midwifery 25 (3):17–21, 1980

Marut JS: The special needs of the cesarean mother. Am J Maternal–Child Nurs 3:202–206, 1978

Moore ML: Realities in Childbearing. Philadelphia, Saunders, 1978

Persson JC, Troup WR, Troup RC, et al: Opinions. Should fathers attend cesarean section deliveries? AORN J 28:434–35, 438–39, 442–43, 446–47, 450–51, 454, 1978

Reeder SR, Mastroianni L Jr., Martin LL, Fitzpatrick E: Maternity Nursing, 13th ed. Philadelphia, Lippincott, 1976

Reynolds CB: Updating care of cesarean section patients. J Obstet Gynecol Neonatal Nurs 6 (4):48–51, 1977

Roy C: Introduction to Nursing: An Adaptation Model. Englewood Cliffs, N.J., Prentice–Hall, 1976

SECTION IV

Facilitation
of Adjustment

CHAPTER 8

Preparing Expectant Parents for a Cesarean Birth: The Role of the Childbirth Educator

Nancy Newport

The primary aim in preparing couples for cesarean birth is to promote feelings of safety and comfort concerning body, self, and the family's anticipated experience. Bolstering the parents' independence and confidence in their ability to solve problems encourages them to make use of their own inner resources in coping with the anticipated birth and resultant parenthood.

PREPARED CESAREAN CHILDBIRTH CLASSES

Who Attends Classes?

Most expectant parents who participate in cesarean childbirth classes are multiparas who have experienced one or more previous cesareans. However, there are some primiparas who either suspect a cesarean delivery or who want to be prepared for birthing no matter which route it takes. There are also those expectant mothers with no previous cesarean history who have been told by their obstetricians that cesarean delivery will probably be necessary. Included in that group are diabetic mothers and mothers with babies in breech or transverse lie positions, suspected pelvic insufficiency, or placenta previa. As more and more physicians openly question the advisability of vaginal delivery and express these concerns to the expectant family, many parents-to-be choose to prepare for the possibility of a cesarean delivery. This creates a unique situation for the cesarean childbirth educator. She faces a group of parents ranging from multiparas, who may have a history of more than one cesarean delivery, to primiparas, who are totally unprepared for this mode of delivery.

Due to the didactic content, there is a certain structure and form to the classes, but each series must be tailored to accommodate the needs of the couples enrolled in that particular series. With skill and flexibility, the cesarean childbirth educator can bring this diverse group together (Donovan and Allen 1977).

Group Needs of Cesarean Parents

Instructors in prepared cesarean childbirth classes find that the needs of the group vary from class to class, but that each group demonstrates to some degree the following universal needs in addition to the needs felt by couples expecting vaginal delivery. Couples should always be contacted before the series begins to assess the felt needs of each individual class member.

The Need to Air Feelings—Most class participants in cesarean classes have already had at least one cesarean birth. Because their previous cesarean experiences were probably unplanned, they may have many unresolved feelings. These feelings may have been suppressed until the current pregnancy and the hormonal changes inherent in the childbearing process brings them to the surface again. The need to sort out these ambivalent feelings is great, and yet many couples do not begin this process until they are in a group setting. Some couples discover things they did not know about each other in the process of interacting with other group members.

The Need for Support—Support derived from sharing experience and concern with other mothers and fathers is more valuable than that given by the instructor. Classes should provide ample time for group exchange and discussion. It is comforting for class members to see that others share many of the same fears and concerns. Of even more significance is the realization that many of the strong feelings of guilt or anger that the couples may have harbored since their previous birth experiences are normal and very common. The realization that they are not alone provides enormous relief and support. This exchange is possible when an accepting and supportive atmosphere is created by the instructor.

The Need for Information—The sharing of educational information is important, but this is not the first priority in childbirth preparation. What childbirth preparation should *not* produce is a feeling of anxiety and increased dependence on authority-figure advice due to an information overdose. The information shared in the class should not be so extensive or presented as so essential that the participants feel that they will never make it alone if they cannot assimilate or absorb it all. Many couples come to class already overloaded with information, much of which is confusing and irrelevant. They need assistance in sorting out the information they do have, keeping that which is meaningful for them for their current pregnancies.

There is a need, however, for accurate basic information about what is going to happen to the mother's body, how it will feel, why specific procedures are done and how to best handle the discomfort of some procedures. The more one understands what to expect and why to expect it, the greater one's coping powers are. The fact that some of the couples in the class may have already experienced one cesarean delivery is no reason to assume that they know what happened to them. Many cesarean parents understand very little of what they have experienced. In fact, there may be many misconceptions that need to be clarified.

The Need for Independence and a Sense of Confidence—Perhaps the greatest needs are for independence and a sense of confidence. These needs produce the greatest challenge to the childbirth educator. They are not met with the mere feeding of information, nor are they met solely by an accepting and supportive atmosphere. More is required to make class members independent and confident in solving the problems of cesarean childbirth. Promotion of independence and a sense of confidence lies at the core of effectiveness in cesarean childbirth preparation.

Group Process

Ambience—Cesarean childbirth classes should be structured to include both expectant parents. When the mother is alone, she should be encouraged to bring a significant other to class, preferably one who will be able to share the birth experience with her. Classes should be small—no more than six to eight couples—to allow the group to develop an identity over the short 4-week period. The smallness of the group is also an enticement to greater group discussion.

The ambience of the class setting should be conducive to learning and sharing. An ideal environment would be a large, carpeted room with slightly dimmed lighting, good ventilation, comfortable seating, and easy access to rest-room facilities. Seating should be arranged in a circular pattern, and class participants should feel free to get comfortable by removing their shoes, sitting on the floor, or to do whatever helps them feel relaxed and therefore attentive and receptive.

Couples should be encouraged to wear comfortable clothing; mothers should be reminded to wear slacks, as each class period will devote time to practicing breathing and relaxation exercises. If carpeting is not available, they should also bring a blanket.

Each class period can be from 2 to 3 hours in length. This should be predetermined by the teacher and made clear to the class at the beginning of the course. Classes should begin and end on time. If group discussion continues past the contracted time, the teacher should make it clear that the class is over but that those who wish to continue with the discussion may remain with her. This permits those who have time constraints to depart without feeling that they are disrupting the group.

Principles—Three basic principles of group process should be established by the instructor from the beginning:

1. There are no right or wrong feelings or ideas. Every class member is free to express himself and others can agree or disagree. Each thought expressed is valued and respected.
2. One of the main functions of the class series is to enable parents to make their own decisions and to promote a sense of confidence in their ability to do so. The group will explore ways of problem solving and decision making. There are many alternatives available in any decision. Exploring the consequences of each alternative helps a person to make his own decision.
3. The objectives for the program are set by the group rather than by the leader. If there is disagreement over the discussion topics, each idea is pursued in the order that the group establishes. The leader makes suggestions as needed. (Swendsen et al. 1978).

Communication—Communication involves two different but interdependent kinds of symbols: the deliberate impressions that one gives (verbal communication) and the less deliberate impressions that one creates (nonverbal communication). Verbal communication occurs through the spoken word. It is easier to mask or hide true feelings in verbal communication. Nonverbal communication is the way we influence others without the use of words. We all express ourselves through our actions and these actions make impressions on others. Nonverbal language is partly taught (the handshake, the smile, tiping of the hat, and the bow), partly instinctive (the cry and the laugh), and partly imitative (wearing clothes in the latest fashion). Both verbal and nonverbal communication can be used for deception, but a person cannot sustain deception in both, and eventually will concentrate on the more familiar and controllable aspect of communication—speech. Thus actions—the nonverbal form of communicating—become more indicative of true feeling (Collins 1977 pp. 62-3). Teacher observations take on greater relevance when these principles are understood.

WORKING THROUGH PAST NEGATIVE
BIRTHING EXPERIENCES

There is a tendency to equate parity with experience and confidence. In reality, the mother who has experienced a previous unplanned cesarean birth may be carrying a heavy burden of fear, anger, and guilt. She may have lost confidence in herself and her body. This woman has unfinished business. It is likely that her past experience did not permit her to express her negative feelings and so she pushed them "under the rug," but the present pregnancy causes these unresolved feelings to surface. If these feelings cannot be dealt with and resolved in positive ways, the multipara with poor birthing experience (MPBE) will "hear" the information in the class with a distorted viewpoint and won't learn well. In general, the past will color her expectations for the upcoming childbirth experience (Edwards 1976).

It is the task of the childbirth educator to assist this woman in integrating her past episode into her current consciousness so that her feelings can be resolved (Edwards 1976). The childbirth educator may ask for a synopsis of past birthing experience. Each story will provide the teacher with valuable data. Working through negative feelings is a process that may last throughout the entire class series. But there is a main focus to the process—to say goodbye to the past sad happenings. Only when these feelings have been relinquished can the individual begin to focus on the present and future, and on the process of preparation for the upcoming cesarean birth. The old negative "tapes" or messages must be erased and replaced with positive ones.

To allow this catharsis to take place, the cesarean childbirth educator must first create a safe, nonthreatening environment. However, the temptation to get overinvolved in a sad recounting—and especially in an angry recounting—must be curbed. Eric Berne (1974) has described a "game" which he calls "Aw, Ain't It Awful," sometimes seen operating in childbirth classes. In this game, someone overtly expresses distress but covertly derives some gratification at the prospect of people feeling sorry for his or her misfortune.

It is not productive for the couple involved, for the other members of the class, or for the teacher to dwell on bad experiences by expressing a sense of outrage and injustice at the way past birthings were managed. A more productive way to handle the emotion-charged stories is to acknowledge them with such comments as "It sounds as though you had a very difficult time." or "How did you feel about that?" The class must not be allowed to wallow in pity, and each story should be followed up with a query by the teacher of "Can this experience be improved for you? What aspects do you want to change for the better?"

Emphasis should be on the upcoming birth and on a realization that this time the parents will have tools and support not available to them previously which will help them toward a fulfilling birth experience (Donovan and Allen 1977).

THE PASSIVE INDIVIDUAL

Most couples who take cesarean classes are very consumer-minded and quite verbal and active in their quest for a satisfying birthing experience. However, there are also individuals or couples in classes who do not see themselves as participants, much less activists, in their cesarean childbirth. They do not want choices. They do not want to make decisions. They have placed themselves in their doctors' care and relinquished all responsibility. They do not seek. They do not reach. They passively allow. A passive individual or one who responds passively to this situation is relinquishing control to "doctor knows best" magic.

J. B. Rotter (1966) introduced a theory of locus of control, based on the individual's tendency to perceive life events as being a consequence of his or her own actions (*internal* perspective) or as being beyond personal control (*external* perspective).

Because externals tend to view themselves as controlled by fate or powerful others, childbirth classes may tend to confuse and frustrate them. Being in control is not valued by externals, and classes may even be counterproductive. Using the Rotter scale (internals and externals), it was found that those internals who were prepared for childbirth experienced more satisfying birth experiences. With externals, however, satisfaction may be lowered by preparation classes (Willmuth et al. 1978).

Some research indicates that locus of control is not necessarily a determining factor in a couple's choice of childbirth preparation (Windwer 1977). Therefore, each childbirth preparation class will probably have a mix of both types of personalities. Working effectively with externally oriented individuals is a challenge. The teacher may feel angry and frustrated with such people. She may feel that they are "copping out." She may even want to "rescue" them. The following case is an example of this.

> Susan B., 23 years old, was a 37-week multipara with poorly controlled diabetes. She was hospitalized by her obstetrician to watch her blood sugar and her estriol levels. After several days in the hospital she called her cesarean childbirth instructor in tears. Her doctor would not answer her questions. She didn't know what was going on. She was worried about herself and her unborn baby. She missed her family at home. Her doctor had informed her that her husband could not be with her for the cesarean delivery because she was to be given a general anesthetic. She had counted on having a family-centered birth. She found her doctor cold and unresponsive to her concerns. Although she was ambulatory, and there were other good hospitals in town, and she knew of other supportive obstetricians, she could not bring herself to check out and get another doctor. She called her teacher every day in tears and each day her teacher listened and reinforced her options. But Susan re-

mained hospitalized and eventually delivered. She had a poor birth experience and had not yet recovered from it 8 months later. She eventually separated from her husband.

Susan was overwhelmed and immobilized. She was angry, yet very frightened. And she could not or would not help herself. Yet she asked others for help daily.

Susan was playing "Poor Me" and encouraging others to rescue her from her plight. "Rescue" is tempting for most health care providers, but it must be avoided. Susan B. did not see herself as having any control over her dilemma. She was angry and frustrated with the control her doctor had over her life situation and sought out her childbirth teacher as someone she wanted to "take over" for her.

The following case provides another example.

Margaret J., 28 years old, multipara, was in her 24th week of pregnancy when her blood pressure began to rise from her normal 120/80 to 136/90. Her physician told her she was "nervous" and put her on Valium 2 mg t.i.d. She did not feel nervous and saw no reason to take the medication. She consulted her cesarean instructor about the hazards of Valium to the fetus. But when she called her physician to say that she did not want to take the medication, her doctor informed her that if she did not take the medication, he would no longer be her doctor. She took the Valium.

Margaret J. showed concern regarding the taking of medication during pregnancy, but when forced to make a choice, she could not. There is a limit to the role of childbirth educator. The educator can teach, counsel, listen, and support but in the final analysis the individual must determine the course he or she will follow.

Anxiety

This author has counselled many women overwhelmed by pregnancy and all the consumer issues and choices available. This feeling often presents as passivity. Facts are not the basis of fears and it is inappropriate to present them as a panacea for anxiety. However, facts can help parents cope better with anxiety, and they can make choices less overwhelming (Cassidy 1974).

*The process of childbirth reduces
the strength and cohesion of the
ego, and while the pregnant woman
may dread the physical damage to
her body, she must intuitively sense*

that this damage will go deeper.
These intuitive fears will reinforce
her sense of helplessness; for, again,
something will happen to her that
she cannot control. (Cassidy 1974)

The amount of anxiety exhibited by an individual in cesarean classes depends on many factors. The basic personality organization (which includes the way one looks at the locus of control as discussed earlier) affects the anxiety level. Those with familiar and workable coping mechanisms have more tools at hand to deal with the unique anxieties of pregnancy and impending childbirth. The general adaptation toward the present pregnancy also affects the degree of anxiety, as does the positive or negative attitude toward the conception of the child.

Our society is becoming more consumer-oriented and this increases the pressures on the childbearing family. The move toward more family-centered cesarean birth is very healthy, but it certainly brings greater responsibility for the family.

CONTENT

Beginning (Class One)

The cesarean childbirth educator asks each class participant to introduce him- or herself and to include name, due date, previous cesarean births, ages of children, and reasons for taking the class. Common responses to the last question are: (1) so that the parents can share the delivery; (2) to learn all about the cesarean; (3) to be prepared this time; (4) to be awake for this birth; and (5) to be less afraid.

This sharing of personal information provides the instructor and other group members an initial assessment of each individual and establishes a sense of each individual's dignity and worth (Smith 1978).

The cesarean childbirth educator observes body communication and receives an impression of how the parents feel about themselves and their anticipated experience. Are they enthusiastic, anxious, passive, bored, optimistic, angry, realistic? Within each brief statement, the person conveys something of him- or herself. The instructor should participate in this sharing process by revealing her name, describing her training, and sharing her qualifications with the group. In this way she can begin to negotiate a contract with the members of the group (Smith 1978, p. 51).

Shells and masks are out in full
array during the first childbirth

*class on the part of both the teach-
ers and the learners. It is an occasion for testing. The teacher is
concerned with facilitation; with
informing not too much, not too
little; and with a general lack of
ease common to meeting a new
group of people. Students are not
sure they want to be here. They are
interested in the character of their
attending classmates: are they
square, straight, nuts, people like
them? They wonder if the teacher
knows what she/he's about because
they're not quite sure what a childbirth educator is, unless their
friends have sent them. (Edwards
1976, p. 33)*

Nutrition—Adequate nutrition is important for all pregnant women, but for
women anticipating a surgical birth it takes on even more importance. Tissue
healing after a cesarean birth is directly affected by the mother's eating
habits. The well-being of the baby is also dependent on the mother's prenatal diet (Brewer 1976).

Women need to understand what their bodies need and then *cooperate* with
their bodies. The single most important tool for having a healthy pregnancy is
in the pregnant woman's own hands: the decisions she makes about what she
eats on a daily basis. Ultimately, this decision-making process has to do with
her goals and motivations within her own life. The class discussion of nutrition is not intended to describe how many vitamins and minerals are found in
each food. This is not the way to create interest in and response to the value
of eating good foods. The instructor must deal with the immediate concerns
of the expectant mother: concern about the baby's well-being and concern
about her own life, safety, and ability to recover from the cesarean. Dealing
with women where they are enables the instructor to mesh goals. The discussion about the importance of good eating during pregnancy then takes on
relevance.

Tests of Fetal Maturity—Most cesarean families experience one or more of
these tests before delivery, and a thorough discussion of each is an important
part of the first class. Since many couples in class have had some experience
with these tests in previous deliveries, the instructor may ask for them to
share what they remember with the group. This provides a springboard for
more detailed discussion.

The test that produces the most anxiety and yet one of the most important for scheduled cesareans is *amniocentesis*. Used to determine fetal lung maturity toward the end of pregnancy, it is usually quite misunderstood. Many expectant parents are quite anxious about the fetus "getting stuck or jabbed" by the cannula as it is inserted. Mothers fear the insertion of the cannula into their abdomen. A woman is instinctively protective of her abdomen during pregnancy. Explaining the procedure and the value of the results can alleviate much anxiety. A concept that is generally poorly understood by expectant parents is the difference in fetal age and fetal maturity. Explaining to the class the difference between the two will also clarify the relevance of the L/S ratio done by amniocentesis.

Signs of Labor—Many cesarean mothers are choosing to go into labor before having their babies delivered by cesarean. And labor can occur even for mothers with scheduled cesarean deliveries. It is important, therefore, to cover completely the signs of labor. A discussion of what to do should labor occur will be valuable and hopefully prevent panic on the part of the couple should spontaneous labor or rupture of membranes occur.

Relaxation Breathing Techniques—Learning to relax and release muscle tension is important to cesarean parents. There are many occasions during the birth and recovery period when this knowledge is useful, as in:

1. Pelvic examinations.
2. Amniocentesis procedures.
3. Spontaneous labor.
4. The insertion of the catheter for epidural or spinal anesthesia.
5. The insertion of the Foley catheter.
6. The insertion of the IV catheter.
7. Providing fundal pressure during delivery.
8. Coping with pain or discomfort from coughing, moving, gas pains, and removal of sutures or clips in the postpartal period.

Abdominal Tightening—This simple technique, described by Donovan and Allen (1977), is very effective in reducing or eliminating distention. It should be initiated within 1 hour after delivery and done five times an hour every waking hour thereafter. Coaches should learn the technique and be prepared to remind the mother. The first few times this is done the mother may find it difficult, but it becomes easier each time. The technique is as follows.

1. Place both hands over the incision to form a splint. A small pillow may be placed directly over the abdomen to further support the incision, if this makes the mother feel more comfortable and secure. On top of the pillow, both hands should be joined just over the incision.
2. Inhale deeply, exhale completely.

3. Inhale deeply again, holding the breath and tightening the abdominal muscles simultaneously.
4. Count slowly to five before exhaling and releasing abdominal muscles. Relax.
5. Repeat five times an hour when awake. (Donovan and Allen 1977)

Introduction of the Pain Wheel (Figure 1)—The pain wheel can be made of red felt and placed on a board. As the different tools of cesarean childbirth preparation are introduced, corresponding parts of the pain wheel are covered. One segment is left uncovered to realistically demonstrate that some pain will be experienced, although most of the pain can be eased through the use of the already discussed tools.

The Birthday! (Class Two)

This second class focuses on the hospital procedures involved in the preoperative period as well as on the birth procedures. The instructor discusses the hospital admission procedures and all the preparations that are part of predelivery. This discussion should take into consideration the policies and procedures of the particular locale. But changes in policies only occur as a result of consumer pressure. Therefore, discussion of dissatisfaction with present policies should be handled realistically. As the client advocate, the instructor can provide valuable tools for couples to use in discussions with doctors and hospitals to effect change in policies.

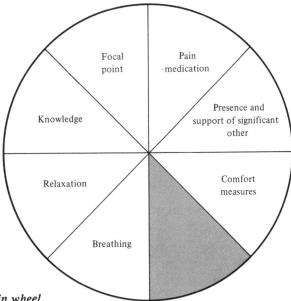

FIGURE 1. The pain wheel.

*Changing Procedures—*A few procedures that have changed drastically in recent years are:

1. Hospital admission policies: many hospitals now allow admission the morning of the scheduled cesarean instead of the night before.
2. Use of premedication: the practice of medicating women with tranquilizers 1 hour or so before delivery is being reevaluated. Research is being done to determine the impact on the newborn. Mothers report feeling "so sleepy" that they do not remember or participate in the birth in any meaningful way. Bonding is difficult if not impossible under this condition. Many mothers are requesting that they have no premedication at all that would alter their sense of awareness.
3. Choice of anesthesia: general anesthesia is no longer routinely used for cesarean deliveries. Epidural and spinal anesthesia is now used more often, allowing the mother to be "present" at birth. The anesthesiologist plays a great role in each family's birth experience. Instructors should discuss the role of the anesthesiologist and encourage parents to request to speak with the anesthesiologist before the delivery.
4. Presence of the father during delivery: more hospitals are becoming aware of the importance of keeping the family unit intact during the birth process. Fragmentation of the family at such a vulnerable time can have far-reaching implications. Fathers are given the opportunity to witness and welcome the birth of the baby and to support and encourage the mother during the delivery. He is the mother's advocate and protects her interests and wishes when she cannot do so for herself. The father's role is discussed at length in classes that have families who plan to remain together during their upcoming cesarean births.
5. Evaluation of each newborn: when not medically contraindicated, the infant is allowed to remain with his or her parents. This enhances closeness and permits bonding of the family to begin. It also allows for increased tactile stimulation of the infant who has not gone through the birth canal.

The delivery procedures are discussed at length and a slide presentation of a cesarean birth is shown. Instructors might find it helpful to bring a Foley and spinal or epidural catheter to class for inspection by couples.

Group discussion should be encouraged by asking the class to explain certain procedures. The following questions are examples of those the instructor might ask about the Foley catheter. "What do you remember about insertion of the bladder catheter? How did you use your breathing in doing that? What type of breathing? Was it helpful? What else helped you relax during this procedure?" The instructor should then talk about the procedure itself. Understanding the procedures and seeing the catheters used for delivery makes it easier to cope with the anxiety and fear that normally accompanies surgical interventions.

When the delivery is described, the time elements for each phase should be included. Many couples think the actual delivery takes hours instead of minutes.

The childbirth educator should not be afraid to say "I don't know" if a class member asks a question that she cannot answer. She can let the class know that she will find the information requested by the next session, making a note of it right away so she does not forget to follow up.

Hospital Recovery (Class Three)

In this class, discussion of the physical changes occuring during the recovery period is coupled with discussion of the realistic expectations women should have of themselves and the hospital staff and of how to facilitate recovery. It is important to stress that each person recuperates differently and at her own rate. The amount of pain and discomfort experienced also varies with the individual.

Relaxation breathing exercises should be rehearsed again and their relevance reinforced.

During this class, exercises are done to increase communication between mother and father. One of the most important exercises is to flush out "hidden agendas." These are defined as preconceived ideas of how events will happen and how people will react to those events. Many times, without realizing it, individuals assume that their partners are aware of how they are imagining the birth, the early recovery, and parenting. When these ideas are discussed, the partners are often amazed at the assumptions that have been made. It is usually very enlightening for the parents to individually fill in open-ended phrases and then discuss their responses in the privacy of their own homes. Following are some examples of such open-ended phrases.

MOTHER

1. When I am in the delivery room, _____.
2. When I am in the recovery room, _____.
3. When I am in the recovery room, the baby _____.
4. While I am hospitalized, _____.
5. When we arrive home, the responsibility for this baby _____.
6. When the baby cries in the middle of the night, _____.
7. The housework _____.

FATHER:

1. When you/we are in the delivery room, _____.
2. When you/we are in the recovery room, _____.
3. When you/we are in the recovery room, the baby _____.
4. While you are hospitalized, _____.

5. When we arrive home, the responsibility for the baby _____.
6. When the baby cries at night, _____.
7. The housework _____.

The possibilities are endless.

The class ends with a showing of a film—such as "A Shared Cesarean Beginning," a family-centered film depicting the joys of the birth of the baby as well as some surgical procedures to clarify the process for the family. A discussion follows the film.

Home Recovery (Class Four)

Postpartum Adjustment—In this class period, the physical and emotional adjustments of the mother and father and other siblings are discussed. Breastfeeding is also covered, as well as sexual readjustment, birth control, and any other topic the group wants to explore. The instructor serves as a facilitator in this class. The group determines the topics discussed. If sexual adjustment is not brought up by the group, the instructor should bring it up. Expectant parents usually have many unanswered questions about sex, but these questions may be difficult or embarrassing to ask. One of the most discussed topics concerns preparation of the older child for the arrival of a new sibling.

Mastering the Parenting Role—Discussion of parenting is an important part of this class. Mastery and integration of the parenting role are not endpoints, but a continuum. Before role mastery can be attained, two intermediate steps must first be taken: role clarity and role taking.

Role clarity requires an understanding of one's parenting role. For couples who are expecting their second or third child, role clarity involves an understanding of their expanding parenting role. This process varies with each individual's own life experiences, needs, and feelings.

Role taking involves the ability to "walk in another's shoes," imaginatively taking the place or point of view of another in order to develop cooperative activity. There are several variations to this theme, as follows:

1. The mother and father assume one another's roles by discussing how each can best assist and support the other while still meeting their own personal needs.
2. Both parents assume the role of the infant and discuss how they might assist their baby in meeting his needs.
3. Both parents assume the roles of their present children to gain insight into their feelings and needs, especially with the arrival of the newborn into the existing family unit.

In working toward these two steps, an effective strategy is role rehearsal, whereby the individual imagines or acts out an experience that may take place in a role and anticipates the responses of the significant others. Situations are presented to the group and the couples discuss how they might respond and react in that situation. In role rehearsal the individual works through the role and identifies several ways of handling specific situations before they happen. This is an important prelude to role taking and helps to plan the course of future actions.

Another useful tool in learning to master the parenting role is the role model. Each person has used role models in the past to form the behaviors and values expected in a given role. The childbirth educator serves as a very significant role model by actively discussing problems and exploring alternatives. Class members learn from this example. Each family may be expected to have internal role models—parents, relatives, friends, and professionals. Most couples have received several different messages about parenting and about expanding the parenting role. By inviting to class a mother and father from a previous series who have recently had a cesarean birth, the educator provides class members with two more role models (Swendsen 1978).

Conclusion of the Class Series—The last class ends with plans for a reunion after each couple has given birth and presentation of certificates to all couples who have completed the series.

Positive Effects of Adequate Preparation

Tools for coping and relaxing and knowledge with which to reduce the unknowns provide expectant parents with the ability to maintain control throughout childbirth. This enhanced ability to cope enables the couple to focus in on present events—to stay "in the now," so to speak. A high level of anxiety would make this focus impossible.

The ability to function in the present frees the parents for a greater appreciation and enjoyment of the childbirth experience. Mothers who are adequately prepared for birthing are often able to remember the experience with more accuracy of detail than mothers unprepared for the sequence of events surrounding their childbirths.

Memories of cesarean childbirth are most positive for parents who have had adequate prenatal preparation for birthing. Families experiencing planned cesarean childbirth that has included prepared cesarean childbirth classes find they have much more positive feelings about their birthings, and they attribute this to their level of preparation for the cesarean and for unexpected events.

Postoperative recovery is usually smoother and less traumatic for the prepared mother. Mastery of the tools of breathing and relaxation makes it easier to cope with anxiety and pain during recovery. For the mother who understands why she feels pain and realizes its limits, there is a decreased tendency to panic or remain immobile in bed. Prolonged use of narcotics, combined with much anxiety and muscle tension, makes for a very unpleasant and unhealthy recuperative period. Realistic preparation provides good preventive as well as therapeutic nursing intervention.

These data concerning new parents' perceptions of the positive effects of adequate preparation were collected by the author through open-ended interviews and through responses from over 60 couples to a questionnaire formulated by the author.

INFORMATION ABOUT CESAREAN BIRTH PROVIDED IN TRADITIONAL CHILDBIRTH CLASSES

Today more expectant parents than ever are taking some type of childbirth preparation class. The growing focus on childbirth as natural and family-oriented has created this demand for couple preparation and involvement. Couples come to classes for many reasons, but one reason many come is to learn how to orchestrate their childbirth experience with a minimum of medical intervention. However, statistics tell us that a certain percentage of these families will experience unexpected cesarean delivery, requiring much medical intervention.

It is doubtful that many expectant parents see themselves in these statistics. The age-old belief that "That won't happen to me; things like that happen to other people." applies to anticipated childbirth experiences as well as it does to getting hit by a Mack truck. So how can we anticipate the unanticipated? First we have to change our thinking—open up to consideration of alternate directions that the childbirth experience might take. Unless a couple can envision many possibilities rather than locking into a preplanned step-by-step birth experience, it is impossible for the childbirth educator to effectively prepare that couple for unanticipated events.

Denial is one of the most frequently encountered defense mechanisms. Denial is used to help us keep a check on overwhelming anxiety. We can only handle so much anxiety at one time without feeling very uncomfortable at best and immobile at worst. The childbirth educator must therefore be aware of what denial is and how it works before she can effectively plan how to "break through." Decreasing the fear of the unknown is a good beginning. This opens the mind to unwanted but possible deviations in the desired "ideal" experience.

Approaches

Some approaches that have been used effectively in traditional class settings to stimulate discussion and absorption of cesarean childbirth possibilities are the following.

1. The childbirth educator discusses the potentiality of a cesarean birth throughout the classes. She weaves information about cesarean childbirth into the class content and discusses it frequently. In the classes that use a simulated labor as part of the content, she carries labor to a certain point and then says, "Now your doctor tells you that you must have a cesarean delivery." This forces the couples' minds to shift gears, so to speak, and they must quickly decide how to deal with this unexpected turn of events. This can generate quite a bit of discussion as each couple then determines what choices to make in the brief period of time available before the delivery. This simulated experience has proven very valuable for many couples who found themselves in exactly that position at the time of the actual delivery. The practice in shifting their thinking helped them to do just that when the time came. This has also been helpful for couples who planned for cesarean birth and had vaginal deliveries at the last minute.

2. Some childbirth educators make it a practice to distribute small squares of paper to each couple. This is done by having each couple blindly choose a square of paper from a box. Each paper has either the words "vaginal birth" or "cesarean birth" printed on it. The percentage of "cesarean birth" papers is closely correlated with the cesarean birth rate in that locality. Group discussion follows as couples share their feelings about the possibility of cesarean birth.

3. Class participants are asked to complete the phrases independently. After completion, the responses are discussed.

   "I probably won't have a cesarean because ＿＿＿＿＿＿＿＿＿＿＿＿＿＿＿
   ＿＿＿＿＿＿＿＿＿＿＿＿＿＿＿＿＿."

   "I might have a cesarean because ＿＿＿＿＿＿＿＿＿＿＿＿＿＿＿＿＿＿＿
   ＿＿＿＿＿＿＿＿＿＿＿＿＿＿＿＿＿."

   "The worst thing about having a cesarean would be ＿＿＿＿＿＿＿＿＿
   ＿＿＿＿＿＿＿＿＿＿＿＿＿＿＿＿＿."

   "The best things about having a cesarean would be ＿＿＿＿＿＿＿＿＿
   ＿＿＿＿＿＿＿＿＿＿＿＿＿＿＿＿＿."

4. Another technique often used by the educator is to invite a cesarean couple from one of her previous classes to speak to her present class. These parents share their birth experience with the group. Of particular importance is the fact that the parents, in their own words, say, "We were in this class, too, and we did not think that we would have a

cesarean, but we did. You can learn from us that it is important to be prepared for alternate experiences."

The childbirth educator should use discretion in choosing the cesarean couple that will speak. The couple should be realistic, cohesive, and healthy. It is not necessary for the couple to have had a totally positive experience, but neither should this be a forum for the unburdening of unresolved anger and hostility.

Content

How much and what kind of information on cesearean birth should be given in traditional childbirth classes? If the information is woven into the fiber of each class period, it is more easily assimilated and also acts as a tool of "de-sensitization." In this fashion much valuable information can be imparted. Essential information includes:

1. Reasons for cesarean deliveries.
2. Types of incisions.
3. Types of anesthesia and the significance of each.
4. Such procedures as starting an IV, use of the Foley catheter, administration of anesthesia.
5. The recovery period.
6. Realistic expectations of family-centered cesarean care in that locality.
7. Cesarean support-group resources.

The Attitude of the Childbirth Educator

In traditional childbirth classes, the childbirth educator who is committed to the goal of preparing couples for birth (no matter what route birthing follows) is faced with the challenge of helping expectant parents to consider alternate directions that the childbirth experience might take. The attitude of the educator plays a vital role in the couples' ability to accept this information. The teacher must be aware of and evaluate her own feelings about childbirth. Does she impart an attitude of success or of failure? Are feelings of success equated with uncomplicated, unmedicated childbirth? Are feelings of failure equated with complicated, medicated, or surgical birth? It should be obvious that negative attitudes are detrimental to the entire purpose of childbirth preparation. To prepare couples for unanticipated events, the childbirth educator must first be comfortable with the reality that an agenda for birthing cannot be planned in advance. No one is granted a guarantee, not even expectant parents who have worked hard and faithfully to master the breathing techniques, followed all the doctor's orders, and read all the books and who feel that they therefore "deserve" a good experience. The childbirth educator must also realize that she is not a coach, the class is not a team, and there is no scorekeeper, because there is no game to win or lose. She assuredly realizes this on an intellectual level but may not have internalized her perceptions. Many times couples are expected to validate the childbirth educators' definition of "success" by having a "successful" vaginal birth. As a result, couples often view their birth experiences as personal failures because of the disappointment expressed by their teachers upon hearing that they had cesareans.

The childbirth educator cannot provide a good birthing experience for her couples. What she can provide are tools which can greatly enhance the experiences they will have.

Terminology

The terminology used in class can be very significant. The educator should avoid such terms as "natural" and "normal" when referring to vaginal birth, since this usage gives cesarean birth, by contrast, the connotation of "unnatural" or "abnormal." In like fashion, cesarean childbirth should not be referred to as cesarean section. While this is accurate surgical terminology, it does not fully reflect the birth process as the total human experience that it is, involving psychosocial as well as biological considerations. This kind of terminology may contribute to the mother's feeling of failure when a cesarean birth becomes an unexpected reality.

Most classes are composed of couples, and the usual couple is composed of the mother and father. The mother and father may not, however, be married. Single mothers often attend classes and bring a friend or relative of either sex. Thus, each class has its own unique set of relationships. The educator should therefore not fall into a pattern of referring to "husband and wife." This will alienate couples to whom this phrase does not apply.

In speaking of the surgical aspects of a cesarean birth, the educator should refrain from using the word "scar." The correct term is "incision." The word "scar" is a loaded word; that is, it brings forth a negative emotional feeling. It reminds one of such expressions as "scarred for life," "deep scars," "painful scars," and "ugly scars." Other loaded words or terms that should be avoided are the following: "knocked out" (general anesthesia), "shot" (injection), and "pain killer" (pain medication).

Technical language should be avoided when other words more familiar will do. The educator should not volunteer unnecessary details. She should weigh each use of technical detail by asking herself these questions:

1. How will this be of value to the discussion?
2. Will it enhance the clarity of the subject?
3. How can couples make use of this information?

The educator should gauge carefully the technical level of each group. This will influence the way the preceding questions are applied.

THE CHILDBIRTH EDUCATOR
AS THE CLIENT ADVOCATE

The instructor of childbirth education is in an excellent position to help the family to use the health care system more effectively. Expectant parents anticipating a cesarean birth need to be especially aware of the importance of being effective health care consumers, because the health care system will directly impact on their birth experience. The extent and amount of intervention by the system into the cesarean birth process will color the family's feelings of satisfaction or dissatisfaction about the birthing.

For expectant parents, the health care system begins with the obstetrician that they choose. As Dr. Marvin Belsky says:

> There are two things to look for
> in a doctor. The first is his compe-
> tence. The second is his compassion.
> They are separate and yet indi-
> visible. There is no competence
> without caring. The noncaring
> physician is a noncompetent physi-
> cian. A doctor who won't hear
> what his patients have to say, who
> can't communicate ideas and inform,
> who can't express emotion and
> empathize with his patients, is an
> incompetent doctor. (Belsky 1975,
> p. 49)

> The demystification of the medical
> mystique is a job for both doctor
> and patient. The assertive informed
> patient must identify and join
> with those doctors who want to do
> away with the priestly, authoritarian
> aspects of the mystique. (Belsky
> 1975, p. 18)

> It's not enough for the doctor to
> stop playing God. You've got to get
> off of your knees. The best advo-
> cate of patients' rights is you, your-
> self, not committees or laws or
> health and welfare programs. The

*best relationship is the simplest rela-
tionship between doctor and
patient—a questioning, assertive
well-informed patient. (Belsky
1975, p. 31)*

A Guide to Making Effective Health Care Choices for Cesarean Birth

*Choice of Medical Doctor—*This includes choice of obstetrician, gynecologist, pediatrician, family doctor, and specialty doctor. These choices include philosophy of care, flexibility, personality, location, schedule, group or individual practice, hospital affiliations, and gender of physician.

*Choice of Hospital Facilities and Health Care Policies for the Particular Service Required—*One hospital may meet the couple's needs for obstetrics but not for pediatrics. One may be adequate for surgery but not for obstetrics. The cesarean couple may find that a hospital progressive in its philosophy of care for vaginal births may not extend that philosophy to the care of the cesarean family. There are hospitals with birthing rooms for vaginal childbirth where the family is treated as a unit, with minimal intervention and separation. That same hospital may regard cesarean childbirth as a surgical event, preventing the father's presence and participation, isolating the baby for an extended period of time, and responding to the mother as a surgical patient rather than as a new mother. At this time in our country, family-centered maternity care does not always refer to all families. It is the responsibility of the health care consumer to investigate these discrepancies before becoming a victim of them.

*Options in Cesarean Childbirth—*Once the consumer has carefully chosen an obstetrician and hospital, there are still options that can and should be negotiated (see Appendix A). If the consumer has chosen wisely, the doctor and hospital will be flexible enough to allow the admission of individual preferences in planning health care. Each family should determine during the pregnancy exactly what options are important. Because some parents are not even aware of cesarean childbirth options, a list of possible choices should be made available to class members with a discussion of what each option entails. Most couples taking cesarean childbirth classes are most interested in *being together* for the delivery. This is usually the top priority. But the family members should be allowed to individually determine their own priorities. One of the most important roles of the cesarean childbirth instructor is to give "permission" for families to choose what seems best for them.

After carefully deciding on personal priorities, the family should be encouraged to discuss them with the obstetrician to determine how they can be implemented. Priorities are set during pregnancy in anticipation of the child-birth experience, but it is important for instructors to note that those priorities could shift at the time of birthing and families should be prepared for that possibility. As one mother said after delivering her second baby by cesarean, "My cesarean childbirth instructor made me feel that it was O.K. to just do and ask for those things I felt up to at the time."

EVALUATION OF THE CLASS AND
THE CHILDBIRTH EDUCATOR

Every childbirth organization or hospital class should have tools for evaluating the effectiveness of childbirth preparation. These tools should be used for continuing growth and improvement of the class series and the childbirth instructor. A class evaluation form and a teacher evaluation form should be distributed to class members at the end of the series. The success the child-birth educator has in getting class participants to complete and return the forms depends upon the educator's attitude. If the instructor has a healthy regard for constructive criticism and a willingness to grow and improve, then the class will sense this. On the other hand, if the teacher communicates to the class that she is unable or unwilling to accept criticism, then this will affect the quality and quantity of feedback. A poor response can be expected by an instructor who distributes the forms saying, "If you get time, fill these out." On the other hand, a cesarean childbirth educator who routinely devotes several minutes to the importance and significance of the evaluations for the continued growth of the childbirth organization, the class series, and herself can expect an effective response. It is best to distribute the forms in an addressed envelope, reminding the couples that they need only affix a stamp in order to mail them.

The forms should not be mailed directly to the childbirth educator. Couples who wish to be forthright and honest in their assessment should be assured of anonymity. The forms should be unsigned and sent to the Education Chairperson or other designated person. Periodically, each childbirth educator should review all evaluation forms recently received from her classes. Some childbirth educators routinely assess each series in writing, including their own feelings about the class and about what went well, what was not well received, how cohesively the group developed, and any problems encountered. When the evaluation forms return, the educators can compare their own assessments with those of their couples. Some cesarean groups also provide questionnaires to class members. There are three different questionnaires, as follows:

1. A class questionnaire is sent to the couple at the time of registration. They are asked to answer the questions and to bring it with them to the

first class. It focuses on the felt needs of the expectant parents. It also provides information useful to the teacher on how she might best be of help to that family.

2. A "history of previous cesarean birth" questionnaire is sent to those families who have experienced a previous cesarean. This can be used to compare past and future experiences, especially if the first experience was unplanned, with no preparation. This is also brought to the first class.

3. A follow-up questionnaire is mailed to couples after they give birth which requests a detailed account of their experiences and their feelings about the birth.

The following are excerpts from two contrasting birth experiences demonstrating the difference between prepared and unprepared cesarean births.

Unprepared Cesarean Birth

"The birth canal was not adequate to allow passage of our baby. The doctor told us that a vaginal birth might mean brain damage for our child. How could I wish for a vaginal birth after hearing that? I wanted a healthy baby. I was hopeful that a cesarean birth would give us just that.

"Then it was time to begin. I said, 'I want to be awake to see my baby.' The doctor replied, 'Oh, no, I always put my cesarean patients to sleep.' I collapsed in tears. I reached for my husband. The doctor walked out of the room. I then realized I was on a merry-go-round that I was not at all prepared for. I had not asked questions. I had assumed answers. And now it was too late.

"My husband was asked to leave. Leave? This was our baby's birthday. It was time to meet her face to face. And neither of us were to be there. I would be anesthetized. My husband would be outside. Our daughter was to be greeted by strangers.

"In the delivery room I ceased to exist. No one spoke to me. I was trembling. I was cold. I was heartbroken. And I was very scared. My arms were strapped, my body exposed and washed, and a mask comes down over my face. It's over. They tell me I have a healthy baby. They tell me it's a girl. They tell me she is beautiful. They should not have to tell me. I should have been there to see her, to touch her, to hold her. My husband joins me in recovery. We are no longer on the same wavelength. He is very nervous, doesn't know what to say to me, what to do for me. Childbirth classes prepared him to be my coach, to carry us through the birth process together—to be my support. But they stripped him of that role. They made him feel useless. They made him feel helpless. And now he doesn't know what to do for me. He is not prepared for this any more than I am. He is with me, but we're not together. Our baby lies in a nursery somewhere. I ache for her. I feel empty."

Prepared Cesarean Birth

"The obstetrician came in and a mirror was arranged so I could see the delivery. No screen was hung to block my vision. My hands were laid across my chest and a drape laid over them. Erich, sitting next to me, slipped both his hands under the drape to hold mine. 'Ready?' asked the obstetrician. 'Okay,' we answered. The fluorescent lights were switched off. The room felt very cozy. It was quiet. I looked out the window. The snow was falling harder now.

"As we watched the delivery, Erich and I occasionally looked at each other and said, 'Are you okay?' The amniotic sac was pointed out to us before it was incised. Seconds later we saw our baby's face. It was crying and it looked to me as if the obstetrician were yanking it out by the ears. 'Oh! Be careful!' I said. 'Don't hurt it!' The doctor laughed and told me I had no reason to worry. 'It's a boy.' the nurse said, as she laid him on my legs while the placenta was removed.

"The baby was moved to the examining table, which I could see. Erich stroked the baby's head. In a few minutes he was diapered and wrapped in a warm blanket and was being quieted by Erich, who brought him to me to kiss and touch. Someone asked if we'd chosen a name. 'Peter,' we said in unison. I was experiencing considerable discomfort as they closed and did not wish to hold or nurse the baby. Erich carried him next door to the nursery, where he weighed in at 10 pounds. In a very short time Erich, Peter, and I were in the recovery room, where a nurse assisted me with breast feeding and in beginning my exercises. In an hour we were in our private room. That evening our pediatrician arrived to examine Peter and to leave orders that he was not to be separated from me without my consent. A sleeping cot was brought in for Erich (who spent every night at the hospital), and a nursery crib was brought in for Peter. I dozed while Erich held the baby and telephoned relatives and friends. Peter nursed a few times during the night, Erich getting up to change him and bring him to me each time he cried. The floor nurses were more than supportive. The next afternoon I desperately needed some uninterrupted sleep, but Peter was fussy. Despite his own exhaustion, Erich decided to give me some peace and quiet by walking Peter in the hall. The charge nurse found him there, staggering sleepily back and forth outside my door, and said, 'You two look like you could use some rest. Come with me.' She led them to an unoccupied private room nearby, where Erich and Peter curled up together on the bed and fell asleep. Three hours later I awoke from a wonderful nap, rang the buzzer, and asked where my husband and baby were. They'd been asleep for three hours and were still sleeping down the hall in their own room.

"Late in the afternoon Alexandra came to visit us in a special lounge where she was able to hold her new brother. She was fascinated with him and very excited. Erich took her home to put her to bed and returned to the hospital. Peter slept with me all night that night.

"On the fourth morning we ate breakfast, dressed Peter and me, and then

Erich went home to bring Alexandra to the hospital to help take us home. The scenes passing by the car window were snowy and beautiful. We were happy to be going home. How nice to have been able to plan a birth experience which leaves us with only happy memories."

REFERENCES

Belsky MS, Gross L: How to Choose and Use Your Doctor. New York, Arbor House, 1975

Berne E: Games People Play. Portland, Ore., Castle, 1974

Brewer B: What Every Pregnant Woman Should Know. New York, Random House, 1976

Cassidy JE: A nurse looks at childbirth anxiety. J Obstet Gynecol Neonatal Nurs 3 (1):52–54, 1974

Collins M: Communications in Health Care. St. Louis, Mosby, 1977

Donovan B, Allen RM: The cesarean birth method. J Obstet Gynecol Neonatal Nurs 6 (6):37–48, 1977

Edwards M: Communications: Dimensions in Childbirth Education. New York, Catalyst, 1976

Rotter JB: Generalized expectancies for internal versus external control of reinforcement. Psychol Monogr 80:609, 1966

Smith ED: Group process and childbirth education: A position paper. J Obstet Gynecol Neonatal Nurs 7 (4):51–54, 1978

Swendsen LA, Mileis A, Jones D: Role supplementation for new parents: A role mastery plan. Am J Maternal–Child Nurs 3 (2):84–91, 1978

Willmuth R, Weaver L, Boronstein J: Satisfaction with prepared childbirth and locus of control. J Obstet Gynecol Neonatal Nurs 7 (3):33–37, 1978

Windwer C: Relationship among prospective parents' locus of control, social desirability, and choice of psychoprophylaxis. Nurs Research 26 (4):96–99, 1977

APPENDIX A.
CHECKLIST OF CESAREAN BIRTHING CONSIDERATIONS

PLANNING FOR THE BIRTH EXPERIENCE

Is it possible to meet with the anesthesiologist before the delivery to share concerns about and preferences for the types of anesthesia to be used?

Can hospital admission take place the day of the cesarean delivery?

Is there an attending obstetrical anesthesiologist in the hospital at all times?

Is there an attending neonatologist in the hospital at all times and present for each cesarean birth?

SHARING THE CHILDBIRTH EXPERIENCE

Can preoperative sedation be declined by the mother?

Is regional anesthesia routinely used?

Can the father (or other supportive person) be present for the birth experience if he (or she) wishes?

If an emergency situation arises, can the father remain with the mother if he wishes?

Can the father be present for the birth if the mother must be given a general anesthetic?

Can the birth experience center around the family members, with conversation directed toward or around them and their birthing?

If desired, can a mirror be provided to view the birth?

Can the surgical screen be removed if the mother desires?

Is it possible to allow one of the mother's arms to remain free during delivery?

Can the warming table be moved so the parents will be able to see the baby while any initial care is given to the infant?

Is the mother or father permitted to hold the newborn baby immediately following the delivery?

Can the baby's temperature be maintained with a warmed blanket placed over the mother or father?

Can the baby's first bath be delayed until his temperature has stabilized?

Are pictures and/or recordings allowed during delivery?

Is the father allowed to stay with the mother in the delivery room?

BECOMING A FAMILY

Can silver nitrate instillation be delayed until after the initial parent-baby contact?

If the baby is in satisfactory condition, can he or she remain with the parents?

Is breast feeding permitted for the breast-fed baby in Intensive Care Unit (ICU) if nourishment by mouth is possible?

Can the newborn be cared for at the mother's bedside?

Do fathers have unrestricted visiting hours?

Is sibling visitation on the maternity unit allowed each day of the mother's hospital stay?

CHAPTER 9

Loss and Grieving in Cesarean Mothers

Linda S. Birdsong

This chapter considers the special needs of the cesarean mother in relation to her feelings of loss and her grief responses. Feelings of loss and grief are described in general terms and the feelings experienced by all childbearing women are identified, as well as those peculiar to cesarean mothers. Nursing care strategies that assist the cesarean mother in successfully resolving losses are discussed.

LOSS AND GRIEVING

The pioneering and now classic work on loss and grieving was initiated by Lindemann (1944), who found that the loss or anticipated loss of significant human relationships results in predictable and normal grief responses. Subsequent work has attempted to determine what constitutes loss, how individuals cope with loss, and how health care practitioners intervene with persons experiencing loss.

Loss refers to the disappearance of or failure to keep that which one once possessed. More specifically, it is viewed as an actual or potential situation resulting in inaccessibility of a valued person, some aspect of self, or external objects (Gruendemann 1976; Peretz 1970). Feelings of loss may occur through the death of a significant other, through loss of a relationship with a valued other, or through physical and social changes arising from growth and development or from injury or illness (Benoliel 1979; Clark 1979; Highley and Mercer 1978).

Thus loss means that something has been taken away from the self which is valued or has meaning. While loss is probably an unavoidable aspect of life, it leaves the individual with uncomfortable feelings such as deprivation, sorrow, disorganization, and longing (Benoliel 1979; Clark 1979).

These feelings, as well as a sense of suffering and deprivation, are the reactions to loss that are termed grief. While not all loss results in a grief response, this is the normal and expected emotional reaction exhibited by a person who has experienced significant loss (Benoliel 1979; Engel 1962, 1964; Nolan 1974). Each person's perception of loss and the subsequent response depends on several factors, including (Benoliel 1971, 1979; Gruendemann 1976):

1. The perceived significance or meaning attached to the valued lost object or relationship.
2. The perceived nature of the threat caused by the loss.
3. Environmental supports.
4. Individual coping abilities and adaptive capabilities.
5. The extent of personal or social disruption caused by the loss.
6. Cultural and societal norms.
7. The degree to which the lost object, ideal, or relationship can be replaced.
8. The time in life when the loss is encountered.
9. The meaning of the current loss in terms of past experiences.
10. The actions and reactions of others to any changed state resulting from loss.

Loss and grief reactions tend to be manifested in observable and distinct behavior patterns. Benoliel (1979, p. 86) suggests the following sequential response patterns exhibited by the bereaved:

1. A period of shock and numbness.
2. Feelings of fear and anger.
3. A wish to be helped and a feeling of helplessness.
4. Feelings of despair, guilt, emptiness, and shame.
5. Renewed hope and reorganized behavior directed toward new relationships. It is in this final state that the loss is successfully integrated into the self-system.

During each stage, individuals may exhibit predictable behaviors which serve as indications of the progress of grief work. For example, in the numbness stage they may appear to be withdrawn and immobile, while in the anger and fear stage they are aggressive, irritable, and anxious. In the helplessness stage they exhibit increased dependency needs, which give way to morbid comments and withdrawal behaviors in the fourth stage. Finally they are able to resolve and talk about the loss and feelings and to find enjoyment in life (Clark and Affonso 1979, p. 726).

The outcomes of grieving are generally categorized as successful or unsuccessful. In successful grief resolution, individuals are able to relinquish emotional ties, personal investments, and strong dependencies upon the lost object. Furthermore, they arrive at a comfortable attitude toward the actual loss experience and are able to release feelings, emotions, and expressions of pain surrounding the loss event (McCawley 1977, p. 66). Those who have successfully resolved loss once again find enjoyment in life's activities and comfortably remember events surrounding the loss. Indeed, these people have added to their coping repertoires for dealing with losses, have mastered their feelings, and have experienced psychological and emotional growth.

In unsuccessful grief resolution, individuals do not successfully complete grief work and may manifest maladaptive reactions, including prolonged depressions, acting-out behaviors, alcoholism, psychosomatic disorders, hypochondriasis, and neurotic or psychotic states (Benoliel 1979, p. 87). These people attempt to deny the loss but appear to be intensely anxious about separation from the lost person, object, or ideal. If they are not assisted in the recognition and resolution of the grief, the uncomfortable and intense feelings associated with the loss are carried into future life experiences. Consequently, future loss or stress may initiatie a severe anxiety reaction or breakdown which is actually a reenactment of the original unexpressed and unresolved grief (McCawley 1977, p. 65).

Anticipatory Grief

In his classic studies of bereaved persons, Lindemann (1944) has noted that there is a process designated as anticipatory grief in which a person grieves over a potential or expected loss. If loss is perceived as imminent, the person anticipating the loss traverses the phases of grief, including depression, preoccupation with impending loss, a mental review of forms of death which may occur, and anticipation of modes of necessary personal readjustment following the loss. Lindemann claims this premature grief reaction may serve as a safeguard against the impact of a sudden loss, but he warns that if grief work is totally successful and the expected loss does not occur, it may be difficult, if not impossible, to reincorporate the perceived-as-lost object or person into the self-structure.

Anticipatory grief, then, is the grief expressed prior to any significant loss, a rehearsal of what one may expect after an impending loss. As in conventional grief, the nature and extent of this early response is determined by many variables, including significance of the loss to the individual, the person's developmental level, and the ability to cope with current internal and environmental stressors (Wilson 1977). Furthermore, as in conventional grief, some clients are better able to resolve anticipated loss before loss becomes reality than are others.

In summary, loss represents removal of a person, object, experience, or ideal from one's self-system and it is significant if the lost item had meaning and value in a person's perception and definition of self. Furthermore, loss as a concept is meaningless without an understanding of the grieving process through which people acknowledge, accept, and integrate loss into their lives.

Loss and Grieving of the Childbearing Woman

It is probable that loss and grieving are experienced by all childbearing women and their families (Clark 1979). Losses for the woman include loss of former roles, loss of control, loss of body image, and loss of self-esteem (Clark 1979; Doering and Entwisle 1975; Grace 1978; Highley and Mercer 1978; Lesh 1978; Rubin 1967, 1968). Rubin (1968) observed that women experiencing labor and delivery and the physical and psychological postpartum processes experience loss or threatened loss of control of bodily functions. This loss of bodily control is termed loss of body image, which is intricately intertwined with one's sense of self. Consequently, Rubin (1968, p. 22) maintained that loss of body-image results in loss of self-esteem.

Other types of loss occurring in childbearing women include loss of a pregnant body, with its accompanying status, privileged societal position, and increased attention by physician and family (Clark 1979; Grace 1978); loss of the perfect, painless childbearing/childrearing experience (Grace 1978); loss of the baby from one's body (Lesh 1978); loss of the model figure, physical attractiveness, and special worth (Clark 1979, Grace 1978); loss of self-definition in societal roles (Clark 1979); and loss of one's interpersonal environment (Lesh 1978). Benoliel (1979) notes that the childbearing woman loses her freedom to pursue her own interests as a woman. The new mother may also experience loss of her ideal mothering capabilities, including loss of her ability to feel instant love and affection for her newborn (Lesh 1978).

Especially important is loss of optimal support of the childbearing woman by her family members, who are also experiencing loss and grieving. Clark (1979, p. 508) noted that childbearing fathers experience loss or anticipated loss, including his former relationship with his wife; sexual gratification; comfortable patterns of daily living (e.g., sleep, recreation, food); and financial stability. Likewise, siblings experience loss of mother; loss of familiar surroundings, if they are sent to stay with someone; loss of status in the family; and loss of a lively, energetic mother (Clark 1979, p. 508). In addition, the neonate loses the warm, secure womb and total, constant fulfillment of needs. In each of these situations, the person experiencing loss is attuned to meeting his or her own needs and is therefore not able to lend support to other family members. Consequently, while the child bearing woman is in extreme need of support from her family, the family is itself in need of support.

While each childbearing woman's perception of loss and her response to this perception do depend on the factors noted earlier, they also depend on her attitude toward pregnancy, her life situation at the time of the pregnancy, and the specific roles ascribed to her by her family and by society (Colman and Colman 1971).

Loss and Grieving in Cesarean Mothers

A review of the cesarean birth literature reveals that many of the reported feelings experienced by cesarean mothers can be interpreted as loss and grieving. Table 1 presents a frequency count of feelings reported by authors who interviewed or collected data from cesarean mothers. Those feelings indicative of loss and grieving are marked with an asterisk.

Table 1 shows that feelings of loss and grieving in cesarean mothers are, in order of frequency of occurrence, failure, anger, depression, fear, guilt, pain, self-blame, "negative feelings," shame, sadness, fatigue, feeling abnormal, withdrawal, defeat, blaming of others, shock and disbelief, anticipation of losing one's life or health or the life or health of the baby, bitterness, powerlessness, abandonment, loneliness, disinterest in one's environment, numbness, a sense of loss of control, and helplessness.

The literature indicates that while the specific object of the cesarean mother's grief often varies, it is invariably related to her perception of her performance during childbirth. However, not all cesarean mothers experience loss. In fact, while Affonso and Stichler (1978) found that most women thought their cesarean births were harder than vaginal deliveries would have been, some viewed the cesareans as being easier. This view seemed especially common when the cesarean was planned in advance and the pain of labor and delivery was therefore avoided. This finding can perhaps be attributed to anticipatory grief work done by the mother prior to the actual delivery.

The literature further suggests that emergency cesareans may engender greater feelings of loss than planned births by this method. For example, Affonso and Stichler (1978) noted that "grieving behaviors" are often observed in women who have undergone unexpected cesarean delivery, since these women have had inadequate time to prepare for the event. Such behaviors include anger, depression, and a need to work through and relive their feelings by repeating the story of their childbirth experience. Affonso and Stichler further maintained that many cesarean birth clients grieve over the loss of their birth right.

Thus the cesarean mother may experience all the losses associated with childbearing as well as the special ones associated with surgical delivery. The

TABLE 1.
LITERATURE REVIEW OF FEELINGS AND BEHAVIORS
COMMONLY EXPERIENCED BY CESAREAN MOTHERS
IN THE INTRAPARTUM AND POSTPARTUM PERIODS

FEELINGS/BEHAVIORS	FREQUENCY	AUTHORS†
Failure*	8	1,2,4,5,6,7,8,9
Anger*	7	2,3,4,6,7,9,10
Depression*	6	2,4,6,7,9,10
Fear*	5	2,3,6,7,10
Resentment*	5	4,7,6,9,10
Guilt*	4	4,7,9,10
Self-blame*	4	1,4,6,7
Inadequacy/incompetence	4	2,4,6,7
Pain*	4	1,2,4,7
Relief	4	2,4,6,7
Negative feelings*	3	4,7,10
Disappointment	3	2,6,10
Jealousy (of vaginally-delivered mothers)	3	2,4,7
Sadness*	2	2,9
Shame*	2	7,8
Defeat	2	1,10
Frustration	2	6,7
Fatigue*	2	1,7
Feelings of abnormality*	2	9,10
Withdrawal*	2	3,4
Blame of others, including baby*	2	7,10
Shock and disbelief*	2	6,10
Anticipation of losing self/baby*	2	1,10
Bitterness*	2	7,9
Powerlessness*	1	2
Abandonment*	1	2
Loneliness*	1	6
Fear of future pregnancies*	1	6
Envy	1	1
Disinterest in environment*	1	3
Intrusion (from surgery)	1	5
Happy	1	2
Numbness	1	10
Dissatisfaction	1	2
Sense of loss of control*	1	6
Helplessness*	1	7
Crying*	2	7,9

TABLE 1. (*Continued*)

FEELINGS/BEHAVIORS	FREQUENCY	AUTHORS†
Talkativeness	*2*	*7,9*
*Denial**	*2*	*4,6*
*Passive/aggressive**	*1*	*9*

Starred terms are indicative of feelings experienced in loss and grief.
†*Authors coded as follows (see References):*
 1. *Affonso 1979*
 2. *Affonso and Stichler 1978*
 3. *Bampton and Mancini 1973*
 4. *Cohen 1977*
 5. *Conklin 1977*
 6. *Conner 1977*
 7. *Donovan 1977*
 8. *Marut 1978*
 9. *Reynolds 1977*
10. *Schlosser 1978*

nature of her losses and the extent of her grief responses seem to depend on all of the factors previously mentioned as well as the degree to which the events surrounding the cesarean birth deviate from her expectations.

AN EXPLORATORY STUDY

Although the literature reveals many indications of loss and grief in cesarean mothers, there are no reports of specific comparisons of the feelings of women who have had vaginal deliveries with those of women who have had cesarean births. Therefore, an exploratory study was designed to determine the differences in frequency, type, and intensity of feelings of loss and grief.

The sample for the study consisted of recently delivered private patients in one urban and one suburban hospital in the Washington, D.C. area, as well as cesarean-delivered women involved in local cesarean support groups and women who had attended childbirth education/preparation classes. The sample included 20 women who had had cesarean deliveries and 16 who had had vaginal births.

Analysis of demographic data revealed that the cesarean and vaginally-delivered mothers were similar when compared on the basis of background variables. The cesarean group was slightly older and had slightly more previous pregnancies not resulting in live births. The mean age of the cesarean mothers was 29.5 years; the range was 23 to 35 years. The mean age of the vaginally delivered mothers was 26 years, with a range of 21 to 34 years.

All cesarean mothers were Caucasian, while the vaginally-delivered group included one black mother and one Indian mother. All respondents were married and all had attended childbirth preparation classes.

Subjects were informed that the purpose of this study was to examine feelings that women experience when undergoing vaginal or cesarean birth. They were told that this information would help health care providers to meet the physical and psychoemotional needs of childbearing families. Furthermore, it was emphasized that anonymity and confidentiality would be maintained.

Each subject received an explanatory cover letter and a questionnaire containing items related to demographic data; seven open-ended questions on feelings experienced before, during, and/or after delivery; and five Likert-scale items reflecting intensity of feelings. The questionnaire was developed with two matched forms with items appropriate for vaginally-delivering mothers (Form V) and for cesarean mothers (Form C). Results from this questionnaire are presented in Appendix A.

The questionnaire was distributed to potential respondents with the instructions that if they wished to participate, they should not sign their names on the questionnaire or the return envelope and should complete and mail the questionnaire to the investigator within 2 weeks. Potential subjects could refuse to participate by not returning the questionnaire. Approximately 50 percent of the potential respondents participated in the study.

Data Analysis

The subjects' responses were tabulated in categories of grief feelings, losses, and positive feelings developed from the categories reported in the literature. For example, the category "loss of optimal birth experience" included loss of the shared birth experience, of normal vaginal delivery, of participation in the delivery experience, and of seeing or feeling the actual birth of the baby. Similarly, the category "loss of optimal bonding experience" included loss of early contact with the baby and loss of a rewarding breastfeeding experience.

The category "loss of control and power over self and situation" included loss of the ability to communicate, of independence, of accurate information, of an expected speedy recovery, and of choices and decision-making abilities. "Loss of self-esteem and self-confidence" included losses related to sexual attractiveness, womanliness, and the ability to adequately care for one's newborn.

Two judges working independently screened each set of open-ended questions and developed frequency counts for reported feelings of loss and grief in the various categories. After independent ratings were completed for open-ended questions, similarity between ratings was checked. An index of inter-rater reliability was constructed, evidencing 77 percent overall agreement. In cases where ratings varied, the items in question were discussed and rated by common consent.

It should be noted that if a single respondent mentioned a particular feeling or loss more than once, that particular loss or feeling was recorded only one time per respondent.

Results

Losses reported by the study subjects are shown in Table 2. Reported grief feelings and behaviors are shown in Table 3. Table 4 presents the positive feelings reported by the subjects. These data indicate that feelings of loss and grief were experienced by both vaginally-delivering and cesarean-delivering mothers, but that cesarean mothers reported greater incidences of these feelings in almost all categories. Moreover, some categories of loss and grief feelings were reported to be experienced only by cesarean mothers. More specifically, the percentage of cesarean subjects who reported grief feelings and behaviors exceeded the percentage of vaginally-delivered subjects in 15 out of 17 "grief feelings and behaviors" categories (Table 3). A higher percentage of cesarean subjects in all "loss" categories (Table 2) and a lower percentage was represented in all "positive feeling" (Table 4) categories, with the exception of the "proud/pleased with baby" category.

Chi-square (χ^2) analyses of the data revealed several statistically significant differences between cesarean and vaginally-delivering mothers' reported losses and grief feelings. These are presented in Table 5. These findings indicate that cesarean mothers experience more losses in relation to optimal birth experiences, self-esteem, and body image, and more feelings of grief in relation to fear and worry, powerlessness, shock and disbelief, disappointment, and distorted body image.

Analysis of the Likert-scale items listed in Figure 1 revealed some significant differences between the two groups of mothers. While most subjects

TABLE 2.
LOSSES REPORTED BY MOTHERS

LOSS REPORTED	WOMEN MENTIONING LOSS*			
	Cesarean		Vaginal	
	N	*%*	*N*	*%*
Optimal birth experience	17	85	4	25
Optimal bonding experience	8	40	3	19
Control and power over self and situation	19	95	9	45
Self-esteem and self-confidence	10	50	2	10
Ideal baby image	6	30	0	0
Fear of surgery and anticipated loss of life	4	20	0	0
Safety and joy in future pregnancies	2	10	0	0
Body image	16	80	3	19

*Cesarean N = 20; vaginal N = 16.

TABLE 3.
GRIEF FEELINGS AND BEHAVIORS REPORTED BY MOTHERS

FEELINGS	WOMEN MENTIONING FEELINGS*			
	Cesarean		Vaginal	
	N	%	N	%
Sadness	3	15	0	0
Anger; resentment; frustration bitterness	7	35	1	6
Fear and worry; anxiety; anticipated loss of self/ baby	15	75	5	31
Failure; inadequacy	5	25	1	6
Pain; soreness	10	50	11	69
Powerlessness; loss of control; helplessness	14	70	4	25
Abandonment; loneliness	2	10	1	6
Shock and disbelief; dis- interest in environment; terrible/traumatic experience	13	65	1	6
Depression; defeat	8	40	2	13
Blaming of others; deceived	6	30	0	0
Disappointment; dissatisfaction	12	60	2	13
Fatigue	5	25	4	25
Distorted body image (intrusion, numbness)	12	60	1	6
Decreased self-esteem (humiliation; less womanly; fear of future pregnancy)	11	55	0	0
Behaviors				
Crying	3	15	0	0
Denial	2	10	0	0
Passive/aggressive behavior	2	10	0	0

*Cesarean N = 20; vaginal N = 16.

disagreed with statements which denigrated cesarean birth, vaginally-delivered mothers tended to agree and cesarean mothers to disagree with the statement reflecting the importance of vaginal delivery to the baby's health and psychological well-being ($t = 5.21$, $p < 0.001$). Conversely, vaginally-delivered mothers tended to disagree and cesarean mothers to agree with the statement,

TABLE 4.
REPORTED POSITIVE FEELINGS

FEELINGS	CESAREAN*		VAGINAL*	
	N	%	N	%
Happy	6	30	15	94
Eager to see baby	5	25	7	44
Prepared	2	10	6	38
Proud/pleased with baby	5	25	2	13
Relieved	11	55	9	56

*Cesarean N = 20; vaginal N = 16.

TABLE 5.
DIFFERENCES BETWEEN CESAREAN AND VAGINALLY-DELIVERED MOTHERS' REPORTED LOSSES AND GRIEF FEELINGS

	χ^2	P
Loss of optimal birth experience	13.17	0.001
Loss of self-esteem	5.63	0.05
Loss of body image	13.38	0.001
Fear and worry; anxiety; anticipated loss of self/baby	6.88	0.01
Powerlessness; loss of control; helplessness	7.20	0.01
Shock and disbelief; disinterested in environment; terrible/traumatic experience	12.92	0.001
Disappointment; dissatisfaction	8.45	0.01
Distorted body image	11.13	0.001

"People often believe that there is something wrong with women who must deliver their infants via cesarean deliveries" ($t = 4.05, p < 0.001$).

The specific comments made by subjects help to illustrate the depth of their feelings about their childbirth experiences. One cesarean mother noted that because she was "put to sleep," she felt she had "missed the ending." Another described her feelings before surgery with one word: "Alone." Other cesarean mothers referred to their childbirth experiences as: "a necessary evil . . . an unfortunate happenstance," "a big disappointment . . . a failure because I couldn't deliver vaginally," "major surgery . . . I was zonked out," "a total lack of the birth experience," "an emotional disaster—a failure—a blank!" One cesarean mother described her birth experience as ". . .

the worst experience I ever had in my entire life—humiliating, shocking, traumatic, painful. I felt as if they tied me to a tree naked and set me on fire while everyone stood around and looked on." Conversely, one mother described her cesarean experience as ". . . good on the whole . . . my husband was there and I was participating fully."

But it wasn't only cesarean mothers who had negative comments about their deliveries. One vaginally delivered mother remarked, "I chafe at the restrictions put on me." Another described her experience as "the pits." In contrast, another mother remarked, "I felt very 'macho' . . . I wanted to try to relive the experience." Interestingly, one mother said she was "grateful I didn't have a cesarean—sweet relief." One other mother noted, "Emotionally, I felt proud of myself. I had accomplished something very important to me— natural childbirth. I've finished a chapter of my life—childbirth, the way *I* wanted it. A very good experience. I'm content."

Discussion

While this study represents only an initial exploratory effort and certainly requires future refinement and replication, the findings indicate that many women experience feelings of loss and grief in relation to their childbirth experiences. Furthermore, it is evident that women undergoing cesarean birth are more likely to report loss and grief feelings, behaviors, and experiences than vaginally-delivered mothers. It is unfortunate that such feelings and losses are experienced by these women at a time when they might be experiencing a most meaningful event in their lives.

Generalization of study findings should be made with great caution. This study was exploratory, involving only a small sample of the studied population. Furthermore, all study subjects had attended childbirth education classes, which may or may not have sensitized them to their own expectations or feelings of failure regarding cesarean birth. Some mothers had, in fact, attended childbirth preparation classes developed for cesarean mothers. These classes may have heightened the consciousness of the expectant cesarean mothers. While cesarean delivery remains, in some settings, an "alone" experience, several cesarean mothers reported partial involvement of fathers, the use of mirrors, and other methods of parent participation. No effort was made in this study to control for differences in cesarean delivery styles.

IMPLICATIONS FOR NURSING

The findings from the study reported here and from the literature review suggest implications for nursing care of cesarean mothers who experience feelings of loss and grief. Ideally, the goal of nursing is to prevent such feelings. The study data indicate that this may be possible when the cesarean birth is planned in advance and when the parents can remain together during the delivery. It is probable in such cases that the parents have experienced some anticipatory grief and were able to successfully resolve their feelings of loss. It is also possible that some couples do not view cesarean birth as a negative experience and thus do not perceive this method of delivery as a loss.

However, the study data and the reports of cesarean experiences in the literature indicate that many cesareans are not anticipated prior to labor and delivery, that few couples have the opportunity to remain together during the delivery, and that most cesarean mothers express profound feelings of loss. Therefore, nurses must understand the phenomenon of loss and grieving in cesarean mothers and must devise plans of care that will promote successful grief resolution. Application of a systematic nursing process with its components of assessment, planning, implementation, and evaluation (Yura and Walsh 1978) will facilitate that goal.

Assessment

In assessing the presence or extent of loss and grieving in cesarean mothers, the nurse must consider each of the following factors.

1. Discrepancies between the mother's expected and hoped-for childbirth and her real childbirth experience, within the perspective of her cultural background.
2. The meaning of the childbearing event to the parents, including preparation, expectations, fears, and concerns.
3. Behavioral expressions of loss and grieving, including such verbal and nonverbal behaviors as sadness, insomnia, fatigue, negative responses to husband and baby, withdrawal, and crying.
4. Progress through the grieving process by determining the present stage of denying, recognizing, feeling, and accepting losses.
5. Availability and utilization of hospital, family, and community support systems within the hospital and for future use at home.
6. Environmental variables—e.g., sensory overload or sensory deprivation, assurance of privacy, and availability of trusted caretakers.
7. Physiological status and physical reserves.
8. The mother's usual coping styles and mechanisms.
9. Her readiness to progress through the grieving stages.

It is important to remember that the mother must not be forced to quickly engage in grief work, since she will only be able to actively grieve when she becomes aware of her losses. Prior to awareness, grief responses are not demonstrated due to denial (Benoliel 1971; Gruendemann 1976). If a mother is not ready to grieve while still in the hospital, she will need anticipatory guidance for feelings which she may later experience (e.g., depression or sadness) and to alert her to community resources which she may utilize (Schlosser 1978).

Assessment may be initiated prior to the cesarean birth. The sense of loss may be diminished greatly if the nurse helps the expectant couple to mentally integrate the possibility of a cesarean delivery prior to labor and delivery. This may be done during childbirth education classes (Cohen 1977; Conklin 1977; Grace 1978; Marut 1978).

Grace (1978) maintained that when the potential for a cesarean delivery is obvious (e.g., in an elderly primiparous woman with a breech presenting part or in a woman with a small pelvis), this information must be shared with the parents. If it is not, grief work is postponed until the time when the mother is experiencing the increased physical and emotional demands of surgery, recovery, and infant care. Furthermore, Grace claimed that withholding this information leads to blocked communication and destroyed trust between parents and health professionals.

Once the possibility of cesarean birth is presented, the nurse can assess each of the couple's responses and identify specific areas in which intervention may be needed if a cesarean delivery does occur. Assessment can be accomplished through observation of the cesarean mother's behavior as well as through interviews with her. Gruendemann (1976) stated that interviewing techniques should include reflection of the client's statements and questions, provision of clues and helps in discerning possible answers to client's questions, and a reassurance that dealing with loss is uncomfortable and difficult. Grace (1978) felt that the nurse should respond to the emotional content of the mother's comments or nonverbal behaviors—e.g., "You look (or sound) angry (or upset)." In so doing, the nurse may unleash an outpouring of feelings indicative of loss and grief which she can then help the mother resolve.

Gruendemann (1976) noted that the nurse must continually reassess the mother's responses for indications of readiness to proceed through the grief stages, but must focus assessment and care on strengthening the mother's own repertoire of problem-solving skills. In so doing, the mother can maintain and indeed enhance her ego-integrity and self-esteem.

Planning

While specific planning of nursing intervention is dependent upon individual assessment findings, general principles in planning to help cesarean mothers to deal with loss and grief include:

1. Allowing ample time to be with and talk with the client.
2. Revising and noting in written care plans all progress or regression.
3. Providing continuity of care through a primary care nurse or through continuous communication with other caregivers.

4. Including family members, significant others, and community support leaders in the plan of care.
5. Reviewing the nurse's own feelings regarding loss and grieving in her past experiences and in the childbearing process (Gruendemann 1976).

This last point is crucial, since health care providers can transfer their own unresolved feelings of loss and grieving into their care of clients experiencing loss and grieving (Benoliel 1979; Gruendemann 1976). Furthermore, if the nurse does not believe that loss occurs in childbearing, she may not be sensitive to the presence of these feelings in clients and thus may not be able to perceive or meet their needs for grief resolution. It is therefore essential that the nurse be aware of her own feelings and attitudes before she attempts to understand the feelings of her clients.

In planning to intervene with cesarean mothers who are experiencing loss and grief, the nurse should consider their needs for safe people, safe places, and safe situations (Grace 1978). Safe people include trusted nursing personnel and significant others who can accept the mother's feelings and behaviors. Safe places are those surroundings which are private enough to cry in and express anger in and which at the same time include familiar objects and safe people. Safe situations are those which offer meaningful and worthwhile activity without taxing the mother's limited coping abilities and which include the presence of caring persons at a difficult time.

Implementation

While what the nurse actually says and does derives specifically from assessment and planning data, the seven general intervention goals and techniques described below are helpful when dealing with cesarean mothers who are experiencing loss and grief.

First, the nurse should ensure privacy and nurse availability. It is essential to spend time with the client as she attempts to recognize, identify, and sort out the objects and feelings of her loss. Given time and opportunities for open communication with a trusted caregiver, the mother can approach and discuss painful issues (McCawley 1977).

Second, it is important to reduce environmental stressors. By manipulating such environmental stimuli as noise, heat, light, proximity of personal belongings, and number of interpersonal contacts, the mother can conserve her energy for the task of coping with loss (Haber et al. 1978). One specific environmental stressor is the absence of the baby. One simple but often neglected nursing intervention is making sure that the cesarean mother has early, extended, and satisfying contact with her newborn. If this is not possible, she should have a picture of her baby and should be taken to the nursery to see and perhaps hold the infant.

Another environmental stressor is a vaginally-delivered roommate. This roommate's greater ability to physically care for herself and her baby may serve as a reminder to the cesarean mother that she cannot presently meet the standards which she set for herself prior to her childbirth experience. Conversely, if cesarean mothers are placed in the same room, they may begin to share their feelings of loss and grieving with each other.

Nurses can be instrumental in eliminating other stressors, such as rules against having fathers in the delivery room, restriction of father and sibling visitation, and failure to keep the client realistically informed of events surrounding her childbirth.

Third, the nurse should assist the cesarean mother in recalling and reexperiencing feelings surrounding her childbirth so that she may accept and incorporate her feelings into her self-image. To do this, the nurse listens for evidence of denial of loss and waits for the mother to indicate her readiness to share and explore her feelings. The nurse may then encourage expression and exploration of feelings in depth while reassuring the mother that her feelings of depression, sadness, etc. are normal and will eventually subside (Joel and Collins 1978).

Also relevant here is Grace's (1978) assertion that the nurse must assist the client in exposing her feelings and beliefs for reality testing through such statements as, "You seem to feel that you are to blame for your cesarean delivery." Grace added that the nurse must utilize clear, accurate, reality-based information so that the mother's inner sense can begin to correspond with her real external situation.

Robischon (1967) noted that nurses can facilitate both the anticipatory or conventional grief process by (1) encouraging open communication and expression of clients' feelings; (2) not supporting clients' denial of reality; (3) not giving false reassurance; (4) accepting and expecting hostile or disturbed behavior, anger, and depression as expressions of loss and grief; (5) respecting cultural, familial, and religious customs in dealing with loss; and (6) observing and noting exaggerated or delayed reactions and responses to loss and grief.

Fourth, the nurse must strive to maintain the new mother's sense of self-control, integrity, and sense of being normal and valuable. While this goal is imperative in all nursing care situations, it is paramount with the cesarean mother, who may be experiencing loss and grief with its concomitant feelings of disorganization and loss of a valued piece of the self. The nurse initiates progress towards this goal by establishing a trusting relationship which assures the mother that she may freely discuss her feelings without guilt, condemnation, or judgment. By conveying a sense of personal and genuine interest in the mother, the nurse further allows her to feel valued, important, normal, and not alone. The nurse reassures the new mother that her behaviors and feelings are experienced by many childbearing women and that maternal roles, feelings, and behaviors are learned and developed rather than innate and automatic (Lesh 1978).

Marut (1978) contended that in our society, which highly values self-control, there is great pressure to use one's self effectively and efficiently to precisely achieve one's goals. It is not surprising, then, that when control is taken away from the cesarean couple, especially if general anesthesia is used or the father is not permitted to be in the delivery room, the couple may perceive loss and feelings of failure.

To maintain the mother's sense of control, the nurse should include her in decision-making throughout the intrapartal and postpartal periods. Specific interventions that foster control include: (1) having the mother awake throughout the delivery, with arms untied, with the screen down, and/or with a mirror available so that she may see her baby born; (2) showing the baby to his parents while he remains attached to the umbilical cord; (3) letting the parents witness the birth together and see, touch, and hold the baby in the delivery and recovery rooms; (4) preventing postpartal separation of the parents and their infant; (5) providing unlimited visiting hours for fathers; (6) rooming cesarean mothers together and ensuring easy access to lavatories and nurseries; (7) promoting and assisting early breast-feeding; (8) assisting in infant care; (9) providing adequate rest and nutrition; (10) letting the mother know that her feelings and crying are normal; and (11) providing information about local cesarean support groups (Cohen 1977; Donovan 1977).

In each of these situations the nurse attempts to help the mother to set attainable and realistic goals for the care of herself and her baby. Subsequently, the mother may be verbally rewarded for her increasingly successfull abilities to care for herself and her baby, thus increasing her sense of control, her self-esteem, and her coping abilities (Highley and Mercer 1978).

Fifth, the nurse should be attuned to each mother's specific needs and feelings regarding her perceived loss. Each client perceives loss and grief in a unique manner. Indeed, McCawley (1977) noted that the extent of feelings of loss and grief is dependent upon the client's needs. By reflecting back to the mother her statements of unresolved conflict, refraining from quick reassurance, and allowing free expression of feelings of guilt and anger, the nurse enables the grieving cesarean mother to reach her own sense of assurance about and understanding of her childbirth experience (McCawley 1977).

Sixth, it is important to recognize the role of loss and grief in precipitating or intensifying physical symptoms experienced by the grieving mother. While it is difficult to tell whether a cesarean mother's symptoms (e.g., pain, insomnia, fatigue, anorexia, etc.) are due to surgery or to the grief experience, it is important to hypothesize that these symptoms may be connected with the grief experience. If the nurse can then assess perceived loss and assist the mother in confronting and resolving her loss, physical symptoms may decrease or abate.

Seventh, the nurse should help the cesarean mother to make maximum use of available support systems. In the case of the cesarean couple, the father of the baby or another significant other must be included in grief intervention. If the couple had anticipated a shared vaginal delivery but experienced an unshared cesarean, both parents may need to confront their feelings of loss. It is appropriate for the nurse to assist the parents in sharing their feelings and in realizing that these feelings are normal, painful, temporary, and shared by many cesarean families. Couples must also be prepared with the knowledge that feelings of depression, anger, sadness, etc. may continue for a period of time after the family returns home. It is at this point that the nurse might encourage the couple to ". . . call in a couple of weeks and let us know how you're doing and if you have any questions" (Grace 1978). The nurse should also provide the cesarean couple with a list of local cesarean support groups, such as C/SEC or the Cesarean Families Association, and should encourage early contact with someone in the support group.

By utilizing these goals and techniques of grief intervention, the nurse assists the cesarean mother in her efforts to focus upon and deal with those aspects of her childbearing experience which she perceives as a loss and about which she must grieve before accepting herself as a childbearing woman.

Evaluation

If nursing intervention in facilitation of grief work is successful, the nurse will note the client's progression through the various grief stages. For example, if the nurse initially assesses complete denial of loss and later observes the cesarean mother's desire to express and explore her feelings, the mother has made progress in grief resolution. When the mother can freely and openly discuss both the positive and negative aspects of her childbearing experience and can feel "good" about herself as a childbearing woman, then the grieving process has been successfully completed.

CONCLUSION

The purpose of this chapter was to describe the feelings of loss and grief experienced by childbearing women, especially those having cesarean births, and to identify strategies for care which can be used by nurses and other health care workers to help cesarean mothers recognize and successfully resolve their perceived losses.

Marut (1978 p. 202) noted that the childbearing woman's resolution of feelings concerning failure to achieve personal labor and delivery goals may be critical to quality of future mothering. Cohen (1977) claimed that to feel good about one's childbirth experience is to feel good about one's self and one's newborn infant. Kitzinger (1972 p. 17) said that the experience of child-bearing is central to each woman's life and that for years after the baby is born the mother acutely remembers the details and her feelings about the childbirth experience. Through grief intervention, nurses can assist child-bearing clients in recognizing, dealing with, accepting, integrating, and re-membering both the positive and the negative aspects of their experiences. Furthermore, if nurses are aware of the common losses associated with cesar-ean birth, many of these may be prevented or minimized through nursing intervention and changes in hospital policies.

ACKNOWLEDGMENTS

The author gratefully acknowledges the invaluable guidance of her research consultant, Scott K. Birdsong, M.S.W., A.C.S.W., and also Saundra Albrite, R.N., M.S.N. who helped to collect data for this study.

REFERENCES

Affonso DD: Complications of labor and delivery. In Clark AL, Affonso, DD, Childbearing: A Nursing Perspective, 2nd ed. Philadelphia, Davis, 1979

Affonso DD, Stichler JF: Exploratory study of women's reaction to having a cesarean birth. Birth Fam J 5 (2):88–94, 1978

Bampton BA, Mancini JA: The cesarean patient is a new mother too. J Ob Gynecol Neonatal Nurs 2 (4):58–61, 1973.

Benoliel JQ: Assessments of loss and grief. J Thanatol 1 (3):182–94, 1971

Benoliel JQ: Loss. In Clark AL, Affonso DD, Childbearing: A Nursing Per-spective, 2nd ed. Philadelphia, Davis, 1979

Clark AL: Application of psychosocial concepts. In Clark AL, Affonso DD, Childbearing: A Nursing Perspective, 2nd ed. Philadelphia, Davis, 1979

Clark AL, Affonso DD: Childbearing: A Nursing Perspective, 2nd ed. Phila-delphia, Davis, 1979

Cohen NW: Minimizing emotional sequelae of cesarean childbirth. Birth Fam J 4 (3):114–19, 1977

Colman AD, Colman LL: Pregnancy: The Psychological Experience. New York, Seabury, 1971

Conklin MM: Discussion groups as preparation for cesarean section. J Obstet Gynecol Neonatal Nurs 6 (4):52–54, 1977

Doering SG, Entwisle DR: Preparation during pregnancy and ability to cope with labor and delivery. Am J Orthopsychiatry. 45 (5):825–37, 1975

Donovan B: The Cesarean Birth Experience. Boston, Beacon, 1977

Engel GL: Grief and grieving. Am J Nurs 64 (9):93–98, 1964

Engel GL: Psychological Development in Health and Disease. Philadelphia, Saunders, 1962

Grace JT: Good grief: Coming to terms with the childbirth experience. J Obstet Gynecol Neonatal Nurs 7 (1):18–22, 1978

Gruendemann BJ: Problems of physical self: Loss. In Roy C, Introduction to Nursing: An Adaptation Model. Englewood Cliffs, N.J., Prentice-Hall, 1976

Haber J, Leach A, Schudy S, Sideleau B: Comprehensive Psychiatric Nursing. New York, McGraw-Hill, 1978

Highley BL, Mercer RT: Safeguarding the laboring woman's sense of control. Am J Maternal Child Nurs 3 (1):38–41, 1978

Joel L, Collins D: Psychiatric Nursing: Theory and Application. New York, McGraw-Hill, 1978

Kitzinger S: The Experience of Childbirth. Baltimore, Penguin, 1972

Lesh AA: Postpartum depression. In McNall K, Galeener T (eds), Current Practice in Obstetric and Gynecologic Nursing. St. Louis, Mosby, 1978

Lindemann E: Symptomatology and management of acute grief. Am J Psychiatry 101:101–48, 1944

Marut JS: The special needs of the cesarean mother. Am J Maternal Child Nurs 3 (4):202–06, 1978

McCawley A: Help patients cope with grief. Consultant 17 (11):64–67, 1977

Nolan T: Ritual and therapy. In Schoenberg B, Carr AC, Kutscher AH, et al (eds), Anticipatory Grief. New York, Columbia University Press, 1974

Peretz D: Reaction to loss. In Schoenberg B, Carr AC, Kutscher AH, et al (eds), Loss and Grief: Psychological Management in Medical Practice. New York, Columbia University Press, 1970

Reynolds CB: Updating care of cesarean section patients. J Obstet Gynecol Neonatal Nurs 6 (4):48–51, 1977

Robischon P: The challenge of crisis theory for nursing. Nurs Outlook 15:28–32, 1967

Rubin R: Attainment of the maternal role, Part I: Processes. Nurs Res 16 (3):237–45, 1967

Rubin R: Body image and self-esteem. Nurs Outlook 16:20–23, 1968

Schlosser S: The emergency c-section patient. Why she needs help . . . what you can do. RN Vol 41:53–57, 1978

Yura H, Walsh MB: The Nursing Process, 3rd ed. New York, Appleton-Century-Crofts, 1978

Wilson JL: Anticipatory grief in response to threatened amputation. Maternal-Child Nurs J 6 (3):177–86, 1977

APPENDIX A.
MATERNAL–INFANT QUESTIONNAIRE

PART I: DEMOGRAPHIC DATA

Please give the following information about yourself:
1. Age:

2. Number of pregnancies resulting in a live birth:

3. Number of pregnancies not resulting in a live birth:

4. Number of (a) vaginal deliveries: ____ (b) cesarean births: ____

5. Race:

6. Marital status:

7. Childbirth education classes attended? Yes ( ) No ( ) Where?

8. When were you told you must have a cesarean (if appropriate)?

9. How long ago was your first cesarean (if you have already had one)?

PART II, FORM V (VAGINALLY-DELIVERED MOTHERS)

Please respond briefly to the following:
1. Describe your feelings during labor (e.g., frightened, relieved, depressed, happy). What caused these feelings?

2. Describe your feelings just prior to and during your delivery:

3. Describe your main feelings during the first 24 hours following your delivery:

4. Briefly describe how you felt (physically, emotionally) about your vaginal delivery in the days/weeks following the delivery:

5. What aspects of your delivery do you feel were:
   a. Positive (good)?
   b. Negative (not so good)?

6. Briefly, how would you compare your delivery with the vaginal delivery you anticipated (or previously had)?

7. How do you feel now when you think about your labor and delivery experience?

PART II, FORM C (CESAREAN-DELIVERED MOTHERS)

Please respond briefly to the following:

1. Describe your feelings immediately after being told you must have a cesarean birth (e.g., frightened, relieved, depressed, happy). What caused these feelings?

2. Describe how you felt immediately before your surgery (i.e., within a half hour before the cesarean):

3. Describe your main feelings during the first 24 hours following your operation:

4. Briefly describe how you felt (physically, emotionally) about your cesarean birth in the days/weeks following the delivery:

5. What aspects of your cesarean delivery do you feel were:
   a. Positive (good):
   b. Negative (not so good)?

6. Briefly, how would you compare your delivery with the vaginal delivery you anticipated (or previously had)?

7. How do you feel now when you think about your labor and delivery experience?

PART III, (VAGINALLY- AND CESAREAN-DELIVERED MOTHERS)

Pleace circle the number which best describes your feelings about each statement.

1. Being able to deliver your baby vaginally is very important for the baby's health and psychological well-being.

Strongly Disagree	Disagree	Neutral	Agree	Strongly Agree
1	2	3	4	5

2. Being able to deliver your baby vaginally is the full symbolization of what it means to be a woman and a mother.

Strongly Disagree	Disagree	Neutral	Agree	Strongly Agree
1	2	3	4	5

3. People often believe that there is something wrong with women who must deliver their infants via cesareans.

Strongly Disagree	Disagree	Neutral	Agree	Strongly Agree
1	2	3	4	5

4. Any normal, healthy woman should be capable of delivering her baby vaginally.

Strongly Disagree	Disagree	Neutral	Agree	Strongly Agree
1	2	3	4	5

5. Women who experience cesarean deliveries must feel that they have been deprived of the optimal labor and delivery experience.

Strongly Disagree	Disagree	Neutral	Agree	Strongly Agree
1	2	3	4	5

CHAPTER 10

Sexual Adjustment of the Postcesarean Couple

Dorothy deMoya

The absence of scientific investigation into sexual adjustment following cesarean birth is striking. Historically, the guidelines for assisting couples through the normal developmental crisis of childbirth and its impact on sexual functioning have been based on unsubstantiated clinical assumptions. Few studies, except the research of Masters and Johnson (1966), Salberg et al. (1973), Falicov (1973), Kenny (1973), Morris (1975), and Tolor (1976), illuminate sexual functioning throughout the four trimesters of the pregnancy year. The authors cited above reported on sexual adjustment as it specifically relates to genital functioning rather than on the broader aspects of a couple's total relationship. Ongoing, definitive investigations into sexuality during the entire reproductive cycle are still needed in order to provide a data base for clinical nursing practice.

Such a data base is particularly important for nurses who provide support and counseling for childbearing couples whose delivery experiences are perceived as being less than ideal and thus incongruent with their childbirth expectations. There are few existing guidelines for providing support to couples in this category, particularly postcesarean couples. However, experience gained in my own clinical work as a specialist in sexual dysfunctioning and reproductive counseling does offer some insights that other nurses may find useful in working with postcesarean couples.

The sexual adjustment of the cesarean couple is influenced by a variety of interrelated factors. The factors which I have found to be the most relevant in my own work are considered in this chapter. These factors are:

1. Patterns of sexual response during the three trimesters of pregnancy and the first 6 weeks postpartum.
2. Physiology of the postpartum period.
3. Prepregnancy levels of sexual adjustment.
4. Levels of sexual adjustment as they apply to the cesarean couple.

With this information as a data base, the implications for nursing intervention with postcesarean couples are described.

PATTERNS OF SEXUAL RESPONSE
DURING THE FOUR TRIMESTERS

It is interesting to examine the effects that the normal developmental crisis of pregnancy imposes on the sexual functioning of a couple. Masters and Johnson (1966) described alterations in function and libido in relation to parity and the specific trimester of pregnancy. Fluctuations reflecting increases or decreases in sexual desire were considered within the normal range of variation during the first trimester. Decreases in sexual functioning reported in nulliparous women were due to the discomfort of nausea, vomiting, and fatigue, along with fear of harming the fetus. The majority of parous women reported levels of sexual interaction similar to those in the prepregnant period. The second trimester revealed a greater interest and responsivity, regardless of parity, in 82 of the 101 women interviewed. Perhaps this was due to a better overall sense of well-being as nausea and vomiting subsided and increased vasocongestion led to higher levels of sexual tension. The third trimester brought with it the discomforts of an enlarged uterus, fatigue, awkwardness, and changes in body image which influenced the couples' genital expression.

The women believed their husband's withdrawal from sexual encounters to be due to their bodily changes, their not wanting to create discomfort for the wife and lastly their fear of injuring the baby. The nulliparous women withdrew from sexual contacts due largely to somatic complaints, while the parous women reported withdrawal due to the pressure and exhaustion resulting from the care of other children.

Salberg et al. (1973), after questioning 260 postpartum women, reported that the women recalled a continual gradual decrease in coital activity. Morris (1975) concurred with Salberg that coital frequency gradually decreases as pregnancy progresses. Falicov (1973) reported a decrease in coital frequency in the first trimester. Tolor and DeGrazia (1976) and Falicov (1973) observed an increase in sexual desire and function during the second trimester with subsequent declines in the last trimester.

While there is a difference in the results of the investigations as they relate to the first and second trimesters, there is a consensus that there is usually a decline in sexual encounters during the last trimester.

The return to sexual functioning in the fourth trimester or postpartum period was found to be related not to parity but directly to breast-feeding, as greater levels of sexual response in the immediate postpartum period were reported by the group of nursing mothers. Lowered levels of sexual tension were mostly associated with chronic exhaustion, coital discomfort, and fear of injury to the mother due to early resumption of intercourse.

Kenny (1973), in his study of 33 women, reported that almost half of the mothers resumed sexual relations before the fourth week. Interestingly, this was a population of breast-feeding mothers. There was also a positive correlation between the older, more sexually experienced women and an earlier resumption of sexual relations.

In a study of 19 primigravidas, Falicov (1973), using a sexuality index, discovered that resumption of sexual relations in the early postpartum period was influenced more by the physical condition of the women and their partner's desire, than by the women's actual personal interest in sexuality. This contrasts with Kenny's findings (1973) that a woman's prepregnancy sexual investment influences her sexual adjustment during pregnancy and the late postpartum period.

PHYSIOLOGY OF THE POSTPARTUM PERIOD

Research on the physiology of the postpartum period has been conducted by Masters and Johnson (1966). Six women studied by them were examined at 4 to 6 weeks, 6 to 8 weeks, and 3 months postpartum. All six women were reported to have had uncomplicated deliveries and were found to be in good health. Three of the six women were breast-feeding mothers. Pelvic examination at 4 to 5 weeks revealed well-healed episiotomies, closed cervices, and the uteri as abdominal organs. The uteri appeared to be better involuted in the nursing mothers. Significant changes were found in the physiology of the pelvis from the time of the first evaluation to the last check at 3 months.

Despite the fact that four out of six women described a significant degree of eroticism at the initial exam, the physiological parameters did not coincide. The physiological reactions were slowed and of decreased intensity. Vasocongestion was delayed, thus requiring a longer time for vaginal lubrication to occur, and there was a diminution in the quantity of transudate. The typical vagina resembled that of a steroid-deprived woman, as seen in vaginal senility—i.e., smooth consistency of the vaginal walls along with light pink coloration. This was particularly evident in the breast-feeding mother.

Decreased vasocongestion was also evident in the decreased amount of congestion surrounding the orgasmic platform. Although the length and intensity of vaginal contractions was decreased, subjective reporting revealed satisfaction from the orgasmic experience.

Masters and Johnson (1974) found no significant change between the first and second evaluations (6 to 8 weeks); however, by the end of the third month postpartum, vaginal rugae were reestablished (to a greater degree in nonnursing mothers) and vaginal lubrication, vaginal barrel expansion, uterine elevation during plateau levels, orgasmic platform contractions, and reactions of the skin to sexual activity had returned to nonpregnant levels. Lochia, or bleeding from the placental site, lasted from 2 to 4 weeks after delivery, while episiotomies were healed within 2 to 3 weeks.

Although the study subjects reported no significant difference in their orgasmic experiences during all three evaluations, there were significant physiological differences between the first and last testings. Physiologically, there is no need for coital abstinence once bleeding has stopped and the incisions have healed. However, psychologically, women differ in their desire to resume coital activity.

No studies have been reported on the direct effects of cesarean birth on the sexual functioning of couples. John Lamont (1977) observed that obstetrical and gynecological patients undergoing surgical procedure (episiotomy, vaginal and abdominal hysterectomy, laparotomy, and cesarean delivery) did not usually develop sexual dysfunction as a result of these procedures. Relatively few complaints of dyspareunia were associated with painful vaginal or pelvic scarring after surgery. Lamont felt that most of the complaints were of a psychophysiological nature.

THE PREPREGNANCY LEVELS
OF SEXUAL ADJUSTMENT

For the purpose of exploring the sexual adjustment of couples, respective levels of adjustment are here listed for the well-adjusted couple, the fairly well-adjusted couple, and the poorly-adjusted couple.

Well-adjusted couples:

  1. Possess self-esteem and a positive body image.
  2. Have knowledge of their own as well as their partner's body.
  3. Take pride in their ability to respond sexually.
  4. Experience pleasure in any interactions with each other.
  5. Are vulnerable in their expression of feelings.
  6. Have the power and freedom to make choices in a responsible way.

Fairly well-adjusted couples:

1. Possess self-esteem but question their adequacy when sexual goals are not met.
2. Are satisfied with their body images but wish to be able to alter certain characteristics so as to feel completely adequate.
3. Are proud of achieving certain sexual goals and are disappointed when these are not reached.
4. Attempt to communicate but often avoid disclosure of feelings.
5. Limit sexual expression by attempting to fulfill certain expectations and blame themselves or their partners when these are not reached.

Poorly-adjusted couples:

1. Have low self-esteem and poor body images.
2. Are ignorant of bodily processes and rely on myth and misinformation to explain these functions.
3. Are fearful and/or shameful of sexual feelings.
4. Reduce sexual expression to a mere task, with little opportunity for pleasure.
5. Communicate mostly on an intellectual level, with deliberate avoidance of expression of feelings.
6. Feel boxed into a pattern of expression with little room for growth and development of sexual expression.

Masters and Johnson (1974) have made the conservative estimate that at least 50 percent of the married couples in this country are experiencing some form of sexual difficulty. It would not be imprudent to estimate that a majority of the population would fall into the "fairly well-adjusted" category.

LEVELS OF SEXUAL ADJUSTMENT AS THEY APPLY TO THE CESAREAN COUPLE

Self-esteem is one of the cornerstones of effective sexual functioning. The desire to feel pleasure and the ability to give pleasure to oneself as well as to one's partner are paramount in a couple's reciprocal exchange of positive sexual feelings. The opinion that one has of one's anatomy and one's experience of that anatomy affects one's fulfillment as a sexual person.

Cesarean birth, when seen as an "abnormal" means of delivery, may disturb one's self-image, which in turn may decrease self-esteem. Feelings of failure associated with not having a "normal delivery" sometimes plague a woman who invests a great deal of sexual self-esteem in the task of vaginal delivery. Often this image of failure is projected in the form of blame of the husband, physician, or nursing staff. This in turn sets up a treadmill of guilt, anger, and anxiety that can have deleterious effects on a couple's sexual functioning.

This need not happen, however, for a woman with a strong investment in nonprocreative sex and a richly developed sense of self-worth may choose to see cesarean birth as an alternate means of delivery that does not threaten her ability to express herself as a woman giving birth.

The following case studies from my clinical practice illustrate the interaction of cesarean birth and levels of sexual adjustment.

A Well-Adjusted Couple

A primipara named Carol with a graduate degree in nursing was told after several hours of trial labor that because of cephalopelvic disproportion the baby would have to be delivered abdominally. Carol managed to cope well with the change in the plan of delivery. Knowing what options were available, Carol asked for spinal anesthesia so that she could be awake and share the birth with her husband Jim (a urologist). The obstetrician approved this request; however, the anesthesiologist, who had the authority to make the final decision about fathers in the delivery room, disapproved of the husband's presence. The patient, after being wheeled into the delivery room, asked where her husband was. When told he would not be allowed in, Carol refused to move onto the delivery table. Realizing she meant what she said, the anesthesiologist reluctantly called her husband in. Carol and Jim reported feelings of warmth, joy, and intimacy as a couple in greeting their brand new son together. The anesthesiologist apologized to Carol and Jim for his reluctance and was so moved by this couple's experience that he reevaluated his attitude and relaxed his policy on participation of fathers in cesarean birth.

When questioned about resumption of sexual relations, Carol and Jim reported a decrease in sexual tension levels for the first 4 weeks. However, they also reported a great deal of physical contact in the form of cuddling and light caressing. "Making love" through coital contact was not their priority during the early postpartum period, while "feeling loved" was a need they both expressed. By the fourth week postpartum, Jim openly communicated his high level of sexual tension. Carol did not feel the demand or the wish to resume intercourse. Carol consequently used several means of tension release that were totally acceptable to both of them to give release to Jim and pleasure to both. During their first coital contact at 5 weeks after delivery, Carol experienced minor discomfort, not because of penile penetration but as a result of their "playfulness" while caressing and moving about.

This couple demonstrated self-esteem in valuing themselves, their individual needs, and each other's needs in their relationship. Self-esteem played a role in this mother's assertiveness in meeting the need she and her husband felt to share the birth.

Husband and wife were sensitive to their bodily functions and accepted discomfort initially as something to be expected following abdominal surgery. Their greatest assets were their openness and ability to express feelings, and the freedom they both felt in making choices about their sexual expression. They both understood and agreed that this expression was not limited to coital contact.

A Fairly Well-Adjusted Couple

Janice was a 26-year-old primipara who worked as a secretary and was married to Bill, a buyer for a large department store. They both attended childbirth classes and expected a vaginal delivery. Janice's 10-hour labor progressed very slowly. When the fetal heart rate began decelerating, Janice was told that abdominal delivery would be the safest route. An emergency cesarean set-up was begun and there was not much time for Janice to think about anything except the abdominal prep, urinary catheter, and intravenous drip. Bill asked to go with Janice to the delivery room. The obstetrician approved and the anesthesiologist was reluctant but would have yielded, but the delivery room nurses disapproved. The nurses felt that the purpose of the husband in the delivery room was only to support his wife if she were awake, and as general anesthesia was planned they saw no need for him to be there. Besides, that was the policy. Janice felt abandoned, as she had lost her most valued support person. Bill felt helpless in not being allowed to comfort her. In the end, a healthy, 9 pound boy with a tight short cord around his neck was born without either member of the marital unit able to witness the birth.

Janice's postoperative course was uneventful except for allergic dermatitis of unknown origin. The mother chose to nurse the baby with the full support of her husband. While on the postpartum unit, Janice expressed feelings of sadness and disappointment that she could not deliver vaginally. She acknowledged that she felt "cheated" and that she could not fulfill her fantasy of giving birth in the presence of her husband. She expressed pleasure in nursing the baby, which gave her a feeling of closeness and attachment and a sense of power.

When questioned about their resumption of sexual relations, Janice said that she felt her husband was anxious for tension release at 3 weeks after delivery. Janice reported that she felt ambivalent about resuming coital activity. She wanted to, on the one hand, because she had heard stories that some women became frigid after childbirth and was anxious to find out what her response would be. However, she asked her husband to wait another week because she still felt exhausted and was also sensitive around the incision. Bill agreed to her request and used masturbation to relieve his tension. Janice felt somewhat guilty about this and initiated coitus the following week. Because of dryness, Janice used K-Y Jelly. She was not that concerned about this because she had heard in class that there might be a decrease in vaginal lubrication due to hormonal deprivation while nursing.

Janice felt satisfied by this sexual encounter, although she did not experience orgasm. She was relieved that she was capable of responding favorably. Bill asked whether or not Janice had had an orgasm and felt somewhat disappointed that she had not. Janice subsequently began to feel unsure of herself and hoped the next time would bring orgasmic release. Janice failed to respond orgasmically until 7 months postpartum. At her 6-month check she was reassured and counseled to explore the behavior that felt good and pleasurable to her rather than aiming for end-point release.

Janice and Bill demonstrated self-esteem in their preparation for childbirth. They wanted a positive childbirth experience and attempted to follow through on this goal. They attended the classes and Bill accompanied his wife on most of the prenatal visits; he also visited afterward in the hospital for as long as he could. Husband and wife both derived a great deal of pride in observing their healthy son, and Janice's feelings of self-esteem were heightened while nursing her baby. Feelings of inadequacy for Janice were associated with not being able to control the modality of delivery. Janice felt both a loss of control and the loss of her closest support person. Afterward, a feeling of guilt was precipitated by the nursing personnel and friends as they tried to comfort her with the assurance that the most important thing after all was having a healthy baby. Janice felt inadequate but was afraid to express her true feeling and her disappointment out of fear of being put down or not being accepted.

Janice also felt very concerned about having to wait longer before initiating an exercise program in order to get back her prepregnancy figure. She thought the vertical scar from the cesarean birth was ugly and was concerned that her husband would be turned off. The cesarean procedure and its relationship to sexual function was particularly evident in Janice's case, with her own particular body image.

Kleeman (1977) described body image distortion as being dependent on how much self-identifying value a person places on each part of his or her body. Janice felt that anything less than a bikini figure was not attractive. Concurrently, Janice had also to cope with another's response to her change in body image.

Janice did take pride in nursing and enjoyed a sense of power in being able to naturally nourish her child both emotionally and physically. Pride in her ability to respond sexually was somewhat dissipated when her husband expressed concern about her failure to achieve orgasm. Her inability to be orgasmic lasted as long as she set orgasm up as a goal. Initially, she attributed her anorgasmia to the surgery. Then she began to blame her husband for the demands he placed on her. When Janice was able to take responsibility for her own sexual response and felt free to seek those things that felt pleasurable and point out those things that were displeasurable, she spontaneously experienced orgasm. Janice and Bill needed assistance in learning how to level with each other. They made assumptions about each other which were for the most part inaccurate. They needed to express their concerns openly in a safe environment. They also needed to increase their options for sexual expression so that their interaction would reflect the flow of their feelings at any particular moment as opposed to losing that flow to the goal of end-point release every time.

A Poorly-Adjusted Couple

Debbie was a 24-year-old primipara who worked as a telephone operator and was married to George, a 28-year-old roofer. Her prenatal experience was filled with complaints of gastric distress, muscular cramping, and inability to control her appetite. Debbie had gained 35 pounds and complained of not being able to walk for more than short periods of time during the last trimester of her pregnancy.

With the encouragement of the obstetrician, this couple attended prepared childbirth classes. George felt hassled about going to the classes and complained of fatigue due to long hours at work. Debbie felt disappointed in his lack of enthusiasm. After Debbie was in labor for 10 hours with no significant descent, pelvimetry revealed inadequate diameters for the passage of a relatively large infant. Because of the long, nonproductive labor, Debbie felt tired, frustrated, and discouraged. When the doctor informed her of the need to deliver the baby abdominally, Debbie felt "relieved to get it over with." When asked whether she would like to be awake she exclaimed, "No, put me to sleep. I'm tired." George did not wish to go into the delivery room. Debbie delivered a 9½ pound baby girl. Debbie and George were both pleased with their baby and stated, "It was well worth it." Because of the cesarean birth, Debbie's sister volunteered to assist her for the first 2 weeks postpartum. Debbie confided to her sister that she felt she would never look or feel the same. Debbie attempted to breast-feed, but discontinued her efforts after 2½ weeks. She claimed that George felt it was "tiring her out too much," especially after the "surgery." She felt ambivalent about discontinuing nursing but did so because of the pressure from George and the lack of support. She also found breast-feeding to be too confining because she felt uncomfortable nursing the baby outside of the home. George's work commitments continued to increase at this time and Debbie was left alone most of the day. She began to resent George's absence and lack of involvement in the baby's care. When George approached her sexually at 5 weeks postpartum, she felt anger and aversion. Any approach on his part was readily rebuked, as Debbie's expectations of George as a father were in no way met. Debbie felt terribly alone and became depressed. Neither George nor Debbie were able to communicate how they really felt, so that they each resorted to assumptions. This led to continued isolation, which increased Debbie's depression and George's absence. This couple was in need of marital/sexual counseling and were so referred by their obstetrician.

In the counseling sessions they were able to see how they both contributed to their state of affairs. Once blame was removed and communication at a feeling level was established, the feeling of isolation and loneliness was replaced by a feeling of mutuality and acceptance of each other's difficulties. Open communication and vulnerability to their feelings in a "safe relationship" led to openness and mutual satisfaction in their sexual relationship. Knowledge of their capacity to respond and the acceptance of this knowledge liberated them to expand their sexual opportunities.

Sexual adjustment is dependent on three components of sexual functioning: (1) the knowledge one has about oneself, (2) the degree of comfort one feels with that knowledge, and (3) the ability to make choices.

Carol and Jim were pretty clear in their definition of sexuality as it applied to them individually and as members of an intimate relationship. Their definition reflected more than coital congress and was broad enough to include their total interaction. For Carol and Jim, sexuality could be known in moments of silence while holding hands, in joy while experiencing birth, in sadness at not having the full freedom to play whenever they "felt like it." Their sexuality was reflected in their physical and emotional nakedness, allowing each other to be completely exposed without the fear of being rejected. Carol talked openly with Jim about her fears of his not liking the cesarean scar. Jim quietly listened to her concern and then said, "I don't like your scar, but I love you! I don't particularly like your nose, either, but I love you. . . . I like your body and I love you!" They both laughed. Jim did not try to change Carol's fear of possible rejection. To do so would be to discount her true feelings and deny her the freedom to be vulnerable. Instead he accepted her feelings and then felt the freedom to be vulnerable himself. Masters and Johnson (1974) have described fear as one of the chief inhibitors of sexual pleasure. The fear of being viewed as ugly, deformed, or unattractive (physically or emotionally) interferes with the ability to truly reveal oneself.

Janice and Bill's definition of sexuality was more circumscribed and goal-oriented. Bill's notion of sexual pleasure was limited to genital expression. Her fear was that if she lost her ability to be orgasmic she would lose her female sexual identity and be labeled as "frigid." When Bill approached Janice about his sexual tension, her initial reaction was to feel responsible for releasing the tension. However, at the time she had "real" reason to postpone coital contact (fatigue and soreness) and asked that they wait. This might reflect an honest representation of her feelings under the circumstances, except that she felt guilty about it, particularly when Bill was left to resort to masturbation. The following week, when she felt she could physically tolerate coitus, she initiated their sexual contact for "his sake." She fell into the traditional wifely role of providing sex as a service. With this dynamic in effect, a couple gradually comes to the point of diminishing return. Much of the active partner's stimulation is stymied by the passive partner. With some counseling, Janice switched tracks and sought opportunities for her own pleasure. As a result, things started to happen for both of them. They began exploring the possibility of touching as an end in itself, without the standard pattern of having to get somewhere. The pleasure came from living each moment as it came, no matter what it brought or where it led.

Debbie and George's definition of their sexuality was the most limited. It was confined to stereotyped roles which knew no relief. Their relationship became one of two individuals cast into roles which were inflexible. Both felt "boxed in" and isolated from each other. They were committed to fulfilling their prescribed duties, as opposed to committing themselves to each other. The more they worked at fulfilling these duties, the more they lost sight of each other. Frustrated by the overwhelming responsibility of baby and home, Debbie became increasingly depressed and withdrawn. George was unable to understand her feelings of frustration and resented her withdrawal from him, gradually pulling away to protect himself. His hours away from home continued to increase. His attempts at coital contact with Debbie were at first rebuked, and then gradually permitted, as Debbie acted out the traditional female role of passive recipient. At this stage, sexuality could never be anything more than intravaginal masturbation.

Sexual counseling assisted Debbie and George in:

1. Removing blame.
2. Learning how to be responsible for themselves as individuals and members of an intimate relationship.
3. Increasing their knowledge about their capacities to respond sexually.
4. Exploring the many options available within their relationship.
5. Developing a commitment based on mutual respect and regard for the other.

6. Developing an understanding that as an individual acquires more knowledge about himself and his partner and a greater degree of comfort in
sharing this knowledge, more choices become available.

In summary, aside from the first 2 to 3 weeks postpartum, it is my experience
that cesarean couples have physiological adjustments to make in their sexual
functioning that are similar to those required of noncesarean couples. The
postpartum pelvis in either vaginal or abdominal delivery is congested and
demonstrates steroid starvation with decreases in the intensity and rapidity
of sexual response.

Psychosocially, the sexual adjustment of the cesarean couple is highly individual, as is also true of the noncesarean couple. It is my experience that
threats to self-esteem exist in women whose identities are very much tied to
the female task of vaginal birth. Body image distortion and the cesarean scar,
along with the inability of the woman's sexual partner to complete active
participation in the delivery, can influence a couple's resumptions of sexual
interaction. Prepregnancy levels of sexual adjustment, including the degree
of sexual knowledge and comfort and the variety of methods of fulfillment,
along with the degree of open communication also impact on the cesarean
couple's postpartum sexual adjustment.

NURSING IMPLICATIONS

Historically, nursing has been loyal to the concept that its focus is the "total
well-being" of the patient as a member of a family and a society. Yet nurses
as well as other members of the health-care profession have neglected or ignored an aspect of health care that is so important to human personality that
its omission carries the blatant message that sexuality is not a legitimate
nursing concern. The health care profession is struggling to free itself of the
dead hand of the past. . . a grasp that still paralyzes with ignorance, anxiety,
and prejudice. Attempts at correcting this condition have been met with
resistance in the guise of "priority setting," lack of time, and "limited bud-
gets." I know of no other area which is a source of such grave concern as a
person's sense of himself or herself as a man or a woman, except of course
for the ultimate need to survive. A threat to this identity increases the gravity
of the struggle for healthy self-restoration and/or adaptation to a normal
developmental stress (such as pregnancy), which may become unbalanced by
the addition of a major surgical procedure (such as cesarean birth). The impact does not end here; its effect also reaches others, particularly the "loved
and intimate ones."

Kolodny et al. (1979) described the paradox of the nurse who is expected
to address the sexual concerns of the patients but has little preparation to

meet this demand. For years the nurse was the silent companion to the "well-informed" physician. All questions of a sexual nature were deferred to the physician, who suffered some similar gaps in his preparation. The patient therefore was left alone to his/her own devices, based many times on misinformation and poor advice.

Nurses can no longer collaborate in a conspiracy of silence. The nurse does not need permission from the physician to be attentive to the sexual concerns of the patient any more than she needs his permission to obtain a dietary history. Rather, the nurse-clinician serves as a role model, expressing her comfort with sexuality in all interactions with the patient, the family, and other members of the professional staff. Nurses have the opportunity to set the stage for providing a safe environment in which this may occur.

This is possible only when the nurse has assumed responsibility for defining for herself the meaning of sexuality in its broadest sense and as a dimension of the total personality, rather than limiting sexuality to mere genital functioning. Self-knowledge and comfort with one's own sexuality is prerequisite to learning how to assist patients with their sexual concerns.

The nurse is often identified as having a nurturing role. Patients often feel vulnerable and dependent during stressful experiences and elicit the instinctual response of the nurse to be a "professional mother" or "parent." Few nurses have difficulty with this role, except when they have gotten so locked into it that they are unable to recognize the sexual concerns of the patient, much as a parent is oblivious to the sexual concerns of his/her children. An example is found in the nurse who may readily offer comfort measures to a patient in labor—e.g., a cool cloth on her face, clean sheets, holding her hand—but sends the husband out of the room for any pelvic exam because she assumes this may cause embarrassment for him. Rather than protect him from a "danger" that may not exist in the first place, the nurse could encourage his presence if he chooses to stay and assist him to be a support agent for his wife.

The patient protects the health professional just as the child protects the parent, by not asking questions that might elicit an uncomfortable response.

Woods (1975) referred to the privacy, warmth, and time that are so necessary in establishing the rapport essential for patient disclosure. Denial or repression of a sexual concern is often evident when no questions are asked by the patient or no information is volunteered by the professional. Often the nurse draws the conclusion that if the patient doesn't bring up an issue, there is no issue. A common example of this is found in the obstetrical nurse caring for antepartum patients. This nurse instructs the patients about body hygiene, nutrition, exercise, weight gain, the danger signals of pregnancy, and the variations in pregnancy, but often leaves them feeling confused about sexual activity before and after birth. When the patient is not counseled about sexual functioning, she is given the message that sex is a taboo area— not to be pursued. This promotes feelings of confusion and guilt while leaving

224 The Cesarean Experience

the patient ignorant of the effects of sexual expression on herself, her spouse, and ultimately her family.

Nurses often fail to see how difficult it is for a patient to find the right words to express sexual concerns. The way in which a nurse discusses the whole area of sexuality can give encouragement and direction to the patient who needs to discuss sexual concerns. The nurse, in these discussions with the mother and her spouse, serves as a role model for the family, thus facilitating a learning opportunity. In helping parents to broaden their understanding of their sexuality, the nurse enables them to draw from their own uniqueness as individuals and as a couple, freeing them to choose options which might never have been discovered had a stressful experience not occurred.

When genital sex is placed in the context of the person's total sexuality and is not distorted as the "be all and end all" of one's sexuality, the couple does not feel devastated when certain aspects of sexual functioning are restricted.

The nurse's ability to deal therapeutically with the sexual adjustment of a couple following birth requires competence in several areas. She must have:

1. Knowledge of and confidence in her own sexuality, as reflected in a warm, sensitive, and positive attitude toward the patient's sexuality. This attitude allows the nurse to give the patient permission to voice sexual concerns.
2. Knowledge of the anatomy and physiology of sexual response before, during, and following pregnancy, coupled with an awareness of the psychosocial-cultural factors inherent in sexual behavior. This allows the nurse to provide information and anticipatory guidance which may prevent escalating future problems.
3. Knowledge and skill in the counseling process. The nurse is thus able to teach the interpersonal skills necessary for open communication and to act as a catalyst in the promotion of an intimate relationship.
4. Specialized training in the diagnosis and/or treatment of sexual dysfunction or problems. This enables the nurse clinician to stimulate, through the treatment modality, behavioral changes that will affect the couple's sexual interaction.

The many levels on which the nurse contributes to the sexual function of her patients following childbirth, be it vaginal or cesarean, depends on her self-knowledge, her knowledge of the disciplines involved, and her desire to further human well-being through affirmation of healthy sexuality.

REFERENCES

Falicov CJ: Sexual adjustment during first pregnancy and postpartum. Am J Obstet Gynecol 117:991-1000, 1973

Kenny JA: Sexuality of pregnant and breast feeding women. Arch Sex Behav 2:215-29, 1973

Kleeman K: Distortions in Body Image in Illness and Disability. New York, Wiley and Sons, 1977, pp. 81-85

Kolodny R, Masters W, Johnson V, Biggs M: Textbook of Human Sexuality for Nurses, Boston, Little, Brown, pp. 1–7, 1979

Lamont J: Sex problems after gynecological surgery. Female Patient 2 (7): 26–29, 1977

Masters WH, Johnson VE: Human Sexual Response. Boston, Little Brown, 1966

Masters WH, Johnson VE: The Pleasure Bond. Boston, Little Brown, pp. 362–63, 1974

Morris NM: The frequency of sexual intercourse during pregnancy. Arch Sex Behav 4:501–507, 1975

Salberg DA, Butler J, Wagner NN: Sexual behavior in pregnancy. N Eng J Med 288:1098–1103, 1973

Tolor A, DiGrazia PV: Sexual attitudes and behavior patterns during and following pregnancy. Arch Sex Behav 5:539–51, 1976

Woods N: Human Sexuality in Health and Illness. St. Louis, Mosby, p. 210, 1975

CHAPTER 11

Counseling, Self-help Groups, and Telephone Services: A Network of Postpartum Support

Anne Wilson

POSTPARTUM ADJUSTMENT

The cesarean couple, like all other childbearing couples, needs assistance in establishing a network of support systems for the postpartum transition so as to be able to activate nurturing behaviors toward the newborn. Cesarean couples are not unique in needing this kind of assistance. Many of the new cesarean mothers' reactions to the settling-in period at home parallel the reactions of mothers who deliver vaginally (Mercer 1977). What differentiates the cesarean mother is the additional surgical intervention; this may intensify the adjustment difficulties, particularly as concerns her feelings of dependence. The initial 3 months at home after delivery appear to produce the greatest number of stresses for all mothers (Haire 1972; Kramer 1979).

In many Western societies the mobility of the nuclear family has weakened traditional support systems. The contemporary nuclear family must confront the complex adjustment problems of assuming responsibility, sharing, and reworking patterns of family life. The expectations parents have of childbearing and parenting experiences are very high. It is not surprising that frustration results when parents feel unable to fulfill the multiple roles expected of the nuclear family unit (Affonso and Stichler 1980).

Couples who feel that they need or want help may be too embarrassed or unable to actively seek it. The constancy of parenting is seldom understood by couples prior to the actual experience (Rising 1974). Few couples have been stimulated by the health-care system or by childbirth educators to develop a plan of options and responses with which to face an unplanned cesarean birth. The unpreparedness contributes to the vulnerability so often described by them (Boyd and Mahon 1980; Hedahl 1980; Schlosser 1978).

Parents who give birth in anguish and fear, who are isolated and stressed will communicate their experience not only to the members of the family unit but also to a multitude of other individuals with whom they will be in contact in the course of their lives. The intensity of giving and taking and supporting requires energy and time that are at a premium immediately after childbirth (Johnson 1979).

For cesarean couples, the combination of low reserves of emotional energy with lack of physical energy may create a survival-oriented atmosphere. At a time when links to a network of trust and competent care are critical, society sends out many messages that asking for help is a symptom of incompetence. Health-care professionals often contribute to feelings of incompetence by manipulating family decisions rather than sharing relevant information on the basis of the belief that families can and will make responsible decisions (Howell 1975).

What is unique about the initial postpartum adjustment period at home is that it is the first time the family is left alone to cope with the patterns of adjustment. There is no professional expert on hand to give recommendations, and there is no hospital nursery to which to return the fretting newborn when the mother is uncertain of what action to take next. There may be no additional help to relieve the mother when she feels exhausted. During the initial 2 to 3 weeks at home, the mother feels least secure and most stressed. She feels most vulnerable because of the constancy of infant demands, interfaced with her own needs for surgical recovery. Even though additional help may be available during the first few weeks at home, the cesarean mother may describe herself as being in a constant state of panic (Gruis 1977). The posthospital adjustment period focuses on five major response adaptations: (1) responses to the newborn, (2) responses to the father, (3) responses to the newborn's siblings, (4) responses to extended family members, and (5) responses to the community.

During the months of January through April, 1978, mothers who had delivered either vaginally or by cesarean birth and who were attending informal group meetings for new mothers at the third postpartal month were interviewed to attempt to gather information about perceptions and feelings related to postpartum adjustment. The meetings were voluntary and were sponsored by a childbirth education group. Groups generally consisted of 6 to 14 members, most of whom were primigravidas. Mothers who were working stated that they were employed either by choice or in order to maintain a higher standard of living, rather than because of economic necessity. Their pregnancies were desired.

An open-ended interview format was used to allow mothers maximal expression of their feelings. A total of 110 mothers were interviewed, 42 of whom were cesarean mothers. Seven mothers were multiparas (five of the seven were cesarean mothers). Mothers were asked to talk about the days at home immediately after hospital discharge and to describe the support systems they utilized or would like to have had available. The comments made by mothers in this chapter are all products of those interviews.

Responses to the Newborn

Caretaking is a central focus of family life. Feeding represents the epitome of family members taking care of one another. It provides life-sustaining nourishment and comfort. A mother's feeding of her infant is often used as a way of communicating her desire and ability to care for him in a more general way (Donovan 1977; Haire 1972). When the mother has delivered her child surgically, the need to breastfeed, if already present, may increase (Donovan 1977). Concerns about feeding patterns and adjustments generally peak about 1 week after going home from the hospital (Shereshefsky and Yarrow 1973). La Leche offers the cesarean mother an opportunity to receive assistance and encouragement when she most needs it (Brewster 1979). Ways of assisting the cesarean mother to successfully initiate breastfeeding will be discussed later in this chapter.

Concerns about sleeping patterns and crying are felt by mothers whose infants do not sleep well. Mothers often associate increased crying and distress with feeding difficulties and thus with unskilled mothering. The intensity of concern expressed by the interviewed mothers did not appear to differ in accordance with method of delivery. The following sample comments represent the feelings of both cesarean and vaginally-delivered mothers.

"I always try to feed him first when he cries. . . . After that, I'm less and less sure about what the problem is."

"I've never been able to distinguish between the different cries. All the books say that a mother can tell the difference, but I just know that something is making him uncomfortable, and I feel so helpless . . . I know *he's* helpless."

"It makes me nervous and upset. I can't ignore it and sometimes I can't do anything about it, either."

Responses to the Father

Cesarean mothers in the sample expressed appreciation of the fathers' presence and help. When fathers are permitted to participate in parenting from the time of delivery, cesarean newborns receive the benefits of a kind of double attachment. Some mothers attempt to prevent the father from assuming child care tasks or are sharply critical of the father's level of expertise.

The mother may project her own negative feelings onto the father. The nurse needs to be sensitive to such patterns of behavior so that positive patterns can be encouraged and referrals for additional counseling can be made, when appropriate (Donovan 1977).

Responses to the Newborn's Siblings

Delayed physical recovery of the cesarean mother accentuates the adjustments necessary in relation to the baby's siblings. Mothers with other children in the toddler age range seem to feel most frustrated. The following comments were made by cesarean mothers.

"I could never seem to get caught up with even the bare minimum, much less get ahead."

"I'de be up all night with the baby and then after my husband would leave for work the 2-year-old would be up, ready to play. I lived on the brink of hysteria."

"My doctor told me to get lots of rest. My babies are exactly 12 months apart and rest is just out of the question."

Siblings may express concerns about the mother's scar. They may be simply curious or genuinely concerned that the new baby "hurt" Mommy. Assistance in handling the questions of young children can be provided by the nurse and through community resources. Responses which help young children understand that babies can be born in "different" rather than "normal/ abnormal" ways reassure them and help establish a foundation for positive interaction with the newest family member. Honest answers that are direct and reassuring are very important. Such resources as the International Childbirth Association and the Birth and the Family Journal's *Instructional Materials Catalogue* offer children's dolls which deliver babies by cesarean. These may be of help by providing children with the opportunity to express concerns and feelings about cesarean birth.

Responses to Extended Family Members

Most cesarean mothers have some additional assistance at home during the first few weeks after delivery. The helper is often the woman's own mother or mother-in-law or a close family member. Cultural factors may be important in the choice of a helper. If the cesarean delivery was unplanned, help may have to be recruited on short notice. The cesarean mothers interviewed expressed very mixed feelings about helpers. The additional physical help seemed appreciated, yet many mothers expressed difficulty in coping with other helping individuals in the house who did not understand or empathize with what they were feeling. The cesarean mother may feel that the helper's presence augments feelings of dependence and inadequacy and the unsettled state of the family routine. She may resent the physical wholeness of the helper. The mother may need reassurance that the need for help is temporary (Donovan 1977).

The cesarean mother may need to be reminded that her willingness to receive help will promote her rapid and full recovery, enabling her to assume the total mothering role as quickly as possible. It is also helpful to point out ways in which the helper can include the mother in infant care activities while she continues to rest and recover.

When possible, it is very helpful for a nurse to meet with the mother and the designated helper before hospital discharge to explore feelings related to settling-in at home and to provide a setting in which a practical plan can be worked out for the family. If the mother is still physically unable to give her infant routine care, then the helper might care for the infant at the mother's bedside to permit her to observe the routines. The helper may also benefit from a more complete orientation to the possible psychological sequelae to cesarean delivery which are within the normal range of behaviors (Hedahl 1980; Affonso and Stichler 1980). Some written guidelines or suggested reading materials will aid the helper in caring for the new mother and infant. The helper who has been recruited after an unplanned cesarean delivery may be unsure of how to handle the situation and may need such guidelines.

Responses to the Community

The cesarean mother seems to be particularly dependent upon the experience and advice of other cesarean mothers, who serve as her peer group. She is less likely than the vaginally-delivered mother to have many family members or friends who have had delivery experiences similar to her own. The social network from which she expects to receive information and support may be inadequate. The early postpartum period is often perceived by new parents (both cesarean- and vaginally-delivered) as a community encroachment on a private event, a sort of territorial imperative response. Cesarean mothers state that they enjoy the attention of family and friends and recognize the efforts to share in the tasks of settling-in. However, they also find that the need to be sociable is superseded by an intense desire to retreat into the intimate nest of "father, mother, infant." Nervousness, fatigue, depression, difficulty in adjusting to the needs of the baby, difficulty in adjusting to the needs of siblings, too much company, interference by relatives and neighbors, and worries about regaining equilibrium are at their peak during this time (Affonso and Stichler 1980; Hedahl 1980; Larsen 1966; Stranik and Hogberg 1979). Cesarean mothers express the need to overcome the social stigma they associate with cesarean birth (Marut and Mercer 1979). Some perceive the experience as a rite of passage. The mothers do not want to fail, yet their comments indicate that they do not feel successful:

> "Everyone rushed in to admire the baby. I seemed to be suddenly an invisible "after-the-fact." She was cute and cuddly and I felt like a sub-human being, but I still needed someone to tell me *I* was doing okay, too, and that I was still attractive and cuddly. I felt physically maimed. No amount of flowers or cards could erase the sense of failure I felt."

> "Everything fell apart. My incision hurt. I couldn't sleep. The baby didn't sleep. I was mad at myself for feeling so low. I was mad at my husband for not understanding and mad at the baby for being so tranquil and unaffected by it all."

> "Family and friends kept trying to help. They made me feel like an invalid. I sometimes felt they wanted to intrude because they had been intruded upon and now it was their turn."

A few women are very optimistic. Although it is not typical, the following comments from a cesarean mother indicate that not all women view the cesarean experience as a negative one: "We imagined a special child all through this pregnancy. When he decided to be born differently [by cesarean birth], then it was just more evidence for me that he was determined to stand out in the crowd. Who was I to squelch his style!"

Among the cesarean mothers who were interviewed, women who had been employed outside the home prior to delivery stated that the stresses they experienced in the early postpartum were intensified by the need to resolve all conflicts within an acutely limited time frame. Many expressed intense frustration about additional losses of time from work as a result of the cesarean delivery and prolonged recovery. Fears of economic loss, as well as fears of physical and emotional setbacks, were frequently mentioned. The need to rapidly balance the demands of family, employer, and self created additional stress for some.

The need for organization and scheduling for these women may increase their difficulty in accepting the disorganized, irregular pattern of the early postpartum period. The nurse may need to help the cesarean mother who plans to return to employment soon after delivery to set realistic goals for herself.

In interviews with women who have had cesarean births, there is a significant number of references to plans for future pregnancies. Cesarean mothers verbalize reservations about attempting future pregnancies more often than vaginally-delivered mothers do (Donovan 1977). They may fear the physical risks. They may also fear lack of access to physicians and other health care professionals who support genuine family-centered maternity care (Affonso and Stichler 1980). Contraceptive information is important for cesarean mothers, not only to provide an opportunity for full physical recovery but also to allow them adequate time to resolve any negative feelings they may associate with the unplanned cesarean birth. Increasingly, families who have had cesarean births are organizing into community groups, both to offer supportive services to one another and to encourage health-care professionals to become more sensitive to their needs (Donovan 1977; Hedahl 1980).

Because the nurse is a natural link between the family, the medical community, and the social community, her skill in creating a supportive network which joins them all in a cooperative effort is vital. The components which interface to make this possible are counseling skills and organizational structure.

COUNSELING SKILLS

Counseling is distinct from education and advice in that its focus is on feelings. The role of the nurse counselor is to assist the individual(s) to explore, expand, understand, and cope with feelings. Her role is to assist the individual or couple in defining and sorting out alternatives—allowing them to determine the available options and to figure out how each of the potential options fits with his or their self-image, value system, cultural system, and future childbearing goals.

The primary goal of the nurse who is counseling the cesarean mother or couple is to facilitate and support the decision-making process. The goals of the nurse who is working with cesarean couples during the immediate postpartum period are (1) to reduce anxiety, (2) to promote successful decision making in forming postpartal plans, (3) to increase self-confidence and knowledge, and (4) by so doing to promote the growth and nurturing of the family (Benjamin 1974; Haley 1976; Johnson 1979).

It is vital for the parents who have experienced an unplanned cesarean delivery to become sensitive to nonverbal cues (Ekman 1964). The cesarean mother who states that she is very happy to have a healthy baby but who is reluctant to receive and care for her child may be communicating underlying unexpressed feelings. She may be attempting to convince herself that she should be happy. She may be terrified of or angry at the infant who has placed her in this predicament. She may feel totally incompetent to provide care. She may be too physically exhausted to be able to nurture. She may be testing the counselor to determine whether the counselor views her as an acceptable human being.

The cesarean mother who makes statements like "I feel like throwing the baby out the window," or "This will never by my baby," may not be a potential child abuser but is an individual who has difficulty defining and expressing the real source of her anger. Cesarean mothers who utilize hotline services occasionally initiate the telephone conversation with such statements. As they establish a comfortable rapport with the counselor, they verbalize a variety of concerns which center around parenting and sorting out and accepting present feelings.

In order to be helpful, the nurse must be comfortable with her own feelings. She must clarify her values. How does she perceive cesarean delivery? Does she feel that it in some way reflects inadequacy of the mother/couple? How does she feel about her own childbearing experience(s) or lack of them? Can she genuinely accept the value system and feelings of the couple even though these may be radically different from her own? Can she accept her professional limitations? Does she feel comfortable in making appropriate referrals to other health-care providers? If she teaches childbirth preparation classes, does she view the cesarean couple as a sign of her own failure to communicate skills or information?

One of the most difficult tasks of the nurse counselor is to allow the individual being helped to assume control of and responsibility for his own growth and development. Because nurses want to assist, they often succeed best in helping the individual to become dependent upon them. Certainly, one of the basic requirements for effective counseling is the desire to be helpful. However, the counselor must also have a deep-seated trust in the capacity of the individual to handle his or her feelings, to work through them, and to find acceptable solutions to his or her problem (Rogers 1951, 1972; Johnson 1979).

The nurse who is counseling must recognize that feelings are transitory. The cesarean mother who feels anger toward all women whom she views as "whole" frequently projects that anger onto the nurse, who is accessible (Donovan 1977). It is probably not the individual personality of the nurse that is eliciting the anger at that moment, but rather the unwounded person she represents. The cesarean mother will be helped by the nurse's recognition that her feelings are acceptable, whatever they may be.

Counselors are people, too. Health-care providers frequently help themselves through helping others. The recognition that working through one's own feelings is necessary before being able to effectively handle the feelings of others will make the initial stages of establishing a trusting relationship easier. It is important for the nurse to recognize that she is responsible for respecting the perceptions of the woman she counsels and for acknowledging the limitations of her own perceptions. It is vital that she distinguish between short-term stress and long-term pathology (LeMasters 1965).

For the postpartal cesarean mother who is still hospitalized, a rapid assessment of counseling needs can be made when answers to the following questions are available (Haley 1976; Halstead 1974).

1. Is the woman under stress?
2. Is she coping with the situation? This is not necessarily the same as asking if she is coping the way the ideal patient *should* cope!

3. Is she requesting help?
4. Are there other factors which complicate the situation (family, outside stressors)?

In order to assist the new mother in developing or improving positive adaptive behaviors, the nurse needs information about the woman's strengths, her life experiences, and her reactions to them. What kinds of defenses have been at her disposal during illnesses? How were they developed? How strong were or are they? Where and why did they break down? (Benjamin 1974; Johnson 1979).

A detailed review of a particular birth experience may uncover a stabilized personality pattern which has been effective for the mother over a long period of time, even though it may be unpleasant for the nurse who feels she has heard the account numerous times. Cesarean mothers who appear comfortable physically and psychologically may also be responding to the cesarean experience uniquely, in accordance with their respective personality patterns (Boyd and Mahon 1980).

The mother's degree of comfort with the nurse is affected not so much by what is said as by how it is said. What the woman senses through nonverbal behaviors has a decisive influence on her ability to establish a feeling of rapport with the nurse. Body language communicates what words may not (Rogers 1972).

Tone of voice also communicates. Judgmental tones, often unnoticed on the surface by the speaker, are received in full force by the listener. Phrases or responses that begin with "Hasn't it occurred to you that . . .?" or "You are very lucky that . . . " make light of the many fears and concerns the cesarean mother may have (Donovan 1977). Avoidance of episodes of silence prevents the mother from expressing useful information and prevents the nurse from having to deal with difficult feelings she herself may be afraid to handle.

Questions need a purpose. They should provide the nurse with useful information rather than merely filling in episodes of silence. Questions which do not elicit information, or which do not explore the information presented, are better left unasked.

Interviewing skills and counseling techniques are developed, not genetically acquired. They depend primarily on the nurse's desire to understand precisely what the meaning of the other person's statement is to that person. The ability to genuinely accept the individual's feelings—whatever they may be and however different they may be from the nurse's own or from what she thinks should be her own—and the ability to recognize the transitory nature of feelings assist the nurse in supporting the cesarean couple. These abilities also prevent the nurse from assuming the negative feelings of the woman or couple or imposing her own feelings on them (Rogers 1972).

The client-centered or Rogerian approach to eliciting information provides the following benefits for both the mother and the nurse.

1. The nurse does not presume that she is more knowledgeable than the woman with whom she is interacting.
2. The method provides an active mode of dealing with the mother's perceived feelings and assisting her in finding solutions to problems.
3. The woman or couple can maintain control over the content of the conversation because the nurse follows their cues in the interaction.
4. The environment is nonthreatening and supportive.
5. The focus is on the woman and her current perceptions and feelings.
6. There is an implicit trust in the woman's capacity to make decisions. (Benjamin 1974; Clark 1977; Haley 1976; Rogers 1951)

SELF-HELP GROUPS

Self-help groups meet basic human needs. They present a means of assessing both present and future expectations and provide an accepting base from which to practice previously learned and new behaviors (Clark 1966). They allow translation of thoughts and feelings into behaviors which are adaptable to the reality of individual families (Bion 1961). The self-help group can generally be described as a group of individuals who are personally affected by similar psychological or social conditions. Membership is voluntary and is restricted to those who have either past or present experience of the distressing event. Activities of the self-help group evolve around fellowship, crisis assistance, mutual aid, development of self, and social action. The group can support a change in the individual's lifestyle to the extent that it affects the individual's ability to cope with the problematic condition. The goal of the self-help group is to provide a group frame of reference that will support a more constructive resolution of the problem for the individual. Some of the benefits which are provided by this group process include:

1. Sharing one's experience with others in a similar predicament while maintaining self-respect as all members pursue more satisfying solutions to the problem.
2. Receiving relevant information about the specific situation.
3. Providing crisis-related services in recognition of the fact that setbacks may occur before recovery is completed. There is recognition that recovery occurs on a progressive continuum of irregular forward movement.
4. Acquiring a realistic perspective. Members recognize that change involves commitment and requires assessment of priorities.
5. Providing a living demonstration that the problems or problematic

situations can be overcome. Hope is given. The aspiration to become like successful group members often stimulates action.

Self-help groups often have appeal in situations where alternative forms of assistance do not. The group provides immediate social approval of members. There is usually some form of status similarity in the group composition and there are certainly common feelings relative to the problem situation which unite members. The self-help group tends to be readily accessible geographically and provides caring both when and where it is needed (Bion 1961; Dinkmeyer 1971; Glasser 1974; Johnson and Johnson 1975).

The nurse can utilize self-help groups in a variety of ways to facilitate and augment existing support networks or to establish networks where they do not already exist. The self-help group may be used by the nurse as a rich source of information about potential resources in the community. Self-help group members—whose primary focus is on their specific problem—very often have the time and energy to research community resources. The group may also provide practical assistance for the individual who does not desire or is not suitable for professional assistance (Adrian 1980). The group may be used as an adjunct to professional treatment. In areas where obstetric programs are undergoing revision, self-help groups can be used for consultation and collaboration between the professional community and the consumer community (Powell 1975).

Three kinds of self-help groups which are particularly beneficial for the cesarean couple during the postpartum transition are groups which assist with breast-feeding, self-help telephone services or hotlines, and postpartum support groups.

Breast-feeding

Health-care providers assume too frequently that the cesarean mother will not wish to breast-feed her infant because of the additional physical debilitation she may have experienced with cesarean birth. Some women assume that they cannot breast-feed because of surgical delivery. Breast-feeding is not only possible for the cesarean mother but may be very important for her and her infant (Brewster 1979; Grams 1978; Jelliffe 1977). Uterine stimulation resulting from breast-feeding may enhance reversion to normal size and facilitate physical recovery. Babies born by cesarean delivery are deprived of the cutaneous stimulation which is part of vaginal birth (Montague 1971). Breast-feeding provides this type of stimulation. In hospitals where even normal cesarean newborns experience immediate and sometimes prolonged separation from the parents after birth, the infant is further deprived of skin contact and its comforting effect. For babies whose cesarean births resulted from fetal complications or who suffer complications immediately after delivery, the nutritional benefits of breast milk may be especially significant. Because breast-feeding sets up a built-in system of immunization for the infant, it may be preferable for the cesarean newborn to protect him from infection (Henderson 1978; Murdaugh and Miller 1975; Ross Laboratories 1979).

Cesarean mothers may have additional handicaps in relating to their infants initially because of an inability to expel them and because they were separated from their infants immediately after delivery, often for long periods of time. They may develop deep feelings of dissassociation and/or disbelief regarding real "ownership" of the infant: "How can I be sure this baby is really my baby?" Breast-feeding may help the mother to finalize her pregnancy and delivery and to begin to perceive the infant as her own (Marut and Mercer 1979; Mercer 1977). The mother whose self-esteem has been damaged because of the cesarean experience may view breast-feeding as an opportunity to overcome her disappointment or sense of failure. It also augments the visible evidence that she is a competent mother (see Chapter 6).

The role of the nurse is to educate the woman who is undecided about a feeding method and to teach and offer support to women who favor breast-feeding and to those who do not. A woman who does not wish to breast-feed, for whatever reason, will meet with marginal success if she feels coerced. The nurse must avoid inspiring additional guilt feelings in the cesarean mother who opts to bottle-feed her infant by implying that she is increasing the possibility of infection, allergic complications, and ineffective maternal-infant attachment. Instead, the role of the nurse is to assist and support the bottle-feeding mother in finding ways to counter these possible adverse effects (Brewster 1979; Jarkowsky 1980).

Some women assume that if they do not begin to breast-feed immediately they cannot opt to do so at a later time. They need to know that delayed breast-feeding is possible. Some cesarean mothers feel so overwhelmed with the alterations in their idealized birth experiences that they do not feel receptive to breast-feeding immediately after delivery, even though they may have expressed interest during pregnancy. It is important for the nurse to determine whether the change in attitude is a temporary or a permanent one. The mother who desires to breast-feed but is fearful that medications and anesthesia may adversely affect the quality of her early milk production needs to be reassured (Doucette 1978; O'Brien 1974; Rothermel and Faber 1974).

The breast-feeding mother needs to continue to maintain adequate fluid intake at home and to find positions that are comfortable for her (Countryman 1977; Jarkowsky 1980; Goetting 1977). Suggestions for alleviating or preventing nipple discomfort should be provided before hospital discharge (Whitley 1978). The mother should have an opportunity to express concerns about breast-feeding (Grassley et al. 1978).

A breast pump may be helpful for women who have difficulty with manual expression of milk from the breasts (Tibbetts and Caldwell 1980). The cesarean mother who is already physically depleted may derive particular benefit from a breast pump. Lloyd pumps can be obtained from the La Leche League if they are not readily available on the hospital maternity unit. La Leche League International, Inc., publishes a helpful pamphlet entitled *Breastfeeding After the Cesarean Section.* It provides practical information for the cesarean mother, in addition to resource materials. It may be obtained through the local La Leche group or by writing to La Leche at 9616 Minneapolis Avenue, Franklin Park, Ill. 60131. Ross Laboratories also publishes an excellent guide to breast-feeding for cesarean mothers for professionals (Ross Laboratories 1979). Providing the mother an opportunity for contact with a community representative of a breast-feeding support group while she is still in the hospital gives reassurance that help and encouragement are close at hand.

Self-help Telephone Services

Cesarean families, and particularly cesarean mothers, may benefit from the establishment of a self-help telephone service. Utilization of a telephone system permits the new mother to receive assistance rapidly without having to leave her home setting. This is particularly helpful during the first few weeks at home and for mothers of young children who frequently have limited child care assistance. Reassurance that many of the mother's feelings fall within the normal range of responses is comforting (Haight 1977). The cesarean mother may feel too physically taxed to leave the home setting to ask for assistance. She may also prefer anonymity, especially if she feels uncomfortable or embarrassed about asking for help.

In communities where a universal hotline is already operating, it may be convenient to establish the self-help line as part of the services available through the hotline. The service may also be established through the postpartum unit of the hospital or through an independent community agency. The most important factor in developing the system is to be certain that new cesarean mothers receive the appropriate telephone number and information in written form *before* they leave the hospital.

The intent of the self-help line determines its organizational framework. The purposes of a self-help line may include sharing feelings giving medical assistance, and providing referral information for ongoing counseling. The self-help line may offer crisis assistance. It may provide continuity between hospital and home (Deakers 1972).

Where self-help lines are available, many calls come in from women who have just been told by their doctors that they have to have cesarean deliveries. These calls are the result of their need for information as well as their feelings of insecurity because they do not know what to do or what will be happening. The self-help line can assist these callers by giving appropriate information and encouraging the callers to consult in greater detail with their doctors. The self-help line can help prenatal and postpartal women to recognize the normal range of behaviors and can give support to these women in their roles as new parents. Some self-help lines (called "warm lines" in some areas) have parent-to-parent services through which a caller can be referred to volunteers who have had experiences which parallel that being approached by the caller. A cesarean mother who wants to return to work and to continue to breast-feed her baby can be referred to a volunteer who has done just that. Many self-help lines have very detailed, cross-referenced lists of volunteers who have had a broad range of very specific experiences. Conversing with someone who has survived and adjusted to a situation parallel to one's own can be very supportive (Freeman 1980).

The selection of staff members to maintain the self-help line is crucial. Controversy exists over the effectiveness of lay counselors, but the results are generally favorable with careful selection and orientation. Volunteers are usually recruited through word of mouth or through solicitation, often in community centers or neighborhood newspapers. "Self-assessment of attitudes" scales, such as the California Psychological Inventory, may be used at the initial conference to screen interested volunteers. Indicators which appear to correlate with successful volunteer self-help line service include flexibility, desire to help, ability to recognize and focus on feeling patterns, and a positive self-image (Gottsfeld et al. 1970; Rioch et al. 1963).

Clearly defined jobs must exist before it is possible to select staff members for those jobs. Once the services to be offered are specified, then a job description outlining duties and levels of functioning can be written. Considerations should include the following.

1. Will the volunteer have back-up resources or is she expected to be totally self-reliant?
2. Is the volunteer expected to have specific skills, such as crisis intervention experience or medical expertise?
3. In what way will the volunteer be responsible to the self-help line administration?
4. What records will she maintain and how will she maintain them? Is a standardized format to be provided?
5. Is the volunteer expected to provide referral resources or is she limited to a predetermined and previously organized Cardex of information?
6. What specific information derived from expert sources must the volunteer have?
7. How much will she be allowed to deviate from the standard pattern of help outlined in the scope of services offered?

Ordering (by rank) of the importance of the volunteer's qualifications is helpful. A scoring system for priority qualifications may be helpful (Delworth et al. 1972).

The purpose of the self-help line will also determine what skills the volunteer must already have and what skills can be taught later. Providing opportunities for volunteers to participate in role-playing situations and group interview procedures will give those who select and screen volunteers for training a chance to see how potential volunteers interact with peers as well as with agency representatives (Riessman 1967; Loomis 1979). The trainers should be individuals who are already recognized for their communication skills in the specific services the self-help line will provide. The crisis center discrimination index described by Delworth (1972) provides useful guidelines for assessing role playing and response-oriented skills.

The preliminary training period may consist of a single intense meeting or a series of closely spaced meetings which through screening and selection will yield a core of potentially acceptable volunteers. In addition to discussion of role playing and/or procedures for handling difficult calls, policies and organizational framework should be addressed. Written materials should include policies and the organizational framework, referral information, responsibilities of volunteers, specific information to be given callers, limitations of services, and an explanation of when to refer callers. A manual of procedures may be provided, as well as guidelines for active listening, good telephone techniques, and protection of caller confidentiality.

Communication between volunteers and the administering agency is vital. A newsletter for exchange of information is helpful. All volunteers need to feel that they are important links in an actively functioning system. Consultation with agency experts over a particularly difficult call or for assistance in assessing skills is important. Volunteers need to be provided with continuing education opportunities to expand and improve skills. The expected commitment of effort and time to skill improvement should be clearly communicated.

A well-organized program is usually well received by social service agencies and other potential sponsors. If the self-help line is to be a service of the maternity area of the hospital, the hospital administration will need to see that the service meets a need not already being addressed. The advantages and disadvantages of the proposed service will need to be accurately and realistically articulated. The costs of office equipment, training materials, and publicity will account for most of the outgoing funds.

It is possible to operate a self-help line from the homes of volunteers or through a central switchboard. If homes are used, a simple taped message explaining which volunteers on the service are available (giving times and telephone numbers) is usually sufficient. If a meeting room or office is desired, the cost of renting the space will need to be considered. Some groups find a central office preferable, since it allows volunteers to maintain a bulletin board for messages and announcements. An office can also provide a central area for files, for staff meetings, and for continuing-education events. It is also a natural place for volunteers to get acquainted with one another in an informal atmosphere. Simple furnishings and refreshments should be provided, if possible. These can often be obtained through community donations. Funds for operation and maintenance may be solicited directly from the community or from groups who will use the service (such as childbirth education or consumer activist groups or the medical community).

The legal aspects of establishing and maintaining the self-help line must be investigated. All staff members have a responsibility to maintain the privacy and confidentiality of the callers (O'Sullivan 1980). An atmosphere of trust and excellence is essential. The representative agency or group providing the service should give clear guidelines to volunteers about what information they are legally permitted to offer. Information about the legal aspects of self-help operations is best obtained from legal counsel. Staff members must understand that they may not give advice unless they are qualified to give it. Written guidelines with attention to prevention, the difference between advice and diagnosis and treatment, and the legalities of doctor/client privileges are helpful. The agency establishing the self-help line should find out what kind of malpractice insurance protection is needed.

Which agency actually operates the self-help line will be determined by the line's purposes and scope. The board of directors may be composed of community leaders, cesarean parents, maternity nurses with experience in the care of the cesarean family, or any mixture of people who seem appropriate to the needs of the service. Whatever the composition of the governing board, policies will have to be established, the physical set-up will need to be arranged, resources will need to be investigated, staff scheduling will need to be designated to someone, and provisions for ongoing staff education will need to be outlined. Publicity will need to be organized and dispersed and contact with other community agencies will need to be initiated.

The information of a self-help line is not complete without development of tools with which to evaluate its effectiveness. Tools of evaluation should address the following questions:

Does the program provide the services it intends to provide?

Does it reach the individuals it hopes to assist at a time when they need the help most?

Does it make a difference in how the individuals using it adjust to problematic situations?

What statistical information does it provide that may be useful for planning future programs and services (in some areas the information provided by such services has given impetus to the establishment or improvement of family-centered maternity services for cesarean couples)?

How much time and how many people are required to operate and maintain the service efficiently?

Is the program cost-effective?

What staff problems predominate and how can they be resolved?

Where self-help lines exist, they are highly utilized. While research data related to the precise effects of the self-help line on cesarean family adjustment are still limited, the general response to the service, where it is offered, seems quite favorable (Freeman 1980; Haight 1977).

Postpartum Support Groups

The purpose of postpartum support groups for cesarean couples is to provide a nonthreatening group experience in which members feel comfortable sharing concerns and in which members work in a cooperative effort to explore specific issues. The setting for support groups should be comfortable, informal, convenient, and free from outside disturbances. The groups may be composed of couples or of fathers only or of mothers only. A 2-hour time limit facilitates group process while providing definite closure time. This enables group members to work toward a specific goal at each session (Clark 1977; Glasser 1974; Haley 1976). At the initial session, information is obtained which guides the group leader or facilitator in structuring the content and concerns to be addressed in future sessions. The leader should review with members the structural aspects of the support group (how long sessions will continue, what ground rules are to be followed, and what the responsibilities of members and leader are). Although the group leader or facilitator usually wants to limit the sessions to a definite number and frequency—both of which may be determined by members and the leader cooperatively—it frequently happens that the core group members continue to meet independently for an extended indefinite period of time after the formal ending of the support group series. These meetings are most often initiated by the members themselves and provide them with a long-term supportive peer group (Johnson 1979; Howell 1975).

It is generally prudent to allow new members to join the group during the initial two sessions and then to close the group to new members. This is important to the development of group cohesion and trust and to prevent repetition. It is also necessary if specific issues are to be addressed during a structured time period. The number of individuals in a group should be limited. Where one leader is acting as facilitator, eight to ten members may be the best maximum (Adrian 1980; Clark 1977).

The group leader or facilitator should have extensive group experience and expertise. It is helpful if the leader is also a cesarean parent. Leaders may serve the dual function of group facilitator and designer of a training program for paraprofessionals who might serve as small group leaders with some supervision (Smith 1980). As with self-help lines, the ethics of maintaining confidentiality and of adhering to legal guidelines must be predetermined (O'Sullivan 1980).

Issues which predominate in most cesarean support groups include:

1. Exploring details of the birth experience.
2. Exploring the origins of the participants' feelings along with information relevant to understanding previous births or planning subsequent deliveries.
3. Understanding the effects of changing roles and expectations.

The development of community acceptance of fathers as primary nurturers is still in progress. Mothers are still viewed as the primary caretakers (Howell 1975). Women as caretakers are not supposed to ask for help. They are supposed to *be* the ever-present help. Because of this assumption an opportunity to receive positive reinforcement for reaching out for help is important.

The support-group leader actively encourages individual members to assume responsibility for exploring their birth experiences and for defining what is helpful for them (Loomis 1979). Some parents want to have the cesarean experience finished and behind them. Some want to concentrate on the planning and preparation for a subsequent experience. The support group provides the cesarean mother an opportunity to give as well as to receive support, and in the giving she may begin to realize that she is both competent and capable of reaching out to family and to the social network.

Recognition of who needs support-group assistance and who needs more intense assistance is important (Adrian 1980). It is frequently through a participatory role in the support group setting that individual members begin to recognize and accept for themselves the need for additional help from a professionally prepared counselor. A support-group setting can often provide the opportunity to restore confidence in providers of health care and clarify for the consumer of health care ways in which he or she can best articulate family-centered care needs.

The three most essential factors in preventing long-term disturbances include the flexibility of hospital policies in providing individual care, early and frequent parent-infant contact, and a cohesive network of community resources (Donovan 1977). Every cesarean mother should receive resource information before leaving the hospital. Active communication between nurse and the referral resource agencies ensures the helpfulness and accuracy of the information given to the new mothers. Self-help lines or hot lines should always be mentioned.

Colman and Colman (1971) have observed that postpartum couples rarely call attention to their psychological states. This is in part due to the internal, developmental nature of the changes which are occurring. The internalization does not, however, diminish the need for support and caring.

Caring is an important component of the services rendered by health-care experts (such as nurses), but it is all too often seen as a low-priority commodity. The cesarean couple has experienced first-hand the fact that no safe passage or perfect outcome is ever guaranteed. Risks abound. Helping and healing do not occur spontaneously, but must be actively sought by cesarean parents. As the parents receive help, and establish a network of supportive systems, they also gain confidence in their competence, in their ability to deal successfully with choices, and in the wisdom of their own experience. Thus the health-care providers and the couples who are the focus of their care can participate cooperatively and creatively in the healing process that may be needed following cesarean birth.

REFERENCES

Adams M: Early concerns of primigravida mothers regarding infant care activities. Nurs Res 12:72, 1963

Adrian S: A systematic approach to selecting group participants. J Psychiatr Nurs 18 (2):37–41, 1980

Affonso DD, Stichler JF: Cesarean birth, Am J Nurs 80 (3):466–70, 1980

Benjamin A: The Helping Interview, 2nd ed. Boston, Houghton-Mifflin, 1974

Bion WR: Experience in Groups. New York, Basic Books, 1961

Boyd S, Mahon P: The family centered cesarean delivery. Am J Maternal–Child Nurs 5:176–80, 1980

Brewster DP: You Can Breastfeed Your Baby. . .Even in Special Situations. Emmaus, Penn., Rodale, 1979

Clark AL: Adaptation problems and patterns of an expanding family. Nurs Forum 5 (1):93–109, 1966

Clark CC: The Nurse as Group Leader. New York, Springer, 1977

Colman AD, Colman LL: Pregnancy: The Psychological Experience. New York, Seabury, 1971

Countryman BA, et al: Surgery and the breastfeeding mother. J Am Operating Room Nurs 25:1082–84, 1977

Deakers LP: Continuity of family-centered nursing care between the hospital and the home. Nurs Clin North Am 7 (1):85, 1972

Delworth U, Rudow E, Taub J: Crisis Center Hotline: A guidebook to Beginning and Operating. Springfield, Thomas, 1972

Dinkmeyer D, Muro J: Group Counseling. Itasca, Ill., Peacock, 1971

Donovan B: The Cesarean Birth Experience. Boston, Beacon, 1977

Doucette JS: Is breastfeeding still safe for babies? Part II. Am J Maternal–Child Nurs 3:345–46, 1978

Ekman P: Body position, facial expression and verbal behaviors during interviews. J Abnorm Soc Psychol 68:295–301, 1964

Freeman K: A postpartum program that really works. . .help for new mothers is as near as the phone. Can Nurse 76:40–42, 1980

Glasser P, Sarri R, Vintner R (eds): Individual Change Through Small Groups. New York, Macmillan, 1974

Goetting T: Teaching resources for childbirth educators. J Obstet Gynecol Neonatal Nurs JOGN #6: 1977

Gottsfeld H, Rhee C, Parker G: A study of the role and performance of paraprofessionals in community mental health. Community Ment Health J 6:285-91, 1970

Grams KE: Nature's infant nutrition. Breastfeeding: A means of imparting immunity, Part I. Am J Maternal-Child Nurs 3:340-44, 1978

Grassley J, Davis, K: Common concerns of mothers who breastfeed. . . classes being taught at the Group Health Cooperative of Puget Sound in Seattle, Washington, Part III. Am J Maternal-Child Nurs 3:347-51, 1978

Gruis M: Beyond maternity: Postpartum concerns of mothers. Am J Maternal-Child Nurs 2:182-88, 1977

Haight J: Steadying parents as they go—by phone. Am J Maternal-Child Nurs 2:311-12, 1977

Haire, D: The Cultural Warping of Childhood. Seattle, International Childbirth Education Association, 1972

Haley J: Problem Solving Therapy: New Strategies for Effective Family Therapy. San Francisco, Jossey-Bass, 1976

Halstead L: Use of crisis intervention in obstetrical nursing. Nurs Clin North Am 9 (1):69-81, 1974

Hedahl K: Cesarean birth: a real family affair. Am J Nurs 80 (3):471-72, 1980

Henderson KJ: Helping new mothers maintain lactation while separated from their infants, Part IV. Am J Maternal-Child Nurs 3:352-56, 1978

Howell MC: Helping Ourselves: Families and the Human Network. Boston, Beacon, 1975

Jarkowsky MJ: How to prevent breastfeeding problems. Supervisor Nurse 11 (1):43-44, 1980

Jelliffe DB, Jelliffe EFP: Breast is best: Modern meanings. N Eng J Med 297:912-15, 1977

Johnson D, Johnson F: Joining Together: Group Theory and Group Skills. Englewood Cliffs, N.J., Prentice-Hall, 1975

Johnson SH: High Risk Parenting. Philadelphia, Lippincott, 1979

Kramer R: Giving Birth: Childbearing in America Today. Chicago, Contemporary Books, 1979

Larsen VL: Stresses of the childbearing year. Am J Public Health, 56 (1):32-36, 1966

LeMasters EE: Parenthood as crisis. In Parad HJ (ed), Crisis Intervention: Selected Readings. New York, Family Services Association of America, 1965

Loomis ME: Group Process for Nurses. St Louis, Mosby, 1979

Marut JS, Mercer RT: Comparison of primiparas' perceptions of vaginal and cesarean births. Nurs Res 28 (5):260-66, 1979

Mercer R:Nursing Care for Parents at Risk. Thorofare, N.J., Slack, 1977

Montague A: Touching: The Human Significanc of Skin. New York, Columbia University Press, 1971

Murdaugh A, Miller LE: Helping the breastfeeding mother. Am J Nurs 121: 465, 1975

O'Brien T: Excretion of drugs in human milk. Am J Hosp Pharm 31:844-45, 1974

O'Sullivan AL: Privileged communication. Am J Nurs 80 (5):947–50, 1980

Powell TJ: The use of self-help groups as supportive reference communities. Am J Orthopsychiatry 45 (5):756–64, 1975

Riessman F: Strategies and suggestions for training nonprofessionals. Community Ment Health J 3 (2):103–10, 1967

Rioch M, Charmian E, Arden A: National Institute of Mental Health pilot study in training mental health counselors. Am J Orthopsychiatry 33: 678–89, 1963

Rising SS: The fourth stage of labor: Family integration. Am J Nurs 74:870, 1974

Rogers CR: Client-centered Therapy. Boston, Houghton–Mifflin, 1951

Rogers CR: The characteristics of a helping relationship. In Avila DL, Combs AW, Purkey WW (eds), Helping Relationships. Boston, Allyn and Bacon, 1972

Ross Laboratories: Breastfeeding After Cesarean Birth. Columbus, Ohio, Ross Laboratories Publications, 1979

Rothermel BS, Faber MM: Drugs in breast milk: A consumer's guide. Birth Fam J 2 (3):76–88, 1974

Schlosser S: The emergency c-section patient: Why she needs help. . .what you can do. RN 4:53–57, 1978

Shereshefsky PM, Yarrow LJ: Psychological Aspects of a First Pregnancy and Early Postnatal Adaptation. New York, Raven, 1973

Smith L: Finding your leadership style in groups. Am J Nurs 80 (7):1301–1303, 1980

Stranik MK, Hogberg B: Transition into parenthood. Am J Nurs 79 (1):90–93, 1979

Tibbetts E, Caldwell K: Selecting the right breast pump. Am J Maternal-Child Nurs 5 (4):262–64, 1980

Whitley N: Preparation for breastfeeding. J. Obstet Gynecol Neonatal Nurs 7: 44, 1978

SECTION V

Trends and Issues

CHAPTER 12

Cesarean Family Care: Hospital Policies and Future Trends

Cora McGuffie Rodriguez

Until recently, cesarean childbirth was viewed as a surgical procedure having its primary impact on childbearing families during and immediately after the actual delivery of the baby. From a holistic perspective, little thought was given to the effects of this method of delivery on the involved family members. This somewhat restricted view of cesarean birth is evidenced by the fact that the topic received only vague attention in the research and narrative literature prior to 1973.

The holistic approach to cesarean care is one that considers the cesarean experience from a psychosocial as well as a physiological viewpoint before, during, and long after the birthing event itself. Through the efforts of childbirth education groups (such as the International Childbirth Education Association and Parent and Child, Inc.), health professionals and lay persons alike have come to realize that cesarean birth has an extensive effect on childbearing families. By examining a cesarean family group one can see how hospital policies can be influenced in relation to the promotion of healthy family functioning.

In early 1977, several couples with cesarean birth experience began a support group in the District of Columbia area in order to help other parents experience a well prepared, satisfying, and meaningful cesarean birth.* As a result of their efforts, the Cesarean Families Association of Greater Washington, D.C. (CFA) became a reality. With some initial financial assistance from

Nancy Newport, R.N., author of Chapter 8, was one of the cofounders of CFA.

Parent and Child, Inc. and the International Childbirth Education Association, CFA was able to offer prepared cesarean childbirth classes by August, 1977. After growth and expansion, CFA elected its first board of directors in February, 1978, and applied for incorporation as a nonprofit educational organization. Annual dues were $6.00/couple. Cesarean parents operated the business of the association, drawing on the skills of lawyers, teachers, nurses, and others in the association.

Several programs and services are conducted by CFA. A bimonthly newsletter, sent to all members, features articles on cesarean childbirth, parents' accounts of their cesarean births, articles on childbearing, news items, book reviews, and birth announcements. Continuing education programs are offered quarterly on topics of interest and concern to cesarean parents.

Other important services of CFA include cesarean childbirth education classes, postpartum support groups, self-help telephone lines (see Chapters 8 and 11), and a bookstore which makes available to interested couples current selections about cesarean care and birth.

CFA also works with area hospitals, nurses, and physicians to promote and encourage changes in existing hospital policies so as to enable cesarean parents to be together at such a significant occasion in their lives. An initial step toward this goal was to determine and publicize the options available for promoting healthy cesarean birth (CFA 1978).

The following options have been developed by CFA and are recommended for those couples who desire them.

1. Allowing hospital admission for a scheduled cesarean on the day of surgery, with tests performed the day before on an outpatient basis or immediately prior to surgery.
2. Having the option of no extra preoperative medication.
3. Exercising the right to talk to the anesthesiologist prior to surgery.
4. Having the option of remaining awake throughout the entire procedure.
5. Using the Pfannenstiel (bikini) incision whenever possible.
6. Allowing a prepared father in the delivery room.
7. Enabling the father to have delivery room contact with his baby.
8. Having the baby's condition at birth evaluated on an individual basis.
9. Making breast-feeding possible in delivery and recovery.
10. Allowing the father in the recovery room.
11. Providing electrically operated beds for all cesarean mothers.
12. Providing rooming-in as soon as the mother is ready and to the extent she desires.
13. Allowing a helper for rooming-in, such as the husband, a friend, or a relative.
14. Providing a demand feeding schedule for the baby.
15. Allowing sibling visitation.
16. Expanding hospitals' prenatal classes and prepared childbirth classes to provide more information on cesarean birth.

In the winter of 1978-79, CFA conducted a descriptive study to evaluate in-patient cesarean care in the greater District of Columbia area (Wilson and Rodriguez 1979). In this study the options for cesarean care promoted by CFA were compared to existing hospital policies. The results of the study are available to CFA members, as well as to participating hospitals, physicians, and the general public for a nominal fee. Orders are available through the Cesarean Families Association of Greater Washington, D.C. 5110 N. 25th St., Arlington, Va. 22207.

The purpose of this chapter is to describe that study, share the results, and suggest implications derived from the data which are relevant to changing hospital policies for improved in-patient care of cesarean childbearing families.

STATEMENT OF PURPOSE

The CFA survey was undertaken to provide accurate, current information about the status of cesarean family care in the greater District of Columbia area. It was intended that consumers and hospital personnel would be able to use the data in considering policy revisions for their cesarean maternity care. Nurses and interested members could consider future directions for CFA work with hospitals. Needs were to be assessed for future change facilitation by CFA members, using their special knowledge of family dynamics, maternity needs, and hospital policy formation in the improvement of cesarean family care.

STATEMENT OF THE PROBLEM

The problem was to determine the degree to which the policies of hospitals in the greater District of Columbia area comply (or fail to comply) with the promoted options of the CFA.

SIGNIFICANCE OF THE STUDY

It was hoped that, through the survey results, CFA members would be able to seek out hospitals able to assist in a desirable cesarean birth with maximum safety and optimal enhancement qualities (Cirz 1978). The study identified hospitals in need of interpretation of the CFA options and assistance in implementing new policies to achieve family-centered cesarean care. As a result, officers and members of CFA planned their work on objectively derived data. Other cities might find encouragement in knowing what is occurring in Washington, D.C. regarding cesarean care. Ultimate significance may be better family relations for the approximately 15 to 20 percent of American families giving birth annually who experience cesarean birth (Hughey et al. 1977; Jones 1976; Marut 1978).

ASSUMPTIONS

It was assumed that the respondents returning the survey gave honest evaluations of the practices in their hospitals. It was also assumed that conforming to the options of the Cesarean Families Association provided families with a well prepared, meaningful cesarean birth.

LIMITATIONS

The survey was sent only to hospitals in the greater Washington, D.C. area; therefore, the findings cannot be generalized to other metropolitan areas. In addition, biased interpretations of policy by personnel within a participating hospital could lead to survey answers based on false impressions of actual policies of that hospital.

DEFINITION OF TERMS

Good (1973, p. 122) defines compliance as "the act or threat of submitting to the wishes, requests, or dictates of another person or a group." This definition was used to determine whether hospitals were in conformity with the options promoted by CFA. A hospital was deemed to be compliant with a specific option of CFA if its policies allowed conformity to the option in question. Conversely a hospital was seen as noncompliant with a specific option of CFA if its policies did not allow conformity to the CFA option in question.

THEORETICAL FRAMEWORK

The efforts of cesarean family associations today are based on theories of family interaction, group dynamics, parent–child bonding, and change facilitation. Pillitteri (1976) emphasized that parenthood involves the protection of the next generation through nurturing of their physical, social, and emotional needs (p. 113). Parenthood develops within the family, which is the basic unit in society concerned with reproduction, child care, and affectional needs (Clark and Affonso 1976, p. 239). Expectant parents spend much time and energy determining how to carry out their parenting roles (Rubin 1967).

Expectant cesarean parents turn to support groups (such as CFA), to gain greater knowledge and information. Through the group process cesarean parents become better able to deal with cesarean birth (Maier 1973, p. 422). Group participation helps cesarean parents see their feelings as similar to those of others, thus negating feelings of isolation arising from interruptions in their expectation of "perfect" birth (Donovan 1977). Group participation also offers clear skills and principles of use in labor and approaches to health professionals that help gain desired birth options (Hughes 1977).

Murray and Zentner (1975) wrote of the advantages of group participation for expectant cesarean parents. There is a decrease of anxiety about the pending surgery as a result of group support and the airing of accurate accounts of sensations in pre- and postoperative procedures.

When parents face a cesarean delivery, they must make a special effort to ensure opportunities for parent–child bonding. The parents must accept the fact that the cesarean birth is the best choice for the health of their infant (Enkin 1977). Klaus and Kennell (1976) suggested that affectional ties can be easily disturbed during the immediate postpartum period (p. 52). The parents are considered to enter a ". . .unique period during which events may have lasting effects on the family. . ." (Klaus and Kennell 1976, p. 50). For these reasons, cesarean support groups encourage the mother to have regional anesthesia and remain awake during the birth. They also encourage the father's attendance at the birth, early contact between parents and infant in the recovery room, and early breast-feeding, when the mother desires.

Cesarean support groups must use a systematic approach in working with hospitals to facilitate change. These groups can make an impact on the health care delivery system because of the similarity in the members' desires, thus creating in hospital personnel a "greater capacity for empathy" (Havelock and Havelock 1973, p. 68). Hospitals may be willing to listen and give the ideas of the support group a fair chance.

The steps the cesarean support group follows are described by Schein (1965) as follows. The group:

1. Senses a need for change.
2. Acquires information about the change needed.
3. Changes production.
4. Stabilizes internal structures.
5. Exports new product.
6. Obtains feedback about the change.

The cesarean support group must face resistance openly, since the resistance is often based on the hospital's concern for the maintenance of the health-care system (Havelock and Havelock 1973, p. 55). Development of a common language between the subsystems (i.e., support group and hospital) is necessary before new options for cesarean parents can be implemented (Frick 1959, p. 614). The hospital must see reciprocal benefits for itself and the support group must know how to offer its ideas at the right time and in the appropriate way (Havelock and Havelock 1973, p. 61). Bennis et al. (1969) emphasized that dialogue between organizations helps to resolve underlying conflict and is necessary before collaboration or linkage is possible. This problem-solving process can move toward:

> ...the creation of a stable and long-
> lasting social influence network.
> The reciprocal and collaborative
> nature of this relationship further
> serves to legitimize the roles of
> consumer and resource persons and
> it builds a channel from resource
> to user (Havelock and Havelock
> 1973, p. 24).

The varied resources of the support group (skills, time, energy, motivation) can be utilized in linking hospital services to cesarean parents (Havelock and Havelock 1973, p. 62). Thus individuals with special knowledge can facilitate the modification of organizational, technological, and interpersonal factors needed for change to occur (Argyris 1962, p. 54). Members of the support group can work with hospital committees responsible for policy revisions. New equipment which would aid the mother and infant in the recovery room (e.g., warmers) can be introduced. Physicians, nurses, and other hospital personnel can be educated and encouraged to accept new ideas and trends for better cesarean care.

A HISTORICAL PERSPECTIVE ON CESAREAN BIRTH

To understand why cesarean families and support groups like CFA are concerned with efforts to improve the quality of the family-centered birth experience, one must consider the past. The fears of the family relate to the complications of the surgery. The advances of obstetrical medicine have resulted in much manipulation of the natural birth process. The concern about having a perfect baby with each pregnancy puts pressure on the couple and on the medical team. In addition, the consumer movement has brought about more parent involvement in the processes of delivery at a time when medical intervention has been maximized.

From the time of primitive cultures to the Classical Age of Greece, skilled midwives supervised the birth of a child (Lieberman 1976). The well-being of the mother and child was important. The spiritual nature of the child was recognized during the Roman Empire. This led to the practice of removing the child from the body of the woman who died in labor. This permitted the separate burial of the infant. From the Latin *caedere* (to cut) came our term, "cesarean birth" (Enkin 1977, p. 99).

Throughout the Middle Ages, pregnancy was considered to be the result of carnal sin and the pain of childbirth was thought to be woman's punishment

(Lieberman 1976). If the woman died in childbirth, the infant's soul could be saved if baptism was performed. Thus many cesareans were performed on dead women to baptize the infant and save his soul (Lieberman 1976).

In 1500, Jacob Nufer, a Swiss hog gelder, performed the first cesarean on a living woman who was unable to deliver vaginally. Though we know she lived to have other children, the fate of the infant is unknown (Enkin 1977; Lieberman 1976). This was a rare success for those times.

By the late 16th century, the Church had become less influential and physicians began to attend births (Lieberman 1976). Midwives were better educated and royalty demanded improved labor and delivery care (Lieberman 1976).

Only occasionally did women in the 17th through 19th centuries survive cesarean birth. The first successful American cesarean was performed in 1794 by Dr. Jesse Bennet. He performed the operation on his wife, Elizabeth Hog Bennet, in a log cabin at Edom, Virginia, with the aid of anesthesia (Pelton 1976).

Though Oliver Wendell Holmes and Semmelweiss both urged the use of aseptic techniques, the medical profession accepted their advice only gradually. Aseptic measures resulted in a decline in puerperal fever, and as a result more women survived childbirth.

The use of anesthesia in the late 1800s further improved the conditions of childbirth (Lieberman 1976). Women were delighted with the relief of pain in labor and delivery. The success of the extraperitoneal approach further improved the chances of survival for a woman having a cesarean delivery (Douglas and Stromme 1976, p. 618).

During the first half of the 20th century, much was learned about the placental barrier and the effect of anesthesia on the newborn (Weiss 1977). After 1940, advocates for natural, prepared childbirth urged the reduction of pain and the control of fear (Dick-Read 1944, p. 19). People began again to believe that having a baby should be a family affair. Brazelton (1973) identified the abilities of the newborn to react with his environment shortly after birth (Brazelton, 1973). The importance of the early postpartum period in facilitating the parent-child bonding process was suggested (Klaus and Kennell p. 50). Husband and wife began to unite as a team and to dictate trends in obstetrics (Cirz 1978).

There were other changes in cesarean care. Advancements occurred in fetal heart monitoring. Estriol tests for fetal maturity were developed and oxytocin challenge tests for fetal stress were used more often. Safer regional anesthesia was utilized, as were better surgical procedures. Amniocentesis and sonography were used to determine fetal maturity and well-being. New indications for the use of the cesarean operation, such as fetal distress and breech presentation, led to an increase in the incidence of cesarean deliveries (Jones 1976; Smith 1977). The concern was no longer for the mother's well-being alone, but also for the infant, who it was felt, should not have to suffer birth trauma or be denied the help of neonatology (Jones 1976). Physicians became more cautious as the number of law suits increased concerning prenatal and delivery care.

Many couples felt cesarean delivery was a devastating experience (Cohen 1977). They had hospital encounters which led to poor development of interpersonal relationships in the new family. Women expressed the desire to participate in the labor and birth process, to have their husbands present, and to be in control (Cohen 1977; Murphy 1956). Cesarean parents, like other parents, needed help to "have positive, meaningful, fulfilled birth experiences" (Donovan 1977, p. 4).

Formal research on the needs of families at birth has only recently been reported. Scaer and Korte (1978) reported that the primary concern of 645 women was that the fathers be present in labor and delivery. Another concern was unrestricted visitation rights for the father. The mothers also wanted to be awake and have as much visual contact with their babies as possible.

Affonso and Stichler (1978) studied the reactions of 105 women to cesarean births and learned that fear was the major concern for 92 percent. Dissatisfaction, anger, or depression was felt by 50 percent of the women. Relief was felt by 30 percent. Measures considered helpful were: (1) the explanations from doctors and nurses; (2) support from husbands, friends, and relatives; (3) having had a cesarean before. Data confirmed that cesarean parents, like other parents, want to be actively involved in the birth and want their spouses to participate (Affonso and Stichler 1978).

Hayes (1978) found that women anticipating repeat cesarean delivery prefer to plan for the event, even though they regret the coming surgery. Parents anticipating cesarean delivery wanted information on the medical procedures, an open and thorough discussion of anesthesia, explanation of the differences and similarities between cesarean and vaginal postpartum periods, and information about the recovery period. (Hayes 1978).

Conner (1977) advocated the discussion of the possibility of cesarean delivery in all childbirth preparation classes, using specific written handouts and audiovisual aids. He found that the instructor's attitude made the difference in whether couples were able to deal with the possibility of a cesarean birth or simply "tuned out" any potential problems.

From the above-mentioned cultural practices, technical advances, and holistic concerns, a new picture of the needs of the cesarean family emerged. With it arose our central question: just how close did the hospitals in the Greater Washington, D.C. area come to meeting the needs of this family?

METHODOLOGY

To determine which hospitals were in compliance with the CFA options, a descriptive survey was designed to study the cesarean birth practices in hospitals located in the District of Columbia and the greater Washington area.

The CFA options were matched with known practices in labor and delivery units; a multiple-choice format was used for the final questionnaire. The validity of the questionnaire was determined by CFA board members and two graduate maternity nursing instructors at a local university school of nursing.

The population for the survey included the various hospitals providing maternity care in the greater Washington, D.C. area (N=24). Three questionnaires were sent to each hospital: one to the hospital administrator, one to the director of nursing, and one to the medical chief of ob-gyn. Each group of questionnaires was mailed with a cover letter and a stamped, self-addressed envelope to encourage its return.

A pamphlet explaining the Cesarean Families Association's purposes and goals was included in each envelope. This was done to educate those in responsible positions about the work of CFA in cesarean care.

Assurance that the results of the survey would be made available to participating hospitals was included in the cover letter. The final survey results were mailed to all hospitals.

PRESENTATION OF DATA

Of the 24 hospitals surveyed, returns came from 23 institutions. As a result of this high return rate, it was possible to study the cesarean birth options of 95.8 percent of the greater Washington, D.C. area hospitals with maternity services.

The data have been grouped for clarity into the following categories: predelivery policies, delivery policies, infant assessment policies, recovery room policies, infant feeding policies, postpartum policies, and visitation policies. The data are presented as percentages only. There was no attempt to subject the data to more sophisticated statistical procedures.

Predelivery Policies

It was learned that 7 hospitals (29.2 percent) currently offer classes for cesarean couples. Four of these classes are presented by CFA.

It is possible to be admitted to the hospital the same day as the cesarean delivery in 11 hospitals (45.8 percent). The obstetrician decides this in 3 of the hospitals permitting it.

In general, the obstetrician has the responsibility of determining the type of anesthesia to be used for the cesarean birth. In some instances the anesthesiologist makes this decision. Through discussion with her obstetrician, the patient can take part in this decision. Regional anesthesia is routinely used in 33.3 percent of the hospitals, while it is available in all of them.

In 87.5 percent of the hospitals, the anesthesiologist who will be with the patient for the cesarean birth sees the patient before surgery. In the remaining hospitals, some member of the anesthesiology department sees the patient before the cesarean delivery.

Delivery Policies

Fathers may be present for the cesarean delivery in 17 hospitals (70.8 percent). However, each of these hospitals has specific requirements that must be met before this is allowed. The obstetrician must be consulted first in all hospitals. Six (25 percent) hospitals do not allow fathers at the cesarean birth.

In 17 hospitals (70.8 percent), fathers have very early contact with their infants, as long as the baby is well.

Only four hospitals (16.7 percent) allow fathers to be present in the operating room for the cesarean birth when the mother has general anesthesia. Twelve hospitals (50 percent) allow the mother to watch the birth with the placement of mirrors in the operating room. Eight hospitals (33.3 percent) make provisions for the mother to breast-feed in the delivery room.

Infant Assessment Policies

Though infants are assessed individually in all hospitals, only 14 hospitals (58.3 percent) allow the infant to stay with the father or mother immediately after birth.

Recovery Room Policies

The father is allowed in the recovery room in 20 hospitals (83.3 percent). The mother may hold her baby in the recovery room at 14 hospitals (58.3 percent). The mother may breast-feed the baby in the recovery room in 14 hospitals (58.3 percent).

Infant Feeding Policies

Feeding on demand may be practiced by the cesarean mothers in 21 hospitals (87.5 percent). One hospital permits it with rooming-in patients only. One hospital has scheduled feeding every 4 hours only.

Postpartum Policies

Rooming-in is available at 22 hospitals (91.6 percent), although some variations in this policy may occur due to space limitations. The hours for rooming-in vary from the amount of time desired by the mother to 12 hours or 24 hours/day. Fathers are allowed to be present to help with rooming-in at all hospitals that allow rooming-in. A supportive other is allowed for help

TABLE 1. PERCENTAGE OF HOSPITALS OFFERING MAJOR OPTIONS IN CESAREAN CARE IN THE GREATER WASHINGTON, D.C. AREA

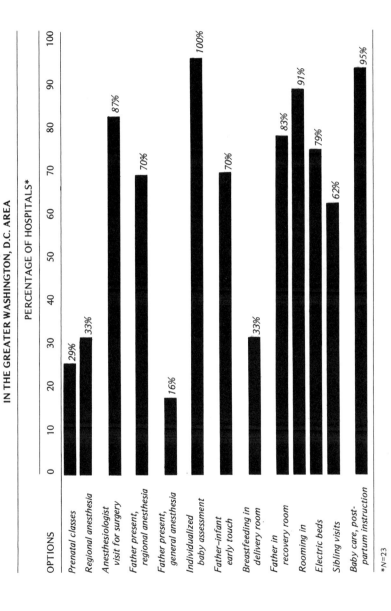

PERCENTAGE OF HOSPITALS*

OPTIONS	Percentage
Prenatal classes	29%
Regional anesthesia	33%
Anesthesiologist visit for surgery	87%
Father present, regional anesthesia	70%
Father present, general anesthesia	16%
Individualized baby assessment	100%
Father-infant early touch	70%
Breastfeeding in delivery room	33%
Father in recovery room	83%
Rooming in	91%
Electric beds	79%
Sibling visits	62%
Baby care, post-partum instruction	95%

*N=23

261

with rooming-in at 20 hospitals (83.3 percent). Cesarean mothers share rooms at five (20.8 percent) of the hospitals. Electric beds are provided for greater mobility in 19 hospitals (79.2 percent). Baby care and postpartum care classes are held in all 23 hospitals (95.8 percent) that responded.

Note that hospitals that did not respond are, in this survey, counted as negative responses. Therefore, the figures given are perhaps somewhat distorted; they might be somewhat higher.

Visitation Policies

Visiting by fathers is permitted at all times in six hospitals (25 percent). Seventeen others offer 12 hours of visitation to the father. The great majority (95 percent) offer 2 to 3 hours visitation for friends per day. Only one hospital limits visits to the father alone. Sibling visits are allowed in 15 hospitals (62.5 percent). Prior arrangements must be made with the nursing staff in all hospitals offering sibling visitation. Designated areas (only) are utilized for sibling visits at all these hospitals.

Visits to the nursery window by siblings are allowed in 19 hospitals (79.2 percent), though some hospitals limit the times. Only 15 hospitals offer special assistance to mothers wishing to be visited by sibling children.

Table 1 is a schematic presentation of the major options of cesarean care offered in the greater Washington, D.C. area.

SUMMARY AND RECOMMENDATIONS FOR CHANGE

From the data gathered, it can be seen that the greatest degree of CFA compliance by maternity units in the District of Columbia is in the provision of baby care and postpartum classes, rooming-in with father participation, and having the anesthesiologist see the mother prior to the cesarean delivery. There is strong compliance with the option of the father being admitted to the recovery room. Three fourths of the hospitals allow fathers to attend cesarean births when regional anesthesia is used. Early father–infant contact is available in nearly three fourths of the hospitals. Electric beds are available in more than 75 percent of the hospitals.

Cesarean support groups need to continue to work closely with hospital administrators, interested physicians, nurses, and concerned parents to make further progress toward the goals of cesarean family-centered care. There are numerous levels at which interested nurses can use their interpersonal skills and knowledge. Within a support group, the nurse can explore the feelings couples had during their cesarean births. She can facilitate resolution of these feelings by encouraging them to help other couples understand similar experiences. The nurse can use her organizational skills to assign interested couples various tasks, such as publicity, the work associated with maintaining membership, hot lines, and bookkeeping.

Further, the needs and goals of cesarean families in each community have to be evaluated. Public interest can be determined only after convening a cesarean support group meeting which has been well publicized in posters, newspapers, radio, and television public service announcements. Even a few dedicated persons can accomplish this initial task. Special talents of those attending the organizational meeting should be tapped for future work. Participants need not be health-care professionals exclusively; persons concerned about improving cesarean care and willing to work toward that goal should also be included.

Individuals within the support group must communicate their needs to health-care providers. An interested nurse can facilitate contacts within the hospital, introducing cesarean support group members to responsible hospital administrators. The nurse's familiarity with the chain of command can help support groups to approach the appropriate individuals at an opportune time. Working with health-planning organizations, nurses can promote optimal hospital staffing with nurses who are educationally prepared, who have the experience to care for cesarean families, and who believe in a family-centered philosophy of maternity care.

Nurses can volunteer to formulate new policies and protocols for implementing desired cesarean support-group goals within their employing agency. The necessary interdepartmental coordination can be assumed by interested nurses in positions of responsibility. An example of this is the head nurse who goes to the department head of anesthesiology and informs that person of the desire of cesarean mothers to be awake for the births of their children. Concerned nurses can work out the details of supplying the needed epidural medications and trays on the delivery unit or they can call the anesthesiologist early enough before the cesarean birth to give epidural anesthesia.

Cesarean support-group members can give nurses information to take back to their hospital staffs. Information can be dispersed at the staff level by working through clinical specialists and maternity coordinators. Desired cesarean family goals can be shared in nursing staff meetings. Local cesarean support-group members can be a valuable resource in teaching nurses what couples want in the birthing experience. Rap sessions are useful in exploring nurses' feelings and their acceptance of such goals.

Audiovisual material is another important tool in the education of hospital staff. Information can be obtained from C/SEC, Inc., c/o Patricia Erickson, 23 Cedar St., Cambridge, MA 02140.

As hospitals develop new protocols, their nurses should share them with interested neighboring hospitals. The cesarean support group can gather data from members who have given birth in various hospitals. Local nursing organizations can share technical and professional data with members of other institutions.

Communication between the hospital and the cesarean support group should be maintained through frequent visits and the written word. Progress should be evaluated periodically. Nurses can study their units for needed changes and policy modifications. Hospitals should have an evaluation tool for determining patients' views on their hospitalizations; this should be used to modify care on an ongoing basis. The support group can inform hospitals of problems reported by members. Through earnest give-and-take, the hospitals, professionals, and parents can provide healthier, happier care.

Figure 1 is an illustration of the various steps involved in changing cesarean family care, as related in the preceding text.

Change takes time and must occur in stages. Interpersonal acceptance often comes more slowly than technical and organizational adjustments, which may be more difficult to accomplish. Individual enthusiasm may be a great asset in the promotion of institutional change. An enthusiastic and energetic nurse can facilitate change among staff members through empathy, by teaching and her ability to function as a role model.

In the future, the increase of communications among cesarean groups in

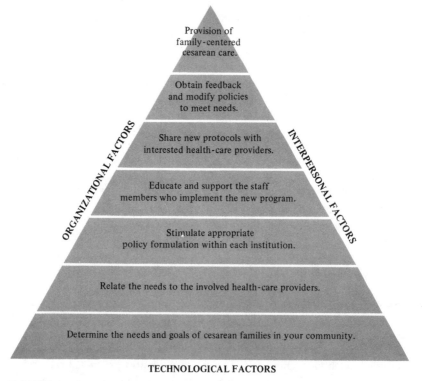

FIGURE 1. *Steps in changing cesarean family care. (Adapted from Argyris, 1962; Schem, 1965.)*

the United States will be necessary. Local and regional policies should be evaluated to determine the status of cesarean care throughout the country. Universal standards for family-centered cesarean care should be formulated and adopted, for instance through the cooperative efforts of the Nurses Association of the American College of Obstetricians and Gynecologists, the American College of Obstetricians and Gynecologists, the American Association of Nurse Anesthetists, and the American Board of Anesthesiology. Dissemination of these standards on a national basis—through workshops, university teaching, and the literature—would be necessary.

Further research by nurses can lead to a sounder understanding of the needs of cesarean families and to more appropriate nursing interventions. Hospitals must utilize advances in technology which permit more patient participation in the birth process—e.g., safer drugs for pain control and more effective anesthesia. In the future, use of closed circuit television could allow the new mother to watch her infant in the observation nursery from her postpartum room. A richer cesarean experience can result from cooperation between nurses and informed couples in cesarean support groups. More meaningful family relationships can develop if cesarean families are better prepared for the experience of cesarean birth, and are more satisfied with their own participation and role performance during that event.

REFERENCES

Affonso DD, Stichler JF: Exploratory study of women's reactions to having a cesarean birth. Birth Fam J 5 (2):88–94, 1978

Argyris C: Interpersonal Competence and Organizational Effectiveness. Homewood, Ill., Dorsey, 1962

Bennis WG, Benne KD, Chin R: The Planning of Change, 2nd ed. New York, Holt, Rinehardt and Winston, 1969

Brazelton TB: Neonatal Behavioral Assessment Scale. Philadelphia, Lippincott, 1973

Cesarean Families Association of Greater Washington, D.C.: Working Toward Family-centered Cesarean Births and Healthy Cesarean Families. Arlington, Va, CFA, 1978

Cirz D: Nurses and the future in childbirth. J Obstet Gynecol Neonatal Nurs 7:25–26, 1978

Clark AL, Affonso DD: Childbearing: A Nursing Perspective. Philadelphia, Davis, 1976

Cohen NW: Minimizing emotional sequellae of cesarean childbirth. Birth Fam J 4 (3): 114–19, 1977

Conner BS: Teaching about cesarean birth in the traditional childbirth classes. Birth Fam J 4 (3):107–13, 1977

Dick–Read G: Childbirth Without Fear: The Principles and Practices of Natural Childbirth. New York, Harper and Row, 1944

Donovan B: The Cesarean Birth Experience: A Practical, Comprehensive, and Reassuring Guide for Parents and Professionals. Boston, Beacon, 1977

Douglas RG, Stromme WB: Operative Obstetrics, 3rd ed. New York, Appleton-Century-Crofts, 1976

Enkin MW: Having a section is having a baby. Birth Fam J 4 (3):99–102, 1977

Frick FC: Information theory. In Koch S (ed), Psychology: A Study of a Science, 2nd ed. New York, McGraw-Hill, 1959, pp. 614–15

Good CV (ed): Dictionary of Education. New York, McGraw-Hill, 1973

Havelock RG, Havelock MC: Training for Change Agents: A Guide to the Design of Training Programs in Education and Other Fields. Ann Arbor, Mich., University of Michigan, 1973

Hayes B: A survey of cesarean childbirth education classes and a hospital parent education program for repeat cesarean delivery. Birth Fam J 5 (2):95–101, 1978

Hughes CB: An eclectic approach to parent group education. Nurs Clin North Am 12 (3): 469–79, 1977

Hughey MJ, LaPata RE, McElin TW, Lussky R: The effects of fetal monitoring on the incidence of cesarean section. Obstet Gynecol 49 (5):513–18, 1977

Jones OH: Cesarean section in present-day obstetrics. Am J Obstet Gynecol 126 (5):521–30, 1976

Klaus MH, Kennell JH: Maternal–Infant Bonding. St. Louis, Mosby, 1976

Lieberman JJ: Childbirth practices: From darkness into light. J Obstet Gynecol Neonatal Nurs 5:41–45, 1976

Maier NRF: Assets and liabilities in group problem solving: The need for an integrative function. In Scott WE, Cummings LL, Readings in Organizational Behavior and Human Performance, rev. ed. Homewood, Ill., Irwin, 1973

Marut JS: The special needs of the cesarean mother. Am J Maternal–Child Nurs 3 (4):202–206, 1978

Murphy P: Expectant mothers organizing for natural childbirth. Am J Nurs 56 (10):1298–1301, 1956

Murray R, Zentner J: Nursing Concepts for Health Promotion. Englewood Cliffs, N.J., Prentice-Hall, 1975

Pelton RW: America's first cesarean section. J Practical Nurs 26 (5):34, 1976

Pillitteri A: Nursing Care of the Growing Family: A Maternal–Newborn Text. Boston, Little, Brown, 1976

Rubin R: Attainment of the maternal role, Part I: Processes. Nurs Res 16 (3):237–45, 1967

Scaer R, Korte D: MOM survey: Maternity options for mothers—what do women want in maternity care? Birth Fam J 5 (1):20–26, 1978

Schein EH: Organizational Psychology. Englewood Cliffs, N.J., Prentice-Hall 1965

Smith BE: Pain relief in labor, delivery and late pregnancy. Controversies in OB–GYN 2:195–98, 1977

Weiss SL: An evaluation of muscle relaxants in cesarean sections. J Am Assoc Nurse Anesthetists 45 (3):306–308, 1977

Wilson A, Rodriguez C: Hospital Survey of Maternity Care Practices for Cesarean Parents in the Washington, D.C. Area. Washington, D.C., Cesarean Families Association of Greater Washington, D.C., 1979

BIBLIOGRAPHY CONCERNING CHANGE

Argyris C: Explorations in consultant–client relationships. Hum Organizations 20:121–33, 1961

Benne KD, Levit G: The nature of groups and helping groups improve their operation. Rev Educ Res 23:289–304, 1953

Benne KD, Sheats P: Functional roles of group members. J Soc Issues 4:41–49, 1948

Bennis WG: Changing Organizations. New York, McGraw-Hill, 1966

Lewin K: Field Theory in Social Science. New York, Deriun Cartwright, 1951

Lippitt R, Watson J, Westley B: Dynamics of Planned Change. New York, Harcourt-Brace, 1958

Rogers CR: On Becoming a Person. Cambridge, Mass., Riverside, 1961

Schein EH: Process Consultation. Reading, Mass., Addison-Wesley, 1969

Schein EH, Bennis WG: Personal and Organizational Change Through Group Methods: The Laboratory Approach. New York, Wiley and Sons, 1965

CHAPTER 13

Effectuating Change: The Maternity Staff Nurse's Role in the Care of Cesarean Mothers

Joanne Sullivan Marut

This chapter describes the strategies used by the author, as a maternity-staff nurse, to bring about changes in the care of cesarean clients on a labor and delivery unit of a large metropolitan medical center. This nurse identified the need to improve the care of her clients while conducting an empirical investigation of the reactions of primigravidas to emergency cesarean births. The results of her study suggested that there are specific factors that facilitate the process of maternal–infant attachment among these mothers, as well as factors that interfere with this process.

The focus of the following discussion is on the ways in which this nurse attempted to apply her research findings on the labor and delivery unit. Her goal was to meet the special needs of the primigravida woman who has had an emergency cesarean delivery.

The author's underlying assumption is that the processes of change, as described here, are illustrative of the multiple factors that must be considered when a nurse attempts to facilitate change in any clinical setting. The dynamics operating within the selected environment of a labor and delivery unit are perceived as representative of the many variables which influence the role of the nurse as a change agent within our vast health-care system.

In this discussion, the term "nurse researcher" refers to the author. It differentiates her activities from those of other staff nurses on this particular labor and delivery unit. The author perceived herself as having dual roles— those of a maternity staff nurse *and* of a nurse researcher. It is hoped that other nursing practitioners will perceive themselves with a similar expanded perspective and will be encouraged to apply nursing research findings within their own clinical settings as a result of the information given in this chapter. As more and more clinical data emerge from research endeavors (such as the one described here), nurses will gradually establish a solid foundation for clinical nursing practice.

DESCRIPTION OF THE PILOT STUDY
AND SUBSEQUENT INVESTIGATION

The cesarean delivery rate in the unit under discussion ranged from 15 to 20 percent yearly. This rate is consistent with the national rate of cesarean deliveries mentioned in earlier chapters of this book. The improvement of the care of cesarean clients should concern nurses in all locales.

Some 80 percent of the maternity clients served by this medical center had attended childbirth preparation classes. The majority of these women expected to be active participants in the vaginal delivery of their children. However, the nurse researcher noted that many of these childbirth-educated women had cesarean deliveries. She wondered what happens to a mother when her expectations for a participatory vaginal delivery are not met. She questioned the effect of a cesarean birth on the maternal–infant attachment processes. Did a cesarean delivery in some way alter the establishment of this essential tie between a woman and her child? If so, how? And most importantly, what strategies could a nurse design to mitigate the adverse influence of a cesarean delivery on the attachment process, if indeed there exists an adverse influence?

Prompted by these and other concerns, a pilot study was begun in the spring of 1977 to determine whether further investigation was warranted. The sample consisted of 9 primigravidas from diverse ethnic and economic groups. All of the clients had unexpected cesarean deliveries. Nursing observations focused on several areas of concern: the client's recollection of her labor experience, with some exploration of her personal goals for labor and delivery; the client's analysis of her delivery experience; and early postpartum experience, with a focus on the maternal–infant attachment process. Finally, there was an attempt to identify factors that make a cesarean birth more fulfilling for some mothers than for others.

Data from the pilot yielded the following information. Cesarean mothers demonstrated a need to integrate their birth experiences and reconstruct events surrounding labor and delivery. Certain factors were found to hasten this assimilative work. One positive factor verbalized by the mothers was the presence of their husbands or labor coaches in the delivery room during surgery. This procedure had only been permitted on a few occasions and was not considered standard practice. Mothers related how the presence of these individuals in the operating room eased the personal trauma of the cesarean birth. These persons welcomed the babies and later filled informational gaps for the often anesthetized women. This appeared to help the mother claim her child and to ease her anxiety over the events surrounding her delivery (Marut 1978).

In an effort to verify these factors, a formal research study was begun in the Fall of 1977 with the assistance of a colleague (Marut and Mercer 1979). The study was approved by the hospital's committee on human research.

Fifty primiparous mothers answered a questionnaire and were interviewed within the first 48 hours postpartum. The questionnaire was based on a study done by Samko and Schoenfeld (1975) but was modified as indicated by the results of the pilot study. In order to validate previous research and provide appropriate comparisons, the sample consisted of equal numbers of vaginally-delivered and cesarean-delivered clients.

Findings suggested that there were differences in the attitudes in the two groups with regard to maternal–infant attachment. The cesarean mothers displayed significantly more hesitancy in claiming their infants. For example, only 50 percent of the cesarean mothers had named their infants by the third postpartum day. In addition, cesarean mothers who had support persons with them in the delivery room seemed to have much less difficulty in attaching to their babies, assuming the maternal role, and performing mothering tasks. These mothers seemed to experience much less ego constriction postpartally than those who did not have their support persons present during delivery (Rich 1973). For instance, the mothers who were alone were much more pre-occupied with their own physical needs postpartally than those who had support persons with them. In addition, those who were alone expressed a greater need to discuss their experiences and tended to display greater hesitancy in independently caring for their infants.

The study was limited in that not all infant–mother pairs could be observed. Even though the use of field notes based on memory of interviews may have skewed results, it was felt that tape-recorded interviews would inhibit client response. The emergent themes evident in the data reinforced the investigator's assumption that cesarean mothers do have specific needs which existing hospital policies did not at that time meet.

On the basis of these findings, it seemed that the inclusion of a labor coach in the operating room during surgery would benefit many clients. However, changing hospital policy in this area would have involved the expenditure of considerable time, due to the number of hospital departments involved—anesthesia, surgery, and obstetrics. This would therefore have been a very difficult procedure to initiate and it was deemed more appropriate as a long-range goal. A more attainable goal and a necessary prerequisite to changing hospital policy was educating the nursing staff about the results of the completed research project. This educational approach would increase the staff's awareness of and sensitivity to the needs of cesarean families.

LITERATURE REVIEW

Review of the literature revealed that only one research study had been conducted to examine the effect of a cesarean birth on the mother-infant relationship. Literature that addressed the needs of cesarean clients had not been based on clinical nursing research. Thus, the only clinical research which supported the need for changing the routine care given to cesarean clients was the empirical research of the nurse-researcher (Marut, 1978). Her investigation validated many of the observations offered in the narrative literature, suggesting that the cesarean mother needs time to review her experience. The more she understands, the sooner she will be able to move beyond concerns for herself and independently mother her infant.

The only research reported in the literature that dealt with issues surrounding a cesarean birth focused on three areas: the anxiety level of the mother; the onset of mothering; and the characteristics of the mother's interaction with her baby (Tryphonpoulou and Doxiadis, 1971). The researchers, Tryphonpoulou and Doxiadis, observed two groups of ten primiparous mothers. One group had an elective cesarean birth under general anesthesia. The other mothers delivered vaginally and all received analgesia for their deliveries.

Pre- and postdelivery interviews were conducted, as well as a third interview before the fifth postpartum day. Each mother's first contact with her infant was observed. The babies all had 5-minute Apgar scores of 8 and were given neurologic exams on the first, fifth, and tenth days of life. The two groups were comparable for age, social status, socioeconomic level, and infant birth weight. The authors did not elaborate on who conducted the interviews or what observational techniques were used to measure mother activity; this limits reader interpretation.

Results revealed that the cesarean babies were neurologically behind the vaginally-delivered babies. The cesarean mothers had a greater anxiety level pre- and postdelivery, and all had delayed infant contact. The authors concluded: "Optimal conditions for the establishment of the mother–infant relationship are not achieved after a cesarean birth due to the surgical stress on the mother and the effects of medication on both baby and mother."

The authors did not offer a review of the literature but did substantiate their use of the postdelivery neurological exam. They utilized previous research on the crisis of neonatal separation and applied this to the cesarean mother. The authors also considered the effect of poor infant health on mothering and controlled for this variable by performing neurological exams.

Research by Lynch (1975) further supported the need for closer examination of the cesarean mother and infant. Lynch compared 25 abused children with 25 nonabused siblings in her retrospective study. The children represented diverse social backgrounds. By using matched pairs from within the same family, the author eliminated many psychosocial variables, thus preserving internal control.

The results revealed that the battered child had a history of an abnormality—either difficulty in pregnancy, difficulty in labor and delivery, neonatal or infancy separation, or illness in the mother or infant in the first year of life. Thus numerous factors not clearly identified in other studies emerged as interfering with successful maternal–infant attachment.

Lynch's work suggests that even events that occur over a short period of time (for instance, during labor and delivery) may have long-term consequences in infant development. This study has been replicated, with similar results (Wolkind et al. 1976; Lynch and Roberts 1977; Koller and Williams 1974).

The mother who has a cesarean delivery can identify with several of Lynch's findings. A cesarean birth frequently is characterized as abnormal, and this perspective often applies to labor, also. The mother is often separated from her infant in the delivery room, and postsurgical recovery may force further extended separation.

Evidence of "attachment failure" may be apparent early. Several studies suggest that this is the result of hospital insensitivity in establishing policy Leifer et al. 1972; Hurd 1975; Lynch and Roberts 1977). Experiments with animals have shown that alteration of this sensitive period immediately after birth can produce deviant behavior in the infant (Dubois 1975; Koller and Williams 1974; Hinde and McGinnis 1977). This may place the infant of a cesarean mother in a precarious situation. Helfer (1975) reported that the rates of prematurity and of delivery by the cesarean method are much higher among abused children than in the general population. Thus, there is a need to investigate the impact of a cesarean birth on maternal–infant attachment and subsequent mothering and to modify existing policy. An emergency cesarean birth is an occurrence that is rarely predicted. Consequently, the cesarean mother is predisposed to numerous medical and surgical hazards, and these may interfere with her early mothering attempts. Furthermore, the mother must fit together all the complex pieces surrounding her delivery before physical and psychological equilibrium can be even minimally achieved (Bampton and Mancini 1973; Tunstill 1977; Levinson 1974).

Through her clinical research, the nurse researcher identified factors that may promote maternal–infant attachment among cesarean mothers. Rubin and Erickson (1977) suggested that, in addition to suggesting measures for immediate use in nursing care, field research should provide a knowledge and understanding of the subjective experiences of clients. Lindeman (1975) recommended that research be used to move the practice of nursing from stereotyped techniques to practice based upon knowledge.

On the basis of her findings in the literature, the nurse researcher selected a problem approach appropriate for this setting, that was designed to make the health professionals who provide care for the woman who has a cesarean delivery more *aware of* and *sensitive to* her special needs.

THE BAILEY AND CLAUS PROBLEM-SOLVING MODEL

According to Bailey and Claus (1975), after a problem or need has been identified (e.g., the need to include a labor coach in the delivery room during a cesarean delivery) and a *goal* has been defined (e.g., to educate the staff to the results of the completed research project), the next step is to identify the constraints, capabilities and resources available. Such a step-by-step procedure enables a decision-maker to think systematically. Bailey and Claus proposed a "problem-solving model" that provides guidelines which make sure that no step in the process is omitted. This model also allows one to begin problem solving at any point in the process, rather than having to start with the first step in all situations.

The steps in the Bailey and Claus model that are referred to in this chapter and that were utilized by the nurse researcher in her attempts to improve the care of cesarean clients are:

1. To define the overall goals and needs of the unit, the cesarean client, and the staff.
2. To define the problem. What is the discrepancy between what should be and what in reality exists?
3. To identify the constraints, capabilities, and resources available to the nurse or decision maker.
4. To choose an approach to the problem. The problem solver is encouraged to view the problem from various perspectives before selecting her approach.
5. To define precisely the goal to be accomplished. (In this particular situation, the ultimate goal was to modify the existing care given to cesarean clients so that the level of care would improve. The nurse researcher was particularly interested in assisting the cesarean mother and infant in the attachment process.)
6. To propose alternative solutions.
7. To analyze the alternatives.
8. To choose the best alternative.
9. To implement the decision.
10. To analyze the effectiveness of the implemented decision.

In addition, the significance of the problem or need must also be firmly established. In reference to the problem of including a labor coach in the delivery room during a cesarean delivery, the nurse researcher examined:

1. How others in similar settings have dealt with this problem.

2. The existing hospital hierarchy and its relationship to the enforcement of policy decisions.
3. The nurse's role within this existing structure.
4. The alternatives existing within the system which allow the nurse flexibility of choice in order to solve the identified problem.

ASSESSMENT OF THE SETTING

The labor and delivery unit under discussion served a diverse social and ethnic consumer group. A majority of the people in the client population had a high school education, and involvement in the birth process was anticipated by most of the parents. Of the women delivered in the labor and delivery unit, 85 percent were seen in the university prenatal clinic, usually by resident staff members. The remainder of the clients were cared for by private physicians.

The nurse researcher was one of 22 staff nurses on the unit. There were three senior staff nurses who functioned as unit leaders. Eighty percent of the nurses had baccalaureate educations and at least 1 year of labor and delivery work experience. The other staff nurses were graduates of diploma programs and has similar work experience. The staff nurses had semimonthly staff meetings where problems were discussed and unit in-service was conducted. The nurses were encouraged to pursue independent research. However, few members of the nursing staff had actually engaged in research, either as participants or as principal investigators.

The unit organization permitted the nurse caring for a maternity client in labor to continue to care for her client during and after the cesarean delivery. The unit's 12-hour work shifts usually provided an opportunity for the nurses to be with their clients for extended periods of time. As a result, the nurse had the chance to assess the needs, expectations, strengths, and weaknesses of her cesarean clients, not only throughout the time prior to the cesarean delivery, but also during the critical period after delivery.

The nurses worked closely with both resident and private physicians. The physicians were ultimately responsible for patient care but relied on the nurses to report client problems. The physicians appeared to listen to nursing suggestions on immediate client concerns. The physicians had weekly in-service meetings which the nurses could but rarely did attend. It is noteworthy that none of the staff nurses had ever been asked to participate in presenting an in-service program for the physicians. However, the physicians regularly instructed the nursing staff. The lack of reciprocity illustrates the subordinate position of the nursing staff within the hospital hierarchy. The nurses rarely were asked by the medical staff to share on a formal basis their ideas on how to improve client care, although as the primary caretakers on the unit they had a great deal of first-hand knowledge.

This delivery unit performed approximately 2,000 deliveries a year. Approximately 18 percent of these were cesarean births, 33 percent of which were performed under general anesthesia. Partners were encouraged to be in the labor room, but were allowed in the delivery room for vaginal deliveries and scheduled cesarean births only.

THE POSSIBLE ALTERNATIVES

Three primary forces operated within the problem setting: the physician staff, the nursing staff, and the consumer or client population. The nurse researcher concluded that the most effective method of communicating her research findings and prompting revision of the routine care given to cesarean mothers was to conduct an educational program to inform and modify the behavior of one of these three groups. The terminal behavior desired was the participation of the selected group in assisting the mother-infant dyad in the attachment process as soon after an emergency cesarean birth as possible.

Alternative 1: Education of the Physician Staff

The obstetrical physician on the delivery unit was primarily in charge of patient management in the delivery room. This physician could therefore easily direct personnel to perform tasks that would benefit mother-infant interaction. Indeed, some of the research recommendations come directly under the physician's responsibility in this setting. Allowing the labor partner in the delivery room, controlling the amount and type of anesthetic for a cesarean birth, and permitting the mother to hold her infant immediately after birth were measures only the physician regulated. Examination of the power structure within the unit and the hospital revealed other factors that made this alternative more substantive.

The hierarchical system in which most work relations occur defines which people are mobile, which people will advance, which positions bow to other positions, and how many opportunities for growth and change occur in a particular chain of positions. Organizational systems also define a network of power relations. The power network defines which people can be influential beyond the boundaries of their positions. Within the realm of the labor and delivery unit under discussion, most of the rules had been made by physicians. Thus, in terms of power, the physician appeared to be in the best position to bring about major policy changes and implement the findings of the nurse researcher's study.

Over the past decade, physicians have demonstrated much interest in the mother-infant unit. Early investigations into the attachment process were carried out by physicians (Barnett et al. 1970; Klaus et al. 1970). Within the past 20 years, physicians have created a medical subspecialty, perinatology, to deal specifically with the needs of the infant in the newborn period (Lozoff et al. 1977).

Physicians have also demonstrated interest in the needs of clients. They have independently investigated consumer satisfaction with their care (Light and Fenster 1974; Zax et al. 1975). This suggests that physicians may be interested in the results of an investigation (such as that conducted by the nurse researcher) which gives some index of maternal satisfaction following an emergency cesarean birth.

The nurse researcher could utilize the weekly physician in-service meetings to present her data. This would involve no cost to her and little loss of time. This setting would also be conducive to discussion.

Alternative 2: Education of the Consumer

Client responsibility and involvement in health care has increased with obstetrical technological progress. The average hospital stay following a cesarean birth was 14 days in 1950, and in most hospitals today the stay averages 5 days (Rubin 1975). Thus, the cesarean client has a greater responsibility to nurse herself back to a healthy state.

Clients who have cesarean births are placed in a precarious situation. With the routine separation of mother and infant following a cesarean birth and the time needed for postoperative recovery, the mother and infant have very little time to get acquainted. The nurse researcher's investigation revealed that the mother perceived the staff as preoccupied with the technical aspects of client care. Therefore, clients felt that they must prepare themselves to do whatever was possible to assist the mother–infant attachment process, for it seemed that this was not a priority of the health professionals in that setting. For some mothers, this meant putting specific desires for infant contact in writing prior to delivery or having advocates state these desires for them.

Analysis of the strengths of this solution revealed that 80 percent of this client population attended childbirth preparation classes. The nurse researcher could therefore integrate her suggestions for cesarean birth preparation into this existing educational model. This approach would allow access to a majority of the clients and would provide them with information that would keep them actively involved in the birth process if a cesarean birth did occur.

The idea of client responsibility for changing health care is not new to maternity care. Few nurses realize that rooming-in, now standard practice in most hospitals, was initiated in response to pressure exerted by mothers (Rubin 1975). The formation of C/SEC in 1973 was sparked by consumers who thought that information, support, and involvement should be provided for the rising number of patients undergoing cesarean birth (Cohen 1977).

There were programs in practice in other hospital settings that the nurse researcher would be able to use as models in planning her own. In these programs, preparation for childbirth included extended discussion of the emergency cesarean birth experience. Expectant mothers were told what their rights were in the event cesarean delivery became necessary. Control of self and environment were seen as key factors in this approach. Proponents of this program felt that a woman searches for information as part of her desire for control in what she anticipates will be a stressful situation (Kimbrough 1977).

Research has validated this emphasis on advance information and later control. Some investigators have hypothesized that extreme fear may lead to arrest of labor and/or loss of fetal well-being (Willmuth 1975; Shainess 1963). Additional studies have shown that women who have attended preparation classes deal with crisis situations that occur in labor and delivery better than those who have not (Doering and Enteviste 1974). Investigations have revealed that preparation classes enhance a woman's self-image and lower her perception of pain (Willmuth 1975).

The nurse researcher could meet with the childbirth instructors to orient them to her research and her suggestions. She could participate in the hospital tours available to all the parents and thus directly speak to them. Through this proposed alternative, the nurse researcher would be employing the services of a powerful group—the consumers of nursing care.

Alternative 3: Education of the Staff Nurses

In the delivery of health care on the labor and delivery unit, the staff nurse appears to be midway between the physician and the client on the health care continuum. Historically, the physicians have given the orders and the nurses have carried them out. However, the traditional role of the nurse is changing coincident with the advances in medical technology. As the physician is pulled further from the client, the nurse assumes greater responsibility for client management (Nettles 1977). Maternity nurses have followed the trend toward greater professional autonomy by the formation of such groups as the Nurses Association of the American College of Obstetrics and Gynecology (NAACOG) (Rielly and Newton 1973). This association of maternity nurses considers the staff nurse to be a peer of the physician in planning and meeting client needs.

Other factors also put the staff nurse in a key position to assist the cesarean mother. The intimacy of the contact between the labor and delivery nurse and her client is without parallel in the care given by any other professional on the health-care team (Kinlein 1977). The nurse has a unique opportunity to see the client and her partner in a crisis situation and to evaluate firsthand their strengths and weaknesses. She is in the best possible position to meet their specific needs and can do this with greater ease than anyone else within the limits of existing hospital policy.

Crisis, defined briefly, is an upset in a steady state. It is provoked when a person faces an obstacle to an important life goal that is not surmountable through customary methods of problem solving. A period of disorganization ensues (Baird 1976). The nurse has a role in crisis intervention that is not available to any other specialist. The primary characteristic of the nurse's role is closeness. Her contact with the client is usually constant and continuous. She is closer than any other health-care provider by virtue of her proximity to clients.

Research on crisis has shown that individuals are usually receptive to intervention, if done at the right time and place, before dysfunctional behavior begins (Dzik 1976). Even separation of ½ hour, as stated earlier, in the initiation of mother–infant attachment may have detrimental effects on mothering behavior (Klaus et al. 1970). The staff nurse can best make sure that this separation does not occur by keeping the baby in the delivery room as long as his condition is stable. The nurse can arrange for the mother to see her baby for a brief moment or describe characteristics of the baby to the mother if emergency resuscitation is required and physical separation is necessary to ensure the infant's survival.

Thus, nurses are placed in the position of knowing the client's desires, expectations, and capabilities better than any other health-care personnel. Nurses can best modify the environment in a crisis to meet mother–infant needs.

ANALYSIS OF THE ALTERNATIVES

The nurse researcher utilized a modified version of the parameters suggested by Bailey and Claus (1975) for her evaluation of the three alternatives. The guidelines selected for evaluation of the alternatives were: cost in time and money, feasibility, acceptability of the suggested approach within the setting, risk to client safety, feasibility of the alternative to monitoring, retrievable data and correction, and overall value of the proposed alternative to patient care.

Quantitative objective analysis of the alternatives, as suggested by Bailey and Claus (1975) and utilized by the nurse researcher, is shown in Table 1. This schematic representation allowed an objective comparison of all the alternatives and the selection of the most feasible solution.

Each alternative may have both strong and weak points. The evaluation scheme or matrix proposed by Bailey and Claus allows the nurse or decision-maker to carefully examine how each alternative measures up with each of the selected criteria. Each alternative is scored or generally evaluated for how well it meets each of the criteria—high, moderate, or low. To aid in the comparison, the ideal value for each criteria is also added to the matrix. Scores are matched and totaled for each alternative, thus permitting one to see which alternative most closely meets the ideal in solving the problem. Table 1 summarizes this process.

TABLE 1. OUTCOME MATRIX

IDEAL	PROPOSED ALTERNATIVES			CRITERIA FOR EVALUATION
	I: Physician	II: Nurse	III: Consumer	
High	Moderate	High*	Moderately Low	Feasibility of implementation
Low	Low*	Low*	Low*	Financial cost
Low	Moderate	Low*	High	Time cost
High	Moderately Low	High*	Moderate	Acceptability
Low	Low*	Low*	Low*	Risk to client
High	Moderate	High*	Moderately Low	Ease of monitoring
High	Moderate	High*	Low	Data retrievability
High	Moderate	High*	Moderate	Ease of correction
High	High*	High*	High*	Value to client care
	3	9	3	Number of matches with ideal score

From Bailey JT, Claus KE: Decision Making in Nursing. St. Louis, Mosby, 1975.
*Matches the ideal alternative.

Eventual establishment of all alternatives would seem to be appropriate. However, the nurse researcher was interested in helping the cesarean clients as quickly as possible. This is why an in-service program for the nursing staff was the most plausible solution to the problem, as the total score of 9 for Proposed Alternative II of Table 1 indicates.

Orientation of the instructors of the childbirth classes might have involved more than one teaching session for the nurse researcher. There might also have been resistance from some instructors, which would consume time. For example, there is some controversy among health educators as to whether the mother should be prepared for negative events in labor (Conner 1977).

Johnson's research on clients' reactions to threatening events suggests that clients should not be told of events that rarely occur (Johnson 1972). Gorsuch and Key (1974) related high anxiety levels during pregnancy to adverse effects on parturition and infant status. Rubin (1975) hypothesized that clients seek and take in only the information they want during pregnancy. Information perceived as harmful or difficult to identify with is often rejected. Interviews conducted by the nurse researcher within her study sample support this hypothesis.

Education of the consumer group might have encouraged clients to request that existing policies for an emergency cesarean birth be changed before the health institution or the staff were prepared to make those changes. In the best interests of client safety, specific guidelines must be established first. There may be situations in which the physician needs to regulate events in the delivery room during an emergency cesarean birth to permit prompt delivery of medical care. This alternative would have taken longer to institute, due to its varying acceptability to involved hospital personnel and due to the required scrutiny and revision of established policies.

The physician could have issued a directive that activities in the delivery room be modified to enhance mother–infant attachment. However, often because of the very nature of an emergency situation, the physician is the most removed from the client on a personal level because he is the person most involved with the technical aspects of the delivery. He may not know the woman's plans or expectations for delivery. Even if he does, these desires may have to be considered secondary when survival of the mother and infant is at stake.

An in-service program conducted by a staff nurse to inform the physicians might also have met with resistance. There is evidence that physicians are reluctant to utilize the professional knowledge of nurses. Since nurses have historically taken a "back seat" to physicians in conducting research, there may be some skepticism about the validity of results (Gaynor and Berry 1973; Henderson 1977; Castles 1975). Nursing has been slow in formulating its own theoretical framework for practice, relying on other disciplines, such as medicine, to guide nursing practices.

The educational program for the physicians would have been novel for the unit. It would have served to redirect the doctors' attention to the emotional needs of the cesarean mother. The main disadvantage was that, due to expected resistance and lack of trust in nursing research, there might have been an extended period of time before active physician participation would have been evident.

On the basis of the considerations outlined above, an in-service program conducted by the nurse researcher to educate the nursing staff seemed to be the most feasible solution. It would involve no cost, and work time could be utilized. There would be minimal risk to client safety, since all of the nurses had experience and could be expected to use sound judgment before taking any specific action. The in-service might also serve as an impetus for others on the unit to initiate nursing research.

One problem with this alternative was the role disparity that often occurs on a unit among nurses. That is, nurses often have different definitions of what their role is and how they should function on a unit. This, however, is often due to a lack of a conceptual framework for nursing practice (Lindeman 1975). The in-service program could, it was hoped, provide an example of an objectively derived basis for nursing practice that all the staff nurses could eventually employ.

IMPLEMENTING THE SELECTED ALTERNATIVE

In planning the in-service program, the nurse researcher considered the concepts of adult education. Knowles (1970) listed four assumptions of the adult learner: (1) the adult needs to be self-directed, (2) adults have a rich source of experiences, (3) adults want to use information immediately, and (4) the adult's readiness to learn is based on the demands of his social role. Knowles suggested that mutual planning is critical for an in-service program. According to this view, if a learner feels a program is being imposed on him, there will be direct conflict with his desire to direct his own behavior.

Although the nurse researcher had in-service objectives, she allowed the instructional aspects of the program to depend on the participants' perceived needs. Therefore, her objectives were to review her study, to discuss crisis intervention and the nurse's role, and to inform the staff about C/SEC and the suggestions it offers for care of the cesarean client. The nurse researcher developed a list of activities which the nurses could carry out in the delivery room with a cesarean mother. The list was based on the suggestions offered in the literature by mothers who have had cesarean births (Enkin 1977) and is reproduced here as follows:

1. If time permits, ask the physician if it would be appropriate for the labor partner to accompany the client to the operating room.
2. Inform the client of what is happening to her. Tell her what will be done to her and why (e.g., insertion of Foley catheter).
3. After delivery of the baby, allow the mother to touch or hold her baby as long as safety needs for both are met. If the mother cannot hold or touch her baby, let her see the baby or let her partner, if present, hold the baby.
4. In case of an emergency with the infant, gather information about the baby for the mother upon her request, if the situation permits. In some emergency situations it might be more appropriate for a member of the pediatric staff to speak to the mother first.

5. If general anesthesia is used, stay with the mother during induction and support her.

6. Following the mother's recovery from anesthesia, inform her of what has happened and try to get feedback from her indicating that she understands you.

7. Make an effort to help the mother breast-feed, if she desires, provided all safety needs are met and the mother is comfortable and not heavily medicated.

8. Try to visit the client postpartally to reconstruct events surrounding the delivery and to answer questions.

Knowles (1970) suggested that participants be allowed to draw from their own experiences and make proposals themselves. Accordingly, the nurses discussed the proposed list, decided as a group which suggestions they felt they could implement, and decided how and when they could evaluate these changes at a future staff meeting. Modification of the activities list was proposed by the staff nurses at the next staff meeting. It was important that consensus be reached, because consistency in nursing care is imperative to ensure client safety and equality of care and to allow proper evaluation of the changes instituted.

Prior to initiating the proposed changes in nursing care, the unit nursing leaders informed the hospital departmental administration. Little resistance was anticipated, because the need for improving the care of the cesarean client was well documented and was supported by the hospital's human research committee. In addition, the proposed revisions involved minimal client risk and no client or hospital cost.

EVALUATION OF THE SELECTED ALTERNATIVE

Criteria for evaluating success were established at the initial in-service program. Behaviors indicating success were: regular use of the proposed behavioral changes by the nursing staff and greater evidence of maternal–infant attachment among the cesarean mother-infant dyads.

The nurse researcher was able to quantitatively measure the use of the suggested role modifications because the nurses charted their activities in their "nurse's notes". Another way of measuring the use of success of the nursing activity changes was to sample a small group of perhaps 20 clients through interviews and use of the questionnaire in the nurse researcher's study (see Appendix A). This provided qualitative as well as quantitative measurements of success.

The nurse researcher also evaluated the in-service program from the perspectives of the learner and the teacher. She needed to know whether learner objectives were met. She measured the effectiveness of her in-service program by seeking verbal evaluations from the staff nurses. She also developed a brief quiz to obtain a more objective measure of whether the in-service program did in fact increase the staff's knowledge of the needs of cesarean clients. Finally, the nurse researcher evaluated her success in meeting her own objectives for the in-service program. Ultimately, success in a program is not really achieved until the suggested role modifications and the behaviors that proceed from these roles become routine practice (Tapper 1976).

REFERENCES

Bailey JT, Claus KE: Decision Making in Nursing. St. Louis, Mosby, 1975

Baird SF: Crisis intervention theory in maternal–child nursing. J Obstet Gynecol Nurs 5 (1):30–39, 1976

Bampton R, Mancini J: The cesarean section patient is a new mother, too. J Obstet Gynecol Nurs 2 (4):55–61, 1973

Barnett CR, Leiderman HP, Grobstein R, Klauss M: Neonatal separation: The maternal side of interactional deprivation. Pediatrics 45 (2):197, 1970

Castles MR: A practitioner's guide to utilization of research findings. J Obstet Gynecol Nurs 4 (1):48–49, 1975

Cohen NW: Minimizing emotional sequelae of cesarean childbirth. Birth Fam J 4 (3):114–19, 1977

Conner BS: Teaching about cesarean birth in traditional childbirth classes. Birth Fam J 4 (3):107–13, 1977

de Chateau P, Wilberg B: Long-term effects on mother–infant behavior of extra contact during the first hour postpartum, I: First observations at 36 hours. Acta Paediatr Scand 66:145, 1977

Doering SG, Enteviste DR: Preparation during pregnancy and ability to cope with labor and delivery. Am J Orthopsychiatry 45 (5):825–36, 1974

Donovan B, Allen RM: The cesarean birth method. J Obstet Gynecol Nurs 6 (6):37-48, 1977

Dubois DR: Indications of an unhealthy relationship between parents and a premature infant. J Obstet Gynecol Nurs 4 (3):21–24, 1975

Dzik R: Transactional analysis in crisis intervention. J Obstet Gynecol Nurs 5 (1):31–36, 1976

Enkin MW: Having a section is having a baby. Birth Fam J 4 (3):99–102, 1977

Gaynor A, Berry RK: Observations of a staff nurse: An organizational analysis. J Nurs Admin 3 (3):43-49, 1973

Gorsuch R, Key M: Abnormalities of pregnancy as a function of anxiety and life stress. Psychosom Med 36 (4):352–62, 1974

Helfer R: The relationship between lack of bonding and child abuse and neglect. In Maternal Attachment and Mothering Disorders: A Round Table. New Brunswick N.J. Johnson and Johnson Baby Products Company, 1975

Henderson V: We've "come a long way," but what of direction? Nurs Res 26 (3):164, 1977

Hinde RA, McGinnis L: Some factors influencing the effects of temporary mother–infant separation: Some experiments with rhesus monkeys. Psychol Med 7 (2):1977

Hurd JM: Assessing maternal attachment: First step toward the prevention of child abuse. J Obstet Gynecol Nurs 4 (4):25–32, 1975

Johnson J: Effects of structuring patient's expectations on their reactions to threatening events. Nurs Res 21 (6):499–503, 1972

Kimbrough CA: The search for labor information during pregnancy. Maternal–Child Nurs J 6 (2):107–16, 1977

Kinlein ML: The self-care concept. Am J Nurs 77 (4):598–601, 1977

Klaus MH, Kennell JH: Mothers separated from their newborn infants. Ped Clin North America. 17:1015–37, 1970.

Knowles M: Gearing adult education for the seventies. J Continuing Educ Nurs 1:11–16, 1970

Koller KM, Williams WT: Early parental deprivation and later behavioral outcomes: Cluster analysis study of normal and abnormal groups. Aust NZ J Psychiatry 8 (99):89–96, 1974

Leifer AD, Williams JA, Leiderman PH, Barnett CR: Effects of mother–infant separation on maternal attachment behavior. Child Dev 43 (4):1203–18, 1972

Levinson G: Valium, innovar and ketamine in obstetrics. In Shnider SM, Moya F (eds), The Anesthesiologist, Mother, and Newborn. Baltimore, Williams and Williams, 1974

Light H, Fenster C: Maternal concerns during pregnancy. Am J Obstet Gynecol 118 (1):46–50, 1974

Lindeman C: Nursing practice research: What's it all about? J Nurs Admin 5 (3):5–7, 1975

Lozoff B, Brittenham GM, Trause MA, et al: The mother–infant relationship: Limits of adaptability. J Pediatr 91 (1):1–12, 1977

Lynch M: Ill health and child abuse. Lancet 16:317–19, 1975

Lynch M, Roberts J: Predicting child abuse: Signs of bonding failure in the maternity hospital. Br Med J 624–26, 1977

Marut JS: The special needs of the cesarean mother. Am J Maternal Child Nurs 3 (4):202–206, 1978

Marut JS, Mercer RT: A comparison of primigravidas: Perceptions of their vaginal and cesarean births. Nurs Res 28 (5):220–66, 1979

Nettles JB: Changing influences on practice of obstetrics. South Med J 70 (6):648–50, 1977

Nunnally DM, Aquiar MB: Patients' evaluation of their prenatal and delivery care. Nurs Res 23 (6):469–74, 1974

Ob Gyn News. 12 (13):1, 1977

Rich OJ: Temporal and spatial experience as reflected in the verbalizations of multiparous women during labor. Maternal–Child Nurs J 2 (4):1973

Rielly P, Newton M: The role of the obstetric, gynecologic and neonatal nurse. J Obstet Gynecol Nurs 2 (4):23, 1973

Rubin R: Maternity nursing stops too soon. Am J Nurs 75 (10):1680–84, 1975

Rubin R, Erickson R: Research in clinical nursing. Maternal–Child Nurs J 6 (3):150–64, 1977

Samko MR, Schoenfeld LS: Hypnotic susceptibility and the Lamaze childbirth experience. Am J Obstet Gynecol 121:631–36, 1975

Shainess N: The psychologic experience of labor. NY State J Med 29:23–32, 1963

Tapper M: Evaluation of inservice programs. AORN 23 (7):307–14, 1976

Tryphonopoulou Y, Doxiadis S: The effect of elective cesarean section on the initial stage of mother–infant relationship. Psychosomatic Med Obstet Gynecol 3 14–17, 1972

Tunstill ME: Detecting wakefulness during general anesthesia for caesarean section. Br Med 6072 (1):1321, 1977

Willmuth LR: Prepared childbirth and the concept of control. J Obstet Gynecol Nurs 4 (5):38–46, 1975

Wolkind SN, Kruk S, Chaves L: Childhood separation experiences and psychosocial status in primiparous women. Br J Psychiatry 128:391–93, 1976

Zax M, Sameroff A, Farnum J: Childbirth education, maternal attitudes, and delivery. Am J Obstet Gynecol 123 (2):185–90, 1975

APPENDIX A*

PLEASE NOTE: This questionnaire should be filled out voluntarily. You
may refuse to fill it out at any time. All data will remain
confidential and all respondents are to remain anonymous.

Please *circle* the number on each scale that best describes the feeling state referred to in each question.

EXAMPLE: How relaxed were you during labor?

Not at
  all   Moderately   Extremely

1   2   3   (4)   5

(This answer would indicate that you were very relaxed, though not extremely relaxed.)

1. How successful were you in using breathing or relaxation methods to help
with contractions?

Not at
  all   Moderately   Extremely

1   2   3   4   5

2. How confident were you during labor?

Not at
  all   Moderately   Extremely

1   2   3   4   5

3. How confident were you during delivery?

Not at
  all   Moderately   Extremely

1   2   3   4   5

4. How relaxed were you during labor?

Not at
  all   Moderately   Extremely

1   2   3   4   5

5. How relaxed were you during the delivery?

Not at
  all   Moderately   Extremely

1   2   3   4   5

6. How pleasant or satisfying was the feeling state you experienced during delivery?

Not at
all   Moderately   Extremely

1   2   3   4   5

7. How well in control were you during labor?

Not at
all   Moderately   Extremely

1   2   3   4   5

8. How well in control were you during delivery?

Not at
all   Moderately   Extremely

1   2   3   4   5

9. To what extent did your experience of having a baby go along with the expectation you had before labor began?

Not at
all   Moderately   Extremely

1   2   3   4   5

10. To what extent do you consider yourself to have been a useful and co-operative member of the obstetric team?

Not at
all   Moderately   Extremely

1   2   3   4   5

11. How useful was your partner in helping you through your labor?

Not at
all   Moderately   Extremely

1   2   3   4   5

12. How useful was your partner in helping you through delivery?

Not at
all   Moderately   Extremely

1   2   3   4   5

13. How valuable were classes that you had to prepare for childbirth?

Not at all		Moderately		Extremely
1	2	3	4	5

14. To what degree were you aware of events during labor?

Not at all		Moderately		Extremely
1	2	3	4	5

15. To what degree were you aware of events during delivery?

Not at all		Moderately		Extremely
1	2	3	4	5

16. How unpleasant was the feeling state you experienced during delivery?

Not at all		Moderately		Extremely
1	2	3	4	5

17. Do you remember your labor as painful?

Not at all		Moderately		Extremely
1	2	3	4	5

18. Do you remember your delivery as painful?

Not at all		Moderately		Extremely
1	2	3	4	5

19. How scared were you during delivery?

Not at all		Moderately		Extremely
1	2	3	4	5

20. Did you worry about your baby's condition during labor?

Not at all		Moderately		Extremely
1	2	3	4	5

21. Did you worry about your baby's condition during delivery?

    Not at
     all   Moderately   Extremely

     1   2   3   4   5

22. Did the equipment used during labor bother you?

    Not at
     all   Moderately   Extremely

     1   2   3   4   5

23. Was the delivery experience realistic as opposed to dream-like?

    Not at
     all   Moderately   Extremely

     1   2   3   4   5

24. Did you have choices about interventions, i.e., examinations or treatments during labor?

    Not at
     all   Moderately   Extremely

     1   2   3   4   5

25. Did your partner (or other person) review your labor experience with you?

    Not at
     all   Moderately   Extremely

     1   2   3   4   5

26. Did you feel better after reviewing the labor and delivery experience?

    Not at
     all   Moderately   Extremely

     1   2   3   4   5

27. Were you pleased with how your delivery turned out?

    Not at
     all   Moderately   Extremely

     1   2   3   4   5

28. How soon after delivery did you touch your baby?

    Immediately   2 hours   8 hours or longer

     1   2   3   4   5

29. How soon after delivery did you hold your baby?

Immediately   2 hours   8 hours or longer

1   2   3   4   5

30. Were you able to enjoy holding your baby for the first time?

Not at
  all   Moderately   Extremely

1   2   3   4   5

*Based on Marut JM, and Mercer RT, 1979.

CHAPTER 14

The Rights of Women in Cesarean Birth: A Bioethical Perspective

B. Louise Murray

Changes in the health care of women, especially concerning childbirth, are not likely to be successful unless both nurses and their clients consider the historical and cultural roots of the many inequitable situations which exist in the health care system today. Pressures toward change must come in concert, not only from within but also from outside the system. On the outside, pressures can be integrated most effectively with the current consumer movement by focusing on ethical principles, human rights, and the rights of patients. Within the system, greater recognition can be given to the concomitant duties and privileges of nurses who provide care for patients.

Just as a concentration on ethical principles can help ensure patients' rights, so can an emphasis on the essence of the nurse-patient relationship support such efforts. Nurses who are confident that the care they provide safeguards patients' rights will also be more assertive toward this end. Nurses can help patients learn to deal with the inequities of the system and learn how to insist that their rights be recognized and respected.

Nurses must also be willing to take those risks which are an integral part of any change process, and especially of a change which involves such firmly entrenched ideas, attitudes, and customary ways of behaving as currently exist in the provision of health care to women.

HISTORICAL AND CULTURAL ROOTS

Both historically and culturally, the health care of women and the health field itself has been characterized by a disparity in beliefs, attitudes, and expectations concerning the roles and functions of men and women as both providers and recipients of care (Corea 1977).

In colonial America, for example, physicians came from the upper classes of society and treated primarily the rich. Other people, including the poor, received health care from nonphysician healers or domestic practitioners. These practitioners were men and women who usually came from the same social class as their patients and belonged to "irregular" medical sects.

In the early part of the 19th century, the elite group of male physicians began to organize medicine as an exclusive profession. They attempted to gain control by establishing licensure only for their own group of practitioners—the allopaths of the "orthodox" medical sect. The public, as well as the members of the "irregular" sects, strongly opposed the licensing laws because they favored the rich and excluded both poor men's sons and women from medical schools. As a result, the licensing laws were revoked, allowing the other medical sects to obtain charters for their own schools, some of which were for women.

The elite, male medical group strongly resisted the efforts of women to enter the orthodox medical profession by attempting to obstruct the founding of medical institutions for women and by bitterly opposing the admission of female students to male medical institutions. The few women who were admitted to established male institutions were assailed and insulted by both professors and students.

Physicians went so far as to promote the idea that the functions of menstruation, pregnancy, childbirth, and menopause were in fact disabling illnesses, since men did not experience these events. They advised women to marry for the sake of their health and to let themselves be cared for by their husbands and by their male physicians. They warned women against too much "brain" activity, as it would be detrimental to their reproductive capacity.

As a result, upper class women cultivated their weaknesses. They learned to associate poor health with femininity, for which they were worshipped and pampered by their husbands and cared for by their physicians.

Similar attitudes are still held today, unfortunately. As Corea (1977, pp. 31-32) discusses, Matina Horner in 1968 showed how women were in a double bind because they worried not only about failure, but also about something which unsexes a woman: *success.* She asked male and female college students at the University of Michigan to complete a paragraph which began, "After one semester John finds himself at the top of his medical school class." Another group completed the same paragraph but substituted the name Anne for John. Almost all students wrote that John had a wonderful personality, an active love life, and an outstanding academic and professional career. However, both male and female students described Anne as neurotic, lonely, and a grind. They assumed she was dateless and despised. That she could be both successful in medical school and a normal female was inconceivable.

Health care of women from the 19th century to the present has reflected such attitudes. With this in mind, one can understand how and why childbirth today has been largely taken over by male physicians.

THE MASCULINE AND FEMININE PRINCIPLES AND TRADITIONAL ATTITUDES IN HEALTH CARE

Another explanation of the cultural basis for our traditional views about sex roles in health care can be found in the conception of "masculine" and "feminine" principles presented by Remen, Blau, and Hively in their monograph, *The Masculine Principle, The Feminine Principle and Humanistic Medicine* (1975). According to these authors, constricted role expectations have resulted from an improper understanding of the nature of human energies.

The masculine principle is characterized by such traits as a strong will; strength; power; rigidity; a volatile spirit; independence; a technical approach; ability to analyze; objectivity; rationality; dominance; demonstration of initiative; and a preoccupation with knowledge, with openness, and with things.

The feminine principle, on the other hand, is characterized by compassion; love; concern with the intrinsic significance of people; flexibility; dependence; intuition; emotion; a subjective approach to reality; warmth; receptivity; secretiveness; submissiveness; preoccupation with meaning and the way things are said and with tone of voice, gestures, body language, and relationships.

These characteristics and attitudes are essentially human in scope, in that they are possessed to some degree by everyone. Culturally, however, the principles have been dichotomized. The masculine principle has been accorded relative ascendancy in our mainly technological society. The feminine principle, on the other hand, has been depreciated and repressed. The many problems and limitations women face today can be thought of as the inevitable consequences of the loss of balance between these two principles.

Patterns of behavior which embody the masculine principle have not only been held in great esteem in our society, but have also been considered to be essential for achievement and for the validation of the individual by society. Feminine traits, on the other hand, have been looked upon as weaknesses and equated with inability to achieve, especially in fields in which masculine traits are valued and traditionally have been dominant.

The disproportionate respect accorded to masculine principle traits, as contrasted with feminine principle traits, has had a significant influence on how people tend to behave, both in general and in relation to specific endeavors. We have been enculturated in accordance with this view to think that the different principles are related primarily to success in different fields of endeavor—for instance, to think that the masculine principle characterizes professional behavior, whereas the feminine principle characterizes effective parenting. In the health field, these principles have had a profound effect on accepted physician and nurse behaviors.

Careers, once they have been recognized as such by society, seem to take on the more prestigious aspects of the masculine principle and divest themselves of the less desired aspects of the feminine principle.

Since most nurses are female, they find themselves in a conflicting situation. The nursing role embodies feminine principle traits, for the most part. However, outward manifestation of these traits is very difficult in an environment which tends to repress as well as show disrespect for the expression of these traits. Thus nurses are made to feel that their profession is not as highly regarded, and indeed is even subservient to medicine.

These role conceptions can also be identified in the image of the "good patient," who is expected to trust and cooperate fully with his doctor, accept medical ministrations without question, have a calm and trusting family, provide an objective and exact account of his major complaints and medical history, and above all have a physical disorder which can be diagnosed and treated successfully.

Thus physicians, nurses, *and* patients may never achieve their potential, either in function or in self-actualization, because repression of either principle requires a tremendous and unproductive expenditure of energy. This is especially true as concerns the patient, since his or her total resources may be unavailable for either the maintenance of health or the healing process.

It would seem, then, that nurses, as a significant group of health-care professionals, along with their patients, must become acutely aware of sex role-related expectations and their marked influence on human behavior. We must learn to function as self-determined persons if we are to maximize our health care potential. And, most important, we must recognize that the mere existence of repressive attitudes and behavior can be expected to result in a concomitant repression of human rights, not only for ourselves but also for patients and their health care.

Nurses who are knowledgeable about the inequities which characterize the health care of women today and who are aware of the cultural roots of such unjust attitudes and beliefs are in a more favorable position to decide on the direction of the changes which need to be made. Moreover, nurses who are familiar with the ethical principles and rules upon which human rights and the rights of patients rest can be successful in identifying those practices which need to be changed and in securing support and agreement toward progressive action, not only from their professional colleagues but also from the women consumers of health care. The remainder of this chapter deals with the ethics involved in the care of women during childbirth, especially with respect to a cesarean birth.

BIOETHICS AND CESAREAN BIRTH

In the field of biomedical ethics, according to Beauchamp and Childress (1979), health care delivery problems can be analyzed by applying general ethical theory; the moral principles of autonomy, beneficence, nonmaleficence, and justice; and the rules of veracity, fidelity, and confidentiality. These principles and rules govern the practices of both medicine and nursing.

Drawing on the ethical theory of rule deontology and the principles and rules cited above, the needs, claims, or rights of cesarean patients and the duties or privileges of the nurses who care for them are here discussed.

The Theory of Rule Deontology

Rule deontological theory is concerned with ongoing relationships between people, which create certain obligations, and with the moral principles and rules by which one can judge actions to be right or wrong, morally binding or prohibited (Beauchamp and Childress 1979).

The rule deontologist believes that the objectives of a moral life are not achieved merely by doing good as an end in itself. There is also a greater obligation to find a way to meet the claims or champion the rights of others. Moral theory must be in harmony with one's moral convictions.

Rules grounded in moral principles justify actions as right or wrong. Rules facilitate the process of going from fundamental principles to final decisions. Principles are more general and basic and serve as the foundation for rules. The consideration of morality vis-à-vis predetermined rules of behavior requires different perspectives. Each depends on a separate understanding of moral terms. Each implies different degrees and kinds of weight and stringency. Some rules are "rules of thumb" which summarize the wisdom of the past. Other rules may be, on their face value, binding; these can be overridden if they are in conflict with stronger duties. Still other rules are absolute and cannot be overriden under any circumstances (Beauchamp and Childress 1979, pp. 33–46).

The Principle of Autonomy

Autonomy is a basic human right characterized by self-determination—that is, the individual freedom to consider, to decide, and to act on one's own volition without significant physical or psychological restrictions (Beauchamp and Childress 1979).

An autonomous person acts independently and with self-confidence on the basis of his or her own moral convictions, which are harmonious with generally accepted moral principles. A person who is autonomous is physically, mentally, and emotionally competent to make self-determined, voluntary choices.

The Rule of Informed Consent—The rule of informed consent is absolute for the autonomous person. It gives one the right to decide matters affecting one's life and encourages one to think and act on one's own initiative. Informed consent must be given to any procedure or treatment carrying a significant risk or having a questionable purpose (Beauchamp and Childress 1979, pp. 63-64).

A Discussion of Autonomy in Cesarean Birth—In applying the principle of autonomy set forth by Beauchamp and Childress (1979, pp. 63-70) to the cesarean mother, a number of important elements must be taken into account. A woman is a person of unconditional worth, with all the basic human rights of any person. During pregnancy, and at the time of childbirth, she has a right to choose her own goals for health care, with the assistance of health care providers. Her goals may differ from those which the provider believes to be good for health, but if providers have explained their rationale for their views and the mother fully comprehends what she has been told, she has a right not to be coerced to change her mind.

If, however, her particular health goals or her beliefs about medical treatment actually place the life of her infant in jeopardy, then that fact must be explained to her so that she can appreciate her responsibility in the matter. If her health should deteriorate and she still refuses treatment, legal measures may be necessary to protect the infant.

An autonomous mother-to-be is a person who is competent—i.e., mature, rational, not acutely ill or in marked distress, and not uninformed, retarded, or otherwise vulnerable. She has a right to know the reasons; the pros and cons; the alternatives; the benefits, risks, and costs to herself, her infant, or her family of any proposed or intended obstetrical treatment, procedure, test, drug or diagnostic technique. This is particularly true of any invasive procedures, such as internal fetal monitoring, intravenous infusions, or operative procedures such as cesarean delivery. Such information should be explained to her logically, in ordinary lay person's language, in a way that any "reasonable person" under similar circumstances would be able to understand. The information should be complete but not so detailed or distorted as to cause confusion. The client has a right to sufficient time to consider the information, to be encouraged to ask questions, and to be given truthful answers. She has a right to demonstrate her comprehension of what she has been told and her ability to think clearly. She has a right to not be "put down," made to feel stupid or inadequate, or to not be put under pressure to make a nonvoluntary decision. She should be free to decide to withdraw from the situation if there is no major risk to her life or to the life of her unborn infant.

If it is clearly demonstrated that a mother is incompetent, is "waiving" consent, or is acceding for "irrational" reasons to any proposed treatment, consideration must be given to protecting her interests by obtaining informed consent from a second trusted party, such as her husband, or from an institutional body such as an ethics committee.

The Principles of Beneficence and Nonmaleficence

Beneficence means moral and professional responsibility for benefiting consumers—that is, the "active promotion of good" (Beauchamp and Childress 1979, p. 135). A beneficial provider-patient relationship originates out of human need and must be overtly agreed upon by both parties.

To make rational decisions based on this principle, the benefits, possible harm, and costs of care must be carefully weighed. The merit of a procedure must be clear when measured against the risk. Thus more valid information can be provided to patients when seeking their informed consent (Beauchamp and Childress 1979, pp. 135-42).

According to the principles of nonmaleficence, professional codes and licensure to practice (Beauchamp and Childress 1979) stipulate protection of patients' safety—that is, a responsibility to "above all do no harm." In other words, one is not to engage in or fail to protect clients from willful or negligent practices which might cause physical, mental, or emotional injury or suffering. Major risk, if balanced against a lesser benefit, is not permissible. However, if the risk is small and the benefit great, and if actions are cautious and the result offsets potential harm, violation of this principle may be acceptable (Beauchamp and Childress 1979, pp. 97-102).

Professionals have a duty to know whether a procedure or treatment is obligatory or ordinary; morally optional or extraordinary (Beauchamp and Childress 1979, pp. 117-26).

If a procedure or treatment is obligatory, the duty is to be sure that it will not be detrimental, that it will have a potentially positive result, that it will not cause great suffering, and that it will not be more costly than necessary in terms of time, money, convenience, comfort, and the autonomous desires of the patient.

If a treatment is optional, it is elective; it could be expensive, cause pain or other inconvenience, and would probably not offer a prospect of benefit.

In matters of life and death, competent patients should make their own decisions, provided that no significant harm is brought to another person (Beauchamp and Childress 1979, pp. 127-29). Incompetent patients must be protected against harm by having responsible health-care providers selected as decision-makers to set up procedures and processes designed to protect the interests of these patients. Families may be presumed to act in the patients' best interests and should be primary decision-makers.

Physicians and other health-care professionals are responsible for providing information and moral counseling, for actively preventing abuse of a patient's interests, and for withdrawing when their consciences dictate. Health-care professionals, hospital committees, and the courts must serve a protective function when there are conflicting judgments or evidence of abuse (Beauchamp and Childress 1979, pp. 130-31).

A Discussion of Beneficence and Nonmaleficence—The principles of beneficence and nonmaleficence apply to women in labor and unborn infants who are not "high risk" clients. That is, the principles apply when the mother has no medical or obstetrical complications and/or when her fetus is not small for gestational age, premature, or otherwise unusually vulnerable. Such a mother and unborn infant should not be *routinely* monitored electronically, either externally or internally, when monitoring might give false positive signals of fetal distress in a high percentage of cases, or when the mother has to remain in a supine position because of the attached equipment. In such cases the possible harm and the costs would outweigh the benefit. The merit of the procedure would not be clearly superior when balanced against the risk.

Nurses and other health-care providers have a duty (or privilege) to consider the possible harm or risk of obtaining technical data erroneously indicating fetal distress which might put both mother and infant under undue constraint and subject them to a potentially hazardous surgical procedure because of an iatrogenically caused problem. The possible harm must be weighed against the benefit of obtaining more accurate data by having a nurse skillfully auscultate fetal heart rate with a fetoscope.

Another benefit/detriment assessment would be involved in preventing the mother from walking around and being otherwise occupied during labor. Ambulation, when there are no complications, prevents pressure of the gravida uterus on the great vessels, which pressure can compromise the circulations of both mother and fetus. Ambulation also promotes the progress of labor by allowing (1) the forces of gravity and the pressure of the fetus to gradually cause the pelvis to expand, (2) the presenting part to promote dilatation, and (3) the fetus to descend normally and progressively through the birth canal.

Thus the enforced use of a fetal monitor and a requirement of bedrest and maintenance of a supine position would constitute failure to do "good" as well as failure to prevent harm. This is morally and professionally wrong.

Another circumstance in which the risk or harm might outweigh the benefit would be pressuring a woman to go to a distant high-risk center for obstetrical care, because of either her own condition or that of her unborn infant, when equally good care could be provided in a hospital near her home. Here, the detriment would be to her psychological needs because of potentially stressful emotional reactions to separation from the support and reassurance of her family, both before and during birth. Harm might also result from interference with a healthy maternal–infant (parental–infant) attachment after birth. In addition, the high cost of maternity care associated with such specialized centers could cause the mother and family extreme worry and distress. The value of the care in the high-risk center would have to be weighed against the cost/risk and detriment.

Health professionals who promote the idea of maternity care in distant high-risk centers may be acting in a strongly paternalistic manner, especially if their ideas of the value of the care differ from those of the woman and her family, and if the woman has not given a fully informed and voluntary consent and is reluctant to comply with such advice. This counsel could jeopardize the woman's autonomy, if she is competent, and in such a case would be morally and professionally wrong, since the woman should be assumed to know what is in her own best interests.

When the mother's or fetus's condition is marginal and the benefit of care in a high-risk center is stronger than the potential detriment, a violation of this principle might be acceptable. However, arrangements should be made for the family to be together if the costs are within reach of their economic means.

Where medicaid or other governmental, tax-supported programs or project grants cover the cost of such care, another question arises. Should the taxpayer be required to indirectly support costly care which might not be essential?

The principle of nonmaleficence refers not only to the accidental risk of harm but also to intentional harm. The American Nurses Association Code for Professional Nurses specifies the professional standards which nurses must meet in order to comply with this principle. They should have a sound general education which provides fundamental knowledge and skills. The code also specifies that professional nurses are responsible for continuing their own education, so that their knowledge and skills are up to date. In this way they make themselves less likely to unintentionally harm a patient. Professional training should instill traits of caring, compassion, and concern, among others, to assist the nurse in promoting the well-being of her patients. Such other traits of character as moral integrity, conscientiousness, and diligence are consonant with avoiding negligence, carelessness, and unintentional harm to patients, which could result in charges of malpractice.

Nurses are responsible for determining whether the patient is competent and whether her autonomous wishes are being followed when the care is said to be obligatory or ordinary. One example of obligatory (or ordinary) care would be the recommendation of a cesarean birth for a diabetic mother who is not entirely in control. Another example would be to recommend cesarean delivery when fetal size, stress, and maturity tests and other examinations have indicated that the fetus is close to term but would be at moderate to high risk if the pregnancy were to terminate in a vaginal delivery.

Nurses are also responsible for carrying out the wishes of the autonomous cesarean mother when the care is judged to be optional or extraordinary. An example of optional (or extraordinary) care would be the recommendation of cesarean delivery because the infant has, through various diagnostic studies, been found to have severe congenital defects not usually compatible with survival. Another example would be giving this infant optional (or extra-ordinary) care after birth which must be continuous in order to sustain life.

In the first instance, the mother must be allowed to decide for herself whether or not to have a cesarean after she has been fully informed about the alternatives and about the benefits and risks to herself and to the infant of vaginal delivery. In the second example, the mother should be allowed to make informed and voluntary decisions—first as to whether to have a cesarean (after she understands the alternatives and risks of the procedure) and second as to whether to continue the optional (or extraordinary) care of the infant. If the mother is pressured into having a cesarean without her voluntary consent when the procedure is not likely to preserve or promote the baby's well-being, and if the parents are not given the opportunity to decide whether to give optional (or extraordinary) care to the infant after birth, the nurse involved should discuss her views with the physician and the patient's family. If no changes are made in the proposed care of the mother or her defective infant, the nurse has a right to withdraw from the case, provided the mother and the infant are not left inappropriately unattended. Again, the nurse is responsible for determining whether the patient is competent to make an informed, autonomous decision.

Principles of Justice

Different principles of justice determine what individuals or groups deserve on the basis of needs or claims. (Beauchamp and Childress 1979). In applying the principle of comparative justice, one must balance the value of competing claims to decide what a person deserves. According to the principle of non-comparative justice, established standards are applied to decide a person's due. The principle of distributive justice calls for properly balancing good or benefit, and scarcity or burden. The formal concept of justice requires that people with similar properties be treated similarly (and, consequently, that those with dissimilar properties be treated proportionate to those differences). The material principles of justice call for giving each person an equal share according to needs, effort, contribution to society, and merit (Beauchamp and Childress 1979, pp. 169-77).

Application of the principles of justice (however one is defining them) can result in conflict among competing claims. The concept of "due process" is more likely to result in just decisions, but several steps are required, as follows: identification of the pool of potentially deserving recipients, establishment of acceptable minimum standards which are objective and easily applied, and utilization of the utilitarian principle of "the greatest good for the greatest number" in a final selection. Equal opportunity and access should be assured by some form of chance, and objective standards (such as medical criteria) should be used (Beauchamp and Childress 1979, pp. 192-98).

The Principles of Justice and Cesarean Birth—According to the principles of justice, all women in childbirth deserve to have quality care based on their needs and their legitimate claims or rights. An example of injustice would be to accept women into high-risk maternity centers only if they could afford to go (i.e., only if they had the economic resources to pay in full for costly care), regardless of the degree of risk to the mother or infant. Another example would be to electronically monitor or perform a cesarean on only those parturients who can afford to pay the additional cost of a surgical birth. There is some evidence that women who go to community hospitals have a higher rate of cesarean deliveries than women who are patients in teaching center hospitals (Jones 1976, p. 521). A third example would be a decision to electronically monitor all women, whether they are high-risk or not, because of a high rate of malpractice suits. A fourth would be to have obstetrical residents perform cesareans in teaching hospitals primarily to gain experience.

Throughout this discussion, it is recognized that the principles of beneficence and nonmaleficence apply in such cases in terms of the potential benefit, risk, harm, or detriment to a particular group of women. The principles of autonomy, informed consent, and general human welfare also apply.

According to the principle of fair opportunity, economic circumstances, education, sex, race, and social class should not influence the type of care provided to pregnant women when they are equal to their more affluent sisters in terms of health-care needs and claims. Moreover, those women who have the greatest need from a medical/physical standpoint (i.e., poor nutrition or limited physical stamina due to overwork or an excessive number of pregnancies) may indeed be more deserving of and/or may require the best health-care resources available.

The Principle of Commutative Justice

The principle of commutative justice applies in the voluntary relationships between professionals and patients. This principle focuses on the rights and duties of the individuals concerned and involves the principle of veracity and the duties of fidelity (Beauchamp and Childress, 1979).

The principle of veracity implies a duty on the part of the health professional to tell the truth to patients; compliance with this duty evidences inherent respect. Veracity is expressed through the principles of autonomy and informed consent. The patient has a general right to the truth as well as a special right to a truthful diagnosis, prognosis, and description of the procedures involved in care.

The principle of veracity is, *prima facie,* not absolute. The duty of veracity requires the disclosure of information which a reasonable person would want to know. Forcing information on an unwilling patient is weak paternalism, which violates autonomy. Respect is expressed in allowing the patient the right to not know, if she so chooses. The concept of fidelity or trust is necessary for a productive professional relationship to be established and maintained. It also evidences respect for autonomy and veracity.

Commutative Justice and Cesarean Birth—Fidelity is established when the nurse and the cesarean mother have voluntarily entered into open communication in a professional relationship. In such a relationship a patient feels comfortable or free to tell the nurse whatever is on her mind, because she feels the nurse is trustworthy and will not use what she has said to harm her. Fidelity also rests on the fact that the patient and nurse both believe that the other person will not deliberately act in a harmful way.

Fulfillment of the duty of veracity is manifested when the patient not only views the nurse as trustworthy, but also believes that the nurse will tell the truth and keep her promises.

When trust is established, mutual confidence and willingness to rely on one another follow. The ANA Code spells out the nurse's responsibility to tell the truth and thus reaffirm this ethical principle. This is not only a moral issue, but a professional one.

The duty of veracity, which requires that the nurse tell the patient the truth, can create a dilemma if the patient's doctor and nurse tell her different things. The patient has the autonomous right to ask for or otherwise indicate what information she wants. She also has the autonomous right not to be given information. However, when the best interests of the patient are served, this principle may be violated; it is *prima facie*, not absolute.

Not revealing a patient's confidences demonstrates respect for the patient's autonomy and privacy. Nurses have a duty to keep what the patient tells them confidential unless a greater harm might be brought upon someone else as a result of not telling. Communication of confidential information by the patient is a demonstration of respect for and trust in the nurse. Confidentiality is a *prima facie* duty, not an absolute one.

However, if a patient communicates something which cannot be held in confidence, the nurse has the duty to so inform her. Release of information at the request of the patient is not, of course, a break of confidentiality.

Since confidentiality is a *prima facie* duty, and not an absolute one, the degree and probability of harm resulting from nondisclosure must be weighed against the effects of breaking a confidence in terms of the quality of the professional–patient relationship.

THE NEEDS, CLAIMS, AND RIGHTS OF PATIENTS AND NURSES' DUTIES AND PRIVILEGES

During pregnancy and childbirth, women are less apt to take an assertive stance on their needs, claims, or rights than women who are not pregnant. Thus, it seems imperative that nurses recognize and actively assume their ethical/moral duties when caring for this group. It is only in this way that changes in health care during childbearing can be effected. Nursing care must be geared toward helping women assume greater responsibility for themselves. In addition, nurses must clearly establish and recognize their professional privileges for the improvement of care on the basis of the needs, claims, and rights of their patients.

As established previously, human rights belong to everyone and enable persons to live decent and fulfilling lives. According to Bandman and Bandman (1978, pp. 51-52), the most important of these rights is the right to be free, which is the basis for having any rights at all. The right of freedom means having a right to one's domain, including one's body, one's life, one's property, and one's privacy. It also means having a right *to not do* whatever one has a right to do.

Human rights also include the right not to be brainwashed, lied to, kept ignorant, deceived, tricked, or otherwise coerced. It means having the authority to determine one's own actions without outside interference. The right of self-determination is the expression of freedom. This right enables one to decide for oneself the course of one's life. To do so, one must have the mental and physical capacity to make choices and the freedom to carry them out.

Rights impose duties on the rightholder. Special duties are imposed on those rightholders who are obligated to protect other persons' rights. Duties or privileges have their origins in rights (Bandman and Bandman 1978, p. 53).

Thus, health-care providers can exercise their privileges through action on behalf of their patients *when and only when* the patients cannot act on their own behalf.

By virtue of their knowledge and skill, their professional license, and their relationship to patients, nurses ". . .are 'permitted to carry the keys to the lock on the gate' of a patient's domain of freedom, when this domain includes a patient's body" (Bandman and Bandman 1978, p. 327). Privileges are granted ". . . at the rightholder's request and at the rightholder's pleasure, assuming the rightholder is informed and the consent is voluntary" (Bandman and Bandman 1978, p. 328). A privilege is not guaranteed and does not signify a correlative duty on the part of the patient, who may withhold or withdraw the privilege at any time. Rights include the most important values, needs, and desires of a free society (Bandman and Bandman 1978, p. 328).

Nurses are responsible for meeting or defending their patients' needs, claims, and rights, and thus have the duty or privilege of serving them. When patients cannot do for themselves and *knowingly* transfer the special right of advocacy to the nurse, they empower the nurse to help and sustain them in time of need.

Health professionals do not have any special role-derived rights that supersede the patient's human rights. Exceptions may occur when it is clear that the vital basic interests of the patient are not being served, as when another health professional is in error. The physician's and nurse's rights must always be consistent with the human rights from which they logically derive (Bandman 1978, p. 329).

The fundamental elements of responsibility in the patient–nurse relationship are the needs, claims, and rights of patients and the duties or privileges of nurses.

The Nurse–Patient Relationship

What, then, are the major characteristics of the nurse–patient relationship? Toward what ends should this relationship be directed if nurses are to practice ethically and protect the rights of their patients?

I believe that the nurse–patient relationship is an association between two human beings made possible because one of them (the client, or patient) has claims or rights originating out of human needs, and the other (the nurse) has a duty and privilege to respond to such claims or rights. This duty emerges from the nature of the professional service which the nurse has been prepared to provide to the patient and from the moral commitments which guide her life. The relationship can be maintained for as long as the patient's claims and needs require nursing care *and for as long as the patient agrees to receive the service.* This concept may extend to a family or other group.

The relationship may by its very nature be short-term or long-term; temporary, intermittent, or semipermanent. Maintenance depends on the particular needs of the particular patient and on the nurse's knowledge, skill, and humaneness in meeting these needs. Ideally, nursing care and patient needs should be proportional: the greater the need, the stronger the claim or right to nursing care; the higher the quality (as separate from the amount) of nursing care, the weaker the need or claim by the patient. One can expect that at some point the client/patient's needs will disappear or become self-manageable and the relationship will then be dissolved, unless or until the person's needs again become greater than his ability to meet them.

This view is consonant with that expressed by Curtin (1979), Acting Director for the National Center for Nursing Ethics, which is that nursing should be defined by its philosophy of care rather than its caring functions *per se*—that is, nursing is a moral art, the purpose of which is to enhance the welfare of other human beings who become clients or patients. Curtin also stated that the philosophical foundation of nursing is advocacy.

According to Gadow (1979), advocacy is an existential concept fundamental to the principle of self-determination. In her view, the best interests of the patient can be determined only by the patient himself; therefore, he should be helped to reach health decisions that are truly his own, expressing the entire complexity of his values. Existential advocacy is:

> *. . . the effort to help persons be-*
> *come clear about* what they want *to*
> *do, by helping them to discern and*
> *clarify their values in the situa-*
> *tion; and, on the basis of that self-*
> *examination, to reach decisions*
> *that express their reaffirmed,*
> *perhaps recreated, values.* (Gadow
> 1979, pp. 82–83).

One of nursing's deepest convictions is that each patient is a total human be-ing, each a unity which cannot be fragmented. Each person is a composite of interrelated and interdependent elements. There is a sameness and a uniqueness about every individual with whom the nurse interacts (Curtin 1979, p. 3).

The nurse is in an ideal position to experience the uniqueness, the strengths, and the complexities of the person because she must attend the client as a unity in immediate distress and therefore at a time of greatest vulnerability. This allows periods of sustained contact in which the nurse helps with mun-dane functions which would ordinarily be considered in the realm of self-care (Gadow 1979). Thus, existential advocacy involves the nurse's interac-tion with the client in determining the personal meaning of the client's ex-perience. This is the most profound human freedom—the *right to determine meaning for oneself.*

What is meant by the idea of treating a patient as a unity, a unified human being? In my view, it means that the nurse must recognize and appreciate the nature and extent of the patient's vulnerability to such things as childbirth, illness, or disability, as expressed through sensitivity to such subjective ex-periences as discomfort, pain, malaise, fear, and anxiety. It means that the nurse must not only sense how the patient responds to these experiences, but must see these experiences as she would likely respond to them. The nurse must be able to appreciate how similar circumstances in her own life could create fears about whether one's own condition would worsen, thus decreas-ing one's ability to cope, and how hope that the sensations would disappear could hasten return to a normal or enhanced state—that is, a state of compe-tence and healthy functioning. It means correct estimation of the needs, sen-sations, and resulting perceptions which bring about feelings of vulnerability. It requires ability to use professional, scientific knowledge and skills to con-sciously act in a therapeutic way and thereby reduce needs, untoward sensa-tions, and unhealthy responses, where possible.

Therapeutic action in this context involves judicious interaction with the patient. As the relationship becomes firmly established, more and more of the client's needs and desires begin to surface. The patient becomes increasingly aware that the nurse is "tuned in" to her or to him as an individual and to his particular manner of being. He also realizes that the nurse will not act to further threaten his integirty. As the patient's needs are uncovered, they can be used to formulate the design of the advocacy relationship—i.e., the structural format which makes it possible for the patient to gradually become able to meet his own needs and to protect his uniqueness, unity, independence, self-image, and other aspects of his human nature.

Through this process, the patient can begin to understand and accept his present vulnerability, learn how to move from a state of dependency toward more active resumption of responsibility for himself, and participate in his recovery, moving progressively toward a nonvulnerable state—these are the goals. The process of self-understanding is initiated through mutual sensing—nurse of patient and patient of nurse—with a meaningful interpersonal interaction becoming a model for all other interactions.

The quality of these mutual interactions and perceptions is crucial in setting the tone for the future relationship. The way the nurse enters the patient's environment (personal space) can convey respect for him as a person with dignity. She can indicate a willingness to listen to him, to learn from him, and with his assent to enter into a partnership with him in the enterprise of helping him to become more healthy.

Thus the concept of human advocacy becomes actualized and the foundation is laid for the nurse and patient to freely and cooperatively determine the form of their relationship for future encounters.

The quality of the professional nurse-patient relationship is fundamentally influenced by the moral convictions and characteristics of the nurse herself. That is, a nurse's ability to utilize moral principles and rules to guide her professional actions and solve ethical problems depends upon the extent to which her personal moral values are congruent with these principles and rules.

Pragmatic Implications of Advocacy

If one believes that the philosophical foundation of nursing is advocacy and that this function constitutes the basic nature and purpose of the nurse-patient relationship, then one must consider a number of important pragmatic implications.

Abrams (1978) has raised the question of whether the nurse is best suited to assume the advocacy role and carry out related functions. She specifies these functions as (1) being a counselor or lay therapist, (2) helping the patient reach decisions about his or her health care, (3) providing information about his or her rights and how to exercise them, (4) being a spokesman for the patient, and (5) securing or checking on the quality of the patient's care. The nurse–patient relationship proposed in this chapter is not antithetical to performance of any of these functions. For one thing, in the proposed relationship, the patient must give voluntary (autonomous) consent to formation of a relationship. The patient must also consent to any ministrations which the nurse proposes. In addition, this type of professional relationship presupposes an adequate grounding in ethical theory, principles, and rules, as well as a sound background in other critical aspects of professional knowledge and skill—e.g., ability to provide counseling.

For the nurse to act ethically as a patient's spokesman in the context of the proposed nurse–patient relationship, she must have the patient's informed consent, since the competent patient is assumed to know his own best interests. Therefore, the nurse who respects the autonomy of the client would not make decisions for him (that is, act paternalistically), but rather would assist him in self-determination.

The patient's basic needs are assumed to be the foundation for his claims or rights. Human rights also engender corresponding responsibilities, duties, or privileges in others, including the duty to "do no harm." It would thus be morally wrong, according to the principles of beneficence and nonmaleficence, for the nurse to act on the basis of a patient's wishes if such actions would bring more harm than good to the patient.

The nurse is morally and professionally responsible for helping the patient understand what his rights are in a given situation and showing him how to make decisions and how to act to protect his rights.

Nurses must recognize that their primary responsibility is to the patient and not to the institution or the doctor, except in carrying out the doctor's orders safely and ethically. The nurse's financial dependence on the hospital can be a source of conflict, as can the power and authority exercised by the physician over interpretation of patients' rights.

Health care providers, health institutions, and the health-care system as a whole are all morally responsible for respecting the patient's rights and acting according to ethical principles. This responsibility does not, therefore, rest solely on the nurse. However, the fact is that the patient's rights are not respected in many instances. It is for this reason that nurses need to assume the responsibility of advocacy inherent in their relationship with patients, despite potential conflicts.

Jameton (1977, p. 22) has identified some ethical issues in nursing which show that principled action in the face of conflict is difficult. These are presented here as follows:

1. The threat to the nurse's personal interest; the nurse's subordinate position and complex role; personal power; the conflict between altruism and self-interest; expertise and authority in relation to moral judgments.
2. The difficulties attendant to the nurse's complex role. A clear framework of accountability must be identified.

3. The strictures placed on the nurse's role as patient educator. These are professionally demeaning and must be resolved in terms of nursing's accountability to the patient.
4. The disparity in income, power, decision-making authority, and prestige between medicine and nursing—a source of resentment and conflict.
5. The responsibility of the nurse to give information to the patient and to obtain informed consent. This responsibility must be clearly identified and established.
6. Actions by nurses to promote and secure their social and political responsibilities in terms of their political power.
7. Ethical considerations in nursing which recognize a multiplicity of professional agents. "Politics and power, personal needs and goals, and rules and roles have their impact on ethical decision making" (Jameton 1977, p. 23).

As concerns cesarean mothers, nurses need to work toward continuity of women's health care, so that women have an opportunity before pregnancy, and certainly before birth to learn about their rights in cesarean delivery. This can be done through health education programs and/or in childbirth preparation classes.

I propose that nurses who clearly understand their ethical and moral responsibilities to patients, and who assume their moral and professional duties or privileges vis-à-vis the patient's needs, claims, and rights, will be able to help patients to retain or protect their rights. In addition, nurses who have a basic understanding of ethics as it affects their profession can utilize moral principles and rules to resolve conflicts which arise between professionals in terms of sharing such responsibilities. It is therefore the task of the individual nursing professional to exercise her *right* and *duty* to practice nursing responsibly in accord with ethics, experience, and conscience (Curtin 1978, pp. 9, 10). Thus:

1. Nurses must join and support their professional organizations.
2. The organizations must establish mechanisms to assure quality of practice, provide for arbitration of conflicts, and protect individual nurses from retaliation by institutions, physicians, and others.
3. Autonomous nursing staffs in individual institutions must be developed to establish channels for complaints and grievances.
4. Review boards for nursing practice must be established on local and national levels.
5. No nurse should be compelled to perform any nursing act which violates her good nursing judgment.

Curtin (1978) pointed out that unless there is public support for nursing accountability and for the general moral commitment of nurses to the welfare of individual patients, it will be difficult to implement the above steps. To ameliorate this situation, all nurses should have the opportunity for formal study of the social dimensions of ethics.

BILL OF CLAIMS AND RIGHTS
OF MOTHERS IN CESAREAN BIRTHS

Given an adequate ethical and professional background, nurses can begin to facilitate full patient autonomy by making sure that cesarean mothers know their rights. The following list is not all-inclusive but does cover the most important aspects of this facilitation, since most mothers and families who experience cesarean birth can be expected to have needs similar to those set forth below. The cesarean mother has a right to:

1. Assistance from health-care providers in making her own decisions and setting health-care goals for herself and her infant during pregnancy and childbirth.
2. Understanding, reassurance, and individualized health care before and after the cesarean birth.
3. An empathetic relationship with health-care providers before and after the cesarean birth.
4. Informed consent to hospitalization for childbirth, especially birth by cesarean.
5. Informed consent to cesarean birth necessitated by an existing medical condition which has a deleterious effect on or is affected by pregnancy or parturition.
6. Informed consent to cesarean birth necessitated by an obstetrical condition which would make vaginal delivery hazardous or impossible.
7. Informed consent to cesarean birth necessitated by an obstetrical emergency which makes vaginal delivery hazardous or impossible.
8. Informed consent to all pre- and postcesarean procedures, tests, medical therapy, and physical care proposed by health-care providers.
9. Informed consent to any type of health care which might affect the mother–infant attachment process, the course of postcesarean recovery, and/or future pregnancies and births.

REFERENCES

Abrams N: A contrary view of the nurse as patient advocate. Nurs Forum 17 (3):258–67, 1978
American Nurses Association: Code for Nurses, with Interpretive Statements. Kansas City, Mo., American Nurses Association, 1976

Bandman EL, Bandman B (eds): Bioethics and Human Rights. Boston, Little, Brown, 1978

Beauchamp TL, Childress JF: Principles of Biomedical Ethics. New York, Oxford University Press, 1979

Corea G: The Hidden Malpractice. New York, Morrow, 1977

Curtin L: The nurse as advocate: A philosophical foundation for nursing. Adv Nurs Sci 1 (3): 1–10, 1979

Curtin LL: The nurse as advocate: A philosophical foundation for nursing. 11, 1978

Gadow S: Advocacy nursing and new meanings of aging. Nurs Clin North Am 14 (1):82–83, 1979

Jameton A: The nurse: When roles and rules conflict. Hastings Cent Rep 7 (4):22–23, 1977

Jones OH: Cesarean section in present-day obstetrics. Am J Obstet Gynecol 126 (5):521–30, 1976

Remen N, Blau AA, Hively R: The Masculine Principle, the Feminine Principle and Humanistic Medicine. San Francisco, Institute of the Study of Humanistic Medicine, 1975

Index

RG
761
.C46

The Cesarean experience